Official Journal of the International Society of Neuroendocrinology

Neuro-endocrinology

International Journal for Basic and Clinical Studies on Neuroendocrine Relationships

Founded 1965 by E. Bajusz
Continued by K.M. Knigge (1973–1978), W.F. Ganong (1979–1984), S.M. McCann (1985–1993)

KARGER

Printed in Switzerland on acid-free paper by Reinhardt Druck, Basel

Appears monthly:
2 volumes per year (12 issues)

Neuro
-endocrinology

The Editorial Board of Neuroendocrinology welcomes articles for review that report new observations on interactions between the brain and the endocrine system. Papers that are published deal with both basic and clinical subjects. Editorials, summaries of meetings, and reviews of timely topics in basic and clinical neuroendocrinology are also published, but these items are accepted only at the invitation of the Editor-in-Chief.

Manuscripts and all correspondence pertaining to them should be addressed to the Editor-in-Chief:

Dr. Claude Kordon
INSERM U. 159
2ter, rue d'Alésia
F–75014 Paris (France)

Manuscripts from North America to:

Dr. Richard Weiner
Department of Obstetrics, Gynecology and Reproductive Sciences
Reproductive Endocrinology Center
University of California
San Francisco, CA 94143-0556 (USA)

Manuscripts from Southeast Asia to:

Dr. Hiroo Imura
Department of Medicine
Kyoto University
Sakyo-ku
Kyoto 606-01 (Japan)

Manuscripts should be written in English. They should contain unpublished results of research work, and should be as concise as possible. They should be typewritten or 'letter-quality' printed on one side of the paper only and double spaced with a wide margin. Please send the original and three first class copies of the manuscript. One set of the original illustrations plus three copies is adequate, except in the case of photomicrographs or other illustrations that do not reproduce well in Xerox or related types of copying equipment. In these instances, it will be necessary to submit four clear prints of each illustration for distribution to the reviewers. The following presentation is recommended: Abstract, Introductory statement on the purpose of the studies, Materials and methods, Results, Discussion, and References. Commonly accepted abbreviations (e.g. ACTH, TSH, DNA) may be used throughout the text and tables, but a definition should be provided the first time each abbreviation is used. Please limit abbreviations to those in common use, and avoid other abbreviations and acronyms. Contributions will generally be printed in order of acceptance for publication.

Contributors should know that one of the criteria considered in reviewing manuscripts is the humane and proper treatment of animals. The editors realize that the use of anesthetics, analgesics, and tranquilizers would defeat the purpose of some experiments. However, the use of painful or otherwise noxious stimuli must be carefully and thoroughly justified in the paper. Papers that do not meet these criteria will not be accepted for publication.

Rapid communications: Manuscripts intended for rapid communication must present new findings of sufficient importance to justify their accelerated appearance. Double-spaced manuscripts cannot exceed 7 pages, including figures, tables and references; longer manuscripts will be returned. Rapid communications are subject to the usual editorial review and are published within 2 months following acceptance. Proofs are sent to the Editor-in-Chief and to the authors.

Arrangement:

Title page: The first page of each paper should carry the title, the authors' full first and last names, and the name of the institute or department where the authors conducted their research work. In addition, the following should be put on the title page: 1. A short title for use as a running head; 2. A list of 3–9 key words for indexing purposes; 3. The name and complete mailing address as well as phone and fax numbers of the individual to whom correspondence, galley proofs, and requests for reprints should be addressed; 4. Acknowledgements, including, where relevant, credit to the sources of grant support.

Abstract: Each paper must have a short abstract describing procedures, observations and conclusions, which will appear at the beginning of the article.

Footnotes: Avoid footnotes if at all possible. When essential, they should be numbered consecutively and typed at the foot of the appropriate page.

Tables and illustrations: Tables (numbered in arabic numerals) should be prepared on separate sheets, and each should have a suitable heading. Illustrations should be numbered in Arabic numerals and legends for the figures should be submitted on a separate page. For the reproduction of illustrations, only good drawings and original photographs can be accepted; negatives or photocopies cannot be used. When possible, group several illustrations on one block for reproduction (max. size 181 × 223 mm) or provide crop marks. On the back of each illustration, indicate its number, the author's name, and 'top'.

Color illustrations: Up to 6 color illustrations per page can now be integrated with the text at the reduced price of SFr. 600.– / U$ 400.00 per page. Color illustrations are reproduced at the author's expense.

References: In the text identify references by Arabic numerals [in square brackets]. Material submitted for publication but not yet accepted should be noted as 'unpublished data' and not be included in the reference list. The list of references should include only those publications which are cited in the text. Do not alphabetize; number references in the order in which they are first mentioned in the text. The surnames of all the authors followed by initials should be given. There should be no punctuation other than a comma to separate the authors. Cite all authors, 'et al' is not sufficient. Abbreviate journal names according to the Index Medicus system. (Also see International Committee of Medical Journal Editors: Uniform requirements for manuscripts submitted to biomedical journals. Br Med J 1988;296:401–405.)

Examples

(a) Papers published in periodicals: Kauffman HF, van der Heide S, Beaumont F, Blok H, de Vries K: Class-specific antibody determination against *Aspergillus fumigatus* by means of the enzyme-linked immunosorbent assay. III. Comparative study: IgG, IgA, IgM ELISA titers, precipitating antibodies and IgE binding after fractionation of the antigen. Int Arch Allergy Appl Immunol 1986;80: 300–306.

(b) Monographs: Matthews DE, Farewell VT: Using and Understanding Medical Statistics. Basel, Karger, 1985.

(c) Edited books: Hardy WD Jr, Essex M: FeLV-induced feline acquired immune deficiency syndrome: A model for human AIDS; in Klein E (ed): Acquired Immunodeficiency Syndrome. Prog Allergy. Basel, Karger, 1986, vol 37, pp 353–376.

Papers that have been submitted to a journal but are not yet accepted should not be listed in the bibliography, but the data in them can be referred to in the text as unpublished observations. If details of methods are only available in papers that are 'in press', copies of the papers should be included with the manuscript submitted to Neuroendocrinology, so that the editorial referees can have adequate information to judge the manuscript.

Further details: Authors may consult our leaflet 'Rules for the Preparation of Manuscripts', available on request from the Publisher, S. Karger AG, P.O. Box, CH-4009 Basel (Switzerland).

Galley proofs: Unless indicated otherwise, galley proofs are sent to the first-named author and should be returned with the least possible delay. Alterations made in galley proofs, other than the correction of printer's errors, are charged to the author. No page proofs are supplied.

Reprints: Order forms and a price list are sent with the galley proofs. Orders submitted after the issue is printed are subject to considerably higher prices. Allow five weeks from the date of publication for delivery.

KARGER

General Information

Neuro-endocrinology

Publication data: 'Neuroendocrinology' is published 12 times annually. Volumes 59, 60 with 6 issues each appear in 1994.

Subscription rates: Subscriptions run for a full calendar year. Prices are given per volume.

Personal subscription:

Subscription	*+ postage and handling*	
SFr. 558.60	+ SFr. 16.80	Europe
SFr. 558.60	+ SFr. 25.20	Overseas
US$ 373.10	+ US$ 16.80	

(Must be in the name of, billed to, and paid by an individual. Order must be marked 'personal subscription'.)

Institutional subscription:

Subscription	*+ postage and handling*	
SFr. 798.–	+ SFr. 24.–	Europe
SFr. 798.–	+ SFr. 36.–	Overseas
US$ 533.00	+ US$ 24.00	

Airmail postage: SFr. 36.–, US$ 30.00. (Extra per volume.)

Discount subscription prices:
International Society of Neuroendocrinology;
American Psychological Association.

Advertising: Correspondence and rate requests should be addressed to the Publisher.

Microforms: Please direct all enquiries and orders to:
University Microfilms Inc.
300 North Zeeb Road, P.O. Box 1346
Ann Arbor, MI 48106-1346 (USA)

Subscription orders: Orders can be placed at agencies, bookstores, directly with the Publisher S. Karger AG, P.O. Box, CH–4009 Basel (Switzerland)
or with any of the following distributors:

Deutschland: S. Karger GmbH, Postfach
D–79095 Freiburg

France: Librairie Luginbühl
36, bd de Latour-Maubourg, F–75007 Paris

Great Britain, Ireland: S. Karger Publishers
11 Ravenscroft Road
Beckenham, Kent BR3 4TP

USA: S. Karger Publishers, Inc.
26 West Avon Road, P.O. Box 529
Farmington, CT 06085

India, Bangladesh, Sri Lanka:
S. Karger India Subscription Agency
B–5/132 Safdarjung Enclave
New Delhi-110029

Japan: Katakura Libri, Inc.
36-9 Hongo 3-chome, Bunkyo-ku, Tokyo 113

Change of address: Both old and new address should be sent to the subscription source.

Single issues and back volumes: Information can be obtained through the Publisher.

Bibliographic indices: This journal is regularly listed in bibliographic services, including *Current Contents®*.

KARGER

3rd International Congress of Neuroendocrinology

Budapest
July 3-8, 1994

ABSTRACTS

Guest Editors
Ida Gerendai
Béla Halász
Budapest (Hungary)

Neuroendocrinology
Vol. 60, Supplement 1, 1994

S. Karger
Medical and Scientific Publishers
Basel • München • Paris • London
New York • New Delhi • Bangkok
Singapore • Tokyo • Sydney

Drug Dosage
The authors and the publisher have exerted every effort to ensure that drug selection and dosage set forth in this text are in accord with current recommendations and practice at the time of publication. However, in view of ongoing research, changes in government regulations, and the constant flow of information relating to drug therapy and drug reactions, the reader is urged to check the package insert for each drug for any change in indications and dosage and for added warning and precautions. This is particularly important when the recommended agent is a new and/or infrequently employed drug.

Printed in Hungary on acid-free paper
by AESCULART – DFC DRUCK
ISBN 3-8055-6012-5

3rd International Congress of Neuroendocrinology

Contents

Abstracts: 3rd Int. Congr. of Neuroendocrinology (Budapest, 1994)
Neuroendocrinology 1994;60(suppl 1): 1–104

PL1

PEPTIDE HORMONES AND THE BRAIN. D. de Wied. Rudolf Magnus Institute, Dept. of Pharmacology, Utrecht University, Utrecht, The Netherlands, 3584 CG.

Much of our knowledge on the regulation of anterior pituitary function has come from studies with hypothalamic releasing hormones which followed Geoffrey Harris' brilliant work on the portal vessel system (Harris, 1951). Seldom has the interpretation of results on the physiology of a system been so accurate. The nearly 30 years of research in this area lasted from the development of the first assay for the CRF in the fifties till the isolation and characterization of this releasing hormone in 1983. It held the interest of most neuroendocrinologists. At the same time another area of research developed initially nearly unnoticed which suggested that pituitary hormones as ACTH and MSH and the brainborn neurohypophyseal hormones possessed CNS activity. It lasted more than 10 years before attention was paid to these findings. This occurred after the discovery of the enkephalins in 1975. Many peptide hormones were subsequently found in the brain and numerous studies aimed at elucidating the action of these hormones on brain function were performed. Our studies and those of others on the CNS effect of ACTH/MSH, the endorphins and the neurohypophyseal hormones, indicated effects on learning and memory processes, on social behavior, maintenance, maternal and sexual behavior, on temperature, nociception, rewarded behavior, and drug tolerance. ACTH/MSH neuropeptides possess in addition neurotrophic effects. Some of the endorphins appeared to exhibit neuroleptic-like and others amphetamine-like properties. Our studies in particular revealed that some of the CNS effects of these hormones are independent of their classical endocrine effects. Structure activity studies indicated that the behavioral effect of ACTH is located in the 4-13 portion of the molecule. Such fragments may be generated from the parent hormone in the brain. The neurohypophyseal hormones can be converted to highly selective C-terminal fragments with powerful effects on learning and memory processes. However, certain effects need the whole molecule as in the periphery. In recent years many receptors have been found for ACTH/MSH neuropeptides, the neurohypophyseal and other peptide hormones in the brain. The search for putative receptors for these peptides in relation to their function will be an exciting challenge for research in the next decade.

PL2

GnRH RECEPTORS AND SIGNALING MECHANISMS IN HYPOTHALAMIC AND PITUITARY CELLS. K.J. Catt, L. Krsmanovic, and S.S. Stojilkovic. Endocrinology and Reproduction Research Branch, NICHD, NIH, Bethesda, MD 20892.

The hypothalamic control of gonadotropin secretion is mediated by episodic basal secretion and midcycle surges of GnRH, which binds to specific plasma membrane receptors (GnRH-R) in pituitary gonadotrophs and stimulates phosphoinositide hydrolysis, calcium signaling, and secretion of LH and FSH. The GnRH-R is a 327 amino acid protein with seven transmembrane regions, consistent with its coupling to G protein-mediated activation of phospholipase C. The receptor is structurally distinct from other G protein-coupled receptors in that it does not possess a carboxy-terminal cytoplasmic domain. Activation of GnRH-R in gonadotrophs leads to rapid and biphasic increases in $InsP_3$ and $[Ca^{2+}]_i$, with an immediate spike phase and a subsequent plateau phase. The spike phase is derived primarily by calcium mobilization from intracellular stores. In single gonadotrophs, GnRH stimulates prominent Ca^{2+} oscillations that exhibit dose-dependent modulation of spiking frequency. In addition to providing the calcium signal for exocytosis, the cytoplasmic oscillations activate Ca^{2+}-sensitive K^+ channels in the plasma membrane, leading to episodic waves of plasma-membrane hyperpolarization with alternating bursts of action potentials that promote Ca^{2+} entry through L-type channels. GnRH-R and their mRNA transcripts are also expressed in immortalized hypothalamic neurons. Activation of these neuronal GnRH-R elicits dose-related $[Ca^{2+}]_i$ responses that are dependent on calcium mobilization and entry. Exposure of perifused neurons to GnRH agonist analogs causes transient elevation of GnRH release and subsequent suppression of the basal pulsatile secretion, followed by dose-dependent induction of less frequent but larger GnRH pulses and ultimately by single massive episodes of GnRH release. The ability of GnRH to exert autocrine actions on its secretory neurons, could reflect the operation of the endogenous pulse generator and the genesis of the preovulatory GnRH surge *in vivo*.

PL3

FROM PARTICLE TRAJECTORIES IMAGING TO THE APPLICATIONS IN BIOLOGY AND MEDICINE. **G. Charpak, CERN, 1211 Geneva 23, Switzerland.**

The determination of the trajectories of particles produced in high energy collisions has led to the development of new instruments giving, with a high efficiency, the co-ordinates of any ionising production, as X-rays or any particle emitted by radioactive elements. Many domains in medicine and biology can be fertilised by these methods permitting a large gain in the speed of data taking or in the radiation doses required for accurate measurements.

PL4

BRAIN 11ß-HYDROXYSTEROID DEHYDROGENASE (11ß-HSD) AND CORTICOSTEROID ACTION. C.R.W. Edwards* and J.R. Seckl: Dept Medicine, Western General Hospital, Edinburgh, EH4 2XU, UK.

11ß-HSD catalyses the reversible inactivation of glucocorticoids, providing tissue-specific regulation of access to receptors. Two isoforms exist. 11ß-HSD1 is NADP-dependent, lower affinity and bi-directional, whereas 11ß-HSD2 is an NAD-dependent, high-affinity dehydrogenase, which engenders aldosterone-selective access to renal mineralocorticoid receptors (MR). 11ß-HSD1 mRNA and activity are present in rat CNS neurons (hippocampus, cortex, cerebellum, hypothalamus) and anterior pituitary. 11ß-HSD2 may occur in hypothalamus, amygdala and hippocampus, which represent possible sites for aldosterone-selective actions on blood pressure and salt appetite. Hippocampal 11ß-HSD1 mRNA and activity are increased by chronic dexamethasone treatment and stress, suggesting 11ß-HSD may protect neurons from glucocorticoid excess. Stronger evidence of functionality comes from studies with the 11ß-HSD inhibitor glycyrrhetinic acid (GE). GE alters neuronal metabolic activity in vivo in the hippocampus and hypothalamic PVN (important loci for glucocorticoid negative feedback) and the preoptic area (which may mediate central corticosteroid actions on blood pressure). Indeed, icv 11ß-HSD inhibition mimics the effects of exogenous aldosterone (not corticosterone) on blood pressure, indicating a sub-population of brain MR protected from glucocorticoid by 11ß-HSD. GE also decreases CRF release into hypophysial portal blood, in the presence of unchanged circulating corticosterone, suggesting 11ß-HSD regulates the effective intracellular feedback signal. 11ß-HSD may thus represent a novel and important control of glucocorticoid action in the brain. Whether 11ß-HSD dysfunction occurs in glucocorticoid or stress-related brain disorders remains to be determined.

0028-3835/94/0607-0001
$ 5.00/0

PL5

NEUROENDOCRINE ASPECTS OF THE NATRIURETIC PEPTIDE SYSTEM.
H. Imura, K. Nakao. Kyoto University, Kyoto 606-01 Japan

The natriuretic peptide (NP) system consists of three peptides that are derived from different genes with sequence homology; atrial NP(ANP), brain NP(BNP) and C-type NP(CNP). ANP and BNP are produced predominantly in the auricle and the ventricle, respectively, of the heart. Although BNP exists in relatively high concentrations in the pig brain, both ANP and CNP are major peptides in murine, canine and human brain. There are two subtypes in the bioactive ANP receptor; ANP-A and ANP-B receptors. ANP and BNP preferentially binds ANP-A receptors, whereas CNP has high affinity with ANP-B receptors. ANP-B receptors are more abundant than ANP-A receptors in the brain. Major molecular forms of ANP in the brain is not ANP 1-28 (the major circulating form) but ANP 4-28 and ANP 5-28. Intracerebroventricular injection of ANP or BNP antagonizes the dipsogenic, salt-preferring, hypertensive, vasopressin and ACTH-releasing actions of angiotensin II. Thus there are the NP system and the renin-angiotensin system in the brain which are involved in the central control of water and blood pressure homeostasis. ANP also affects secretion of anterior pituitary hormones other than ACTH. Possible neuroendocrine effects of CNP will be discussed also.

PL6

EXPRESSION OF THE POMC GENE: FROM THE BRAIN TO THE PITUITARY. J. Drouin, Laboratoire de génétique moléculaire, Institut de recherches cliniques de Montréal, Montréal CANADA H2W 1R7

The pituitary gland develops from a territory present, early in development, at the anterior end of the neural ridge. Brain, including hypothalamus, develop from contiguous territories in the neural plate and thus from very early during embryogenesis the development of brain and pituitary are associated. Expression of pro-opiomelanocortin (POMC) occurs early in hypothalamus and pituitary development before most other pituitary markers. Our analysis of the mechanisms responsible for pituitary specificity of POMC gene expression has provided insight into links that may exist between transcription and differentiation of brain and pituitary. Indeed, analysis of the POMC gene promoter has revealed a complex organization requiring the concerted action of many transcription factors binding as many DNA regulatory elements. Some of these transcription factors are ubiquitous and they play important regulatory roles. For example, glucocorticoid receptor-mediated repression involves unusual complexes of GR interacting with the POMC gene negative glucocorticoid response element (nGRE).
A subset of POMC transcription factors impart pituitary specificity of expression and their cloning and analysis have revealed stricking links to brain transcriptional mechanisms. The role of these factors is considered in the context of pituitary and brain gene transcription in relation to differentiation of pituitary and brain.

PL7

MOLECULAR ANALYSIS OF POSSIBLE INTERACTIONS BETWEEN INTERNAL AND EXTERNAL FACTORS CONTROLLING GENE EXPRESSION IN HYPOTHALAMIC NEURONS. D.W. Pfaff. Laboratory of Neurobiology & Behavior, The Rockefeller University, 1230 York Ave., NY, NY 10021, USA.

Gene expression for the progesterone receptor (PR) and for the opioid peptide preproenkephalin have been tied into neuroendocrine mechanisms and circuitry for reproductive behavior (in Knobil & Neill, Physiology of Reproduction, 2nd Ed., 1993). In the rat, hypothalamic mRNA levels for PR are estrogen dependent, tissue specific and sex specific. Gel shift analyses for protein/DNA binding indicate complex interactions between estrogen levels and AP-1 binding proteins. Preproenkephalin expression in ventromedial hypothalamus is also estrogen dependent, tissue specific and influenced by genetic sex. On a consensus estrogen response DNA element (ERE) as well as in the PPE promoter, competition among nuclear receptors for DNA sites is evident. At the mRNA level, the robust estrogenic induction of PPE messenger RNA can actually be reversed by anesthesia at the time of hormone administration, a phenomenon which matches previously reported behavioral results. For both genes studied in hypothalamic neurons, therefore, possible interactions between internal (hormonal) and external factors are evident, providing a level of integration expected for a complex behavioral mechanism.

S1.1

REGULATION OF GROWTH HORMONE-RELEASING FACTOR (GRF), SOMATOSTATIN (SRIF) AND INSULIN-LIKE GROWTH FACTOR-I (IGF-I) GENE EXPRESSION IN THE CNS. Eugenio E. Muller,V. De Gennaro Colonna, A. Torsello, S.G.Cella,D.Cocchi°,V.Locatelli.Dept.Pharmacology,Univ.ofMilano,viaVanvitelli 32,20129 Milano and °Pharmaco-Biological Dept,Univ. of Bari,Italy.

GRF and SRIF are the physiological regulators of GH secretion and most often the terminal effectors for stimuli acting at CNS level. Little is known on the role of CNS messengers on the regulation of GRF,SRIF and IGF-I gene expression ,though reportedly,blockade of histamine synthesis significantly inhibits GRF gene expression in the rat. GH and IGF-I exert feedback effects on hypothalamic GRF and SS neurons. In particular,in normal or starved rats , GH and IGF-I inhibited and stimulated GRF and SRIF gene expression,respectively. Accordingly , in hypophysectomized rats, 2 weeks post-surgery,GRF gene expression was markedly increased but was partially reverted to control levels by a 4 day GH replacement therapy. Neonatal and aged rats present with reduced function of the GH feedback mechanisms. In 10-day-old neonatal rats,given GRF antiserum since birth,hypothalamic GRF and SRIF mRNA were slightly increased and decreased respectively;in these rats, replacement with GH at substitutive doses failed to modify GRF and SRIF gene expression. In 10-day-old intact rats,pharmacological doses of GH given for 5 days reduced GRF gene expression, while physiological doses of GH did not modify GRF mRNA levels. Twenty-month-old male rats have a markedly reduced GRF gene expression while SRIF mRNA levels are slightly decreased when compared to 8-month-old rats. GH administration failed to modify hypothalamic gene expression of both neuropeptides in 20-month-old rats,at a dose clearly enhancing plasma levels of IGF-I. Thus,in addition to a primary dysfunction in GRF-secreting neurons,the aged rat loses the ability to sense the feedback action of circulating GH.

S1.2

ANATOMICAL AND PHYSIOLOGICAL INTERACTIONS BETWEEN GHRH and SRIH NEURONS J. Epelbaum, U.159 INSERM , Paris, 75014, France.

In addition to their direct actions at the pituitary level on somatotrophs, SRIH and GHRH interact in the hypothalamus. In vivo, after a cysteamine treatment which decreases SRIH activity, GHRH mRNA levels are increased in the ventrolateral arcuate nucleus but not in cells located at the outer rim of the ventromedial nucleus. In vitro, SRIH is able to decrease GHRH mRNA levels and GHRH release from perifused mediobasal hypothalamus. In keeping with these findings, a majority of GHRH neurons in the ventrolateral portion of the arcuate nucleus, but not those located at the outer rim of the ventromedial nucleus, express functional SRIH receptors of the SSTR2/SSTR4 subtypes. These SRIH receptors have been visualised in murine species as well as in sheep and human hypothalamus. Combined retrograde tracing-immunohistochemical techniques indicate that the SRIH fibers innervating the arcuate GHRH neurons do not originate in the periventricular hypothalamus cell group but appear intrinsic to the arcuate. Reciprocally, the limited GHRH projections to the periventricular SRIH cell group arise mainly from cells located at the outer rim of the ventromedial nucleus and not from the arcuate population. However, periventricular SRIH perikarya are also innervated by SRIH fibers originating in the arcuate nucleus. Other peptidergic afferents include Galanin fibers arising in the dorsomedial and arcuate nucleus and β-Endorphin fibers originating in the arcuate nucleus. This complex anatomical network has to be **taken into account to interpret the intrahypothalamic interactions** between SRIH and GHRH neurons such as those taking place in GH negative feedback mechanisms.

S1.3

NEUROPHARMACOLOGICAL INTERVENTIONS TO ENHANCE GROWTH HORMONE SECRETION IN MAN. F.F. Casanueva, Department of Medicine, Faculty of Medicine, Santiago de Compostela University. Santiago de Compostela, Spain, 15780.

The molecular and cellular approaches and techniques have greatly changed our insight about several neuroendocrine fields, and particularly on GH regulation and action. As most of the basic findings on GH regulation are derived from animal data, the integrative view make mandatory to show that those animals have a similar physiological regulation of GH than man. At this level, ethical and technical reasons point toward neuropharmacological interventions as the most or only method to gain pertinent information in man. In the last few years, considerable attention has been devoted to study the role played by new agents like the hexapeptide GHRP-6, or old ones like glucocorticoids on GH regulation. GHRP-6 appears as a a tool to unravel the normal regulation as well as the altered GH secretion presented in states like obesity or Cushing's syndrome. On the other hand glucocorticoids in addition to their classical role of inhibiting GH secretion, are able, when administered acutely, to release GH. Glucocorticoid-induced GH discharge is exerted at hypothalamic level, but the implicated mechanisms are not fully understood. Those two GH stimuli are an example of the advantages and limitations of the neuropharmacological approach to neuroendocrinological problems.

S1.SC1

EFFECTS OF GROWTH HORMONE(GH)-RELEASING HORMONE ON GH RELEASE IN ISOLATED PERIFUSED RAT TYPE I AND TYPE II SOMATOTROPHS. P. Lindström*, L. Sävendahl. Department of Histology and Cell Biology, University of Umeå, S-901 87 Umeå, Sweden

There are two types of rat somatotrophs, one heavily granulated (Type II) and one sparsely granulated (Type I). The aim of this study was to test if there are functional differences between the two types. Fractions of isolated somatotrophs were purified from adult male Sprague-Dawley rats by using continuous Percoll density gradient centrifugation in two steps. The first gradient used (1) was formed linearly around the starting density (1.075 g/ml). Type II somatotrophs accumulated in fractions with densities from 1.065 - 1.087 in gradient 1 as analyzed by electron microscopy (>80%). Fractions with densities from 1.055 - 1.065 were put on gradient 2, which was highly sigmoid around the starting density 1.064. Type I cells were predominant in fraction 1.055 - 1.059 in gradient 2 (42 % of all cells being Type I and only 8 % being Type II cells).

Growth hormone (GH) release was measured in perifused three days' cultured cells. Basal GH release was 0.098 ± 0.023 ng GH/μg protein x min^{-1} (mean ± SE, n=13) in Type I cells and 0.105 ± 0.022 ng GH/μg (n=14) in Type II cells (n.s.). Type II cells responded to a low concentration of GHRH (0.1 nM) with increased GH release and both Type I and Type II cells responded to 1 and 10 nM GHRH. The temporal dynamics of stimulated GH release was similar in the two cell types with maximum release reached within 2 min after GHRH exposure. However, Type II cells released more GH in absolute values and in per cent of basal. This may be explained by a higher GH content in the heavily granulated cells.

The conclusions are that both Type I and Type II somatotrophs contribute to basal GH release, and both cell types respond to GHRH but Type II cells release more GH during stimulated conditions.

S1.SC2

SOMATOTROPIC AXIS AND AGING. EVIDENCE OF SEXUAL DIMORPHISM IN RATS. G.L. Rossi*, G.E. Bestetti, D. Adoutte. Div. Exp. Pathology, Inst. Animal Pathology, Univ. of Bern, Bern, Switzerland, CH-3001.

The effect of aging on growth-releasing factor (GRF) and somatostatin (SRIF) axons in the median eminence (ME) as well as on somatotropes was studied by morphometrical and densitometrical immunocytochemistry in young (6 mo) and old (24-25 mo) prolactinoma-free (P-F) male and female Long-Evans rats. Plasma growth hormone (GH) was determined by RIA. Further, we investigated the in vitro basal and K^+-stimulated SRIF-release from the mediobasal hypothalamus (MBH). Finally we measured the secretory function of somatotropes by reverse hemolytic plaque assay (RHPA) and by cell culture. Compared with corresponding young rats, the plasma GH of old P-F rats was similar or reduced. All morphometrical and densitometrical measurements on GRF and SRIF-labeled axons of young and old rats were similar in the two sexes. By comparing the effects of aging on the two neuropeptides we observed reduced GRF and increased SRIF in old animals, female in particular. The K^+-stimulated SRIF-release from the MBH was highly increased in old female and unchanged in old male rats. The GH-labeled somatotrope measurements were mostly decreased in old female and increased in old male rats. By RHPA the GH released from somatotropes was increased in old female and unchanged in old male rats. The GH released into medium during a 3-day stationary culture by the somatotropes of old and young rats, on the contrary, was comparable in the two sexes. Our structural and short-term in vitro studies of the ME and somatotropes in old P-F rats show changes which suggest reduced activity of the somatotropic axis. These changes are sexually dimorphic and more pronounced in female animals.

S2.1

EXPRESSION AND REGULATION OF NEUROHYPOPHYSEAL HORMONE GENES. J.P.H. Burbach. Rudolf Magnus Institute for Neurosciences, Department of Medical Pharmacology, P.O. Box 80040, Utrecht, The Netherlands, 3508 TA.

Over the last 30 years studies on the hypothalamo-neurohypophyseal system (HNS) have revealed many general features of (neuro)peptidergic systems. The availability of an animal model with defective vasopressin (VP) synthesis, the Brattleboro rat, has been of great importance in these studies. Recent molecular and biochemical research focuses on the regulation of the VP and oxytocin (OT) genes as well as on peptide biosynthesis. Concerning the latter, we addressed the function of the association of VP to neurophysin and the identity of novel gene products. Once again the Brattleboro rat appeared to disclose a hitherto unrecognized event: the generation of +1 frameshifted precursors. The HNS thus remains an important system for dissection of molecular and biochemical processes in peptidergic systems.

S2.2

BASIC AND CLINICAL STUDIES OF VASOPRESSIN RECEPTORS. S. Lolait and M. Brownstein. Laboratory of Cell Biology, National Institute of Mental Health, Bethesda, Maryland, 20892. USA

We have isolated cDNAs encoding three mammalian vasopressin receptors: the V1a, V1b, and V2 subtypes. V1 and V2 receptors mediate vasopressin-induced increase in intracellular calcium and cyclic AMP, respectively. All three of the receptor subtypes are present in the kidney, but only V1 receptors are found in the brain. Mutations in the V2 receptor gene, which is found on the X chromosome (Xq28), are responsible for X-linked nephrogenic diabetes insipidus.

S2.3

ROLE OF NEUROHYPOPHYSEAL PEPTIDES IN THE FORMATION OF SOCIAL BONDS. T. R. Insel. Lab Neurophys., NIMH, Poolesville, MD, USA, 20837

Central pathways for the neurohypophyseal peptides have been implicated in several different functions, including the mediation of specific social behaviors. Oxytocin (OT), for instance, facilitates the onset of maternal and reproductive behaviors and vasopressin (AVP) appears important for social memory and territorial displays. To determine if these same systems might mediate specific aspects of pair bonding (ie. longterm, selective social attachments), we have studied the central actions of OT and AVP in the prairie vole (*Microtus ochrogaster*), a small, monogamous rodent. In anatomic studies, the distribution of receptors for both OT and AVP were markedly different in prairie voles relative to the closely related non-monogamous montane vole. Species differences in receptor distribution appeared specific to OT and AVP and could be partially replicated in other vole species selected for analogous differences in social organization. After mating, the highly gregarious male prairie vole undergoes a profound and enduring change in behavior with the emergence of selective aggression (mate guarding) and selective affiliation (partner preference) - behaviors which appear to be instrumental to pair bonding. AVP (but not OT) appears to be both necessary and sufficient for these behavioral changes following mating in the male. However, in female prairie voles (which normally develop a partner preference after mating), AVP appears to have little effect and OT facilitates the emergence of selective affiliation. These behavioral responses to AVP and OT along with the species differences in receptor distribution, implicate these neurohypophyseal peptides in the mediation of pair bonding - although there appear to be important gender differences in both the behaviors and the peptide involved.

S2.SC1

RAPID EFFECTS OF AN OXYTOCIN ANTISENSE OLIGONUCLEOTIDE INFUSED INTO THE SUPRAOPTIC NUCLEUS ON SUCKLING. I. Neumann, D.W.F. Porter, Q.J. Pittman, *R. Landgraf, Dept. of Medical Physiology, University of Calgary, Calgary, Canada, T2N 4N1, *Max Planck Institute of Psychiatry, Clinical Institute, 80804 Munich, Germany

Suckling was used as an *in vivo* model to study the effects of intracerebral oxytocin antisense oligonucleotide (OT-AS) treatment. Lactating rats were implanted with a guide cannula above the left and right SONs, and the jugular vein was catheterized for blood sampling. Two days later, OT-AS (2.5µg/0.5µl) was infused bilaterally into each SON 4 h before a litter of 10 pups was allowed to suckle for 30 min. Compared with control animals treated with either vehicle, mixed bases or vasopressin AS, there was a significant reduction in the number of milk ejection reflexes performed by the pups (to 34.6±4.88 %) as well as in the weight gain of the litter (to 18.8±6.98 %), whereas the time of onset of suckling was unchanged. Compared with presuckling values, plasma OT levels were significantly increased in all 4 groups, but this increase was significantly less in OT-AS treated rats. In contrast, OT content in neural lobes and OT immunoreactivity in the SON, paraventricular nucleus and the neural lobes did not differ among groups 5 h after infusion.
Our data indicate rapid and specific effects of a single OT-AS infusion into the SON on neuroendocrine suckling-related parameters that are not due to depleted stores of OT in the hypothalamo-neurohypophysial system.

Supported by HESPO, MRC, NATO and VW.

S2.SC2

NEUROENDOCRINE CONTROL OF WATER BALANCE AND TRANSEPITHELIAL TRANSPORT THROUGH NEUROHYPOPHYSIAL HORMONE-REGULATED WATER CHANNELS
R. Acher*, J. Chauvet, Y. Rouillé and G. Michel. Lab. Biological Chemistry, University of Paris VI, 96 Boulevard Raspail 75006 Paris, France.

Neurohypophysial hormones, namely vasopressin (mammals) and vasotocin (non-mammalian vertebrates), are involved in the neuroendocrine control of water balance. Water input and output occur at the level of specialized organs through epithelial cells. Transepithelial water transport involves both hormone-regulated (apical membrane) and non-regulated (basal membrane) water channels formed by specific proteins, aquaporins. Vasopressin or vasotocin stimulates osmotically driven water transport by increasing the number of regulated channels through receptor-mediated cytosolic aquaporin recruitement. Adaptive differential processing of pro-vasotocin led in amphibians to hydrin 1 (vasotocinyl-Gly-Lys-Arg) in the aquatic Xenopus and hydrin 2 (vasotocinyl-Gly), in semi-aquatic and terrestrial frogs and toads, along with vasotocin. Hydrins promote water import through frog skin and bladder but not through the kidney. It is assumed that hydrins and vasotocin operate through distinct receptors for the recovery of external (skin) and internal (kidney) water. Reconstitution of processing has been performed in vitro using bovine secretory granule enzymes and synthetic vasopressinyl-Gly-Lys-Arg.

S3.1

MEDIATION OF ESTROGEN AND NEUROTROPHIN ACTIONS THROUGH THEIR INTERACTIONS? C. D. Toran-Allerand*. Dept. of Anatomy and Cell Biology, Columbia University College of Physicians & Surgeons, New York, USA, 10032

The organization of neural circuits controlling a broad spectrum of adult behaviors are critically regulated by early exposure to certain gonadal steroid hormones such as the estrogens and androgens. For example, estrogen permanently influences neuronal structure and function which results in neuroendocrine, behavioral and cognitive sex differences. Estrogen enhances the growth and differentiation of neurons and their neurites (axons and dendrites) in its targets within the developing hypothalamus, preoptic area and cerebral cortex. Despite the profound effects of estrogen in early neural development, the molecular mechanisms underlying these effects are not known: namely, whether estrogen actions are direct and/or indirect [*e.g.* via interactions with endogenous growth factors such as the neurotrophins and/or their receptors]. Estrogen influences on these molecules could alter the responsiveness of its neuronal targets and promote neuronal survival as well as the growth and differentiation of specific neural systems. Evidence will be presented suggesting a critical interplay of estrogen and the neurotrophins in the nervous system, including the finding that regulation of the estrogen and neurotrophin receptor genes may involve differential and reciprocal regulation by their ligands. Supported by grants from NIH (NIA; NIMH); NSF; and AHAF.

S3.2

MOLECULAR BASIS OF NEURONAL PLASTICITY TO GONADAL STEROIDS. **A. Matsumoto* (1), S. Hyodo (2). (1) Dept. Anat., Juntendo Univ. Sch. Med., Hongo, Tokyo 113, (2) Dept. Biol., Coll. Arts & Sci., Univ. Tokyo, Meguro, Tokyo 153, Japan.**

Gonadal steroids are involved in neuronal plasticity in adult gonadal steroid-sensitive neuroendocrine brain. In adult male rats, androgen plays a crucial role in reorganizing the neuronal elements and synaptic connections in motoneurons of the spinal nucleus of the bulbocavernosus (SNB). As one step to clarify molecular mechanisms of androgen for neuronal plasticity, we examined androgenic regulation of the mRNA expression of cytoskeletal proteins such as β-actin and β-tubulin in the androgen-sensitive SNB motoneurons of adult male rats. Adult male rats were castrated and implanted with silastic tubes containing testosterone or nothing. Animals were sacrificed 4 weeks later. Chick β-actin and mouse β-tubulin complementary DNAs were used to detect mRNAs encoding β-actin and β-tubulin of the SNB motoneurons, respectively. The radiolabeled DNA probes were applied to in situ hybridization histochemistry. Motoneurons in the retrodorsolateral nucleus (RDLN), which innervate hindlimb musculature, were also examined. Autoradiographic signals for β-actin and β-tubulin mRNAs were found to be localized on the somata and proximal dendrites of SNB and RDLN motoneurons. Removal of androgen by castration significantly reduced the expression levels of both β-actin and β-tubulin mRNAs in the SNB motoneurons, whereas the changes were prevented by testosterone treatment. On the contrary, castration or testosterone treatment did not induce any changes in the expression levels of these mRNAs in androgen-insensitive RDLN motoneurons. These results suggest that androgen regulates expression of the cytoskeletal protein genes in the SNB motoneurons and may provide evidence for the molecular mechanisms of hormonally-induced neuronal plasticity in the SNB motoneurons. **(Supported by grants from the Ministry of Education, Culture and Science of Japan).**

S3.3

ESTROGEN ENHANCED NEURITE GROWTH AND MICROTUBULE STABILIZING FACTORS. A. Cáceres. Instituto " Mercedes y Martín Ferreyra ", Casilla de Correo 389
5000 Córdoba, Argentina.

We have used dissociated cultures of medial basal hypothalamic neurons to study the effects of estrogen on neurite outgrowth, microtubule dynamics and the pattern of expression of several microtubule-associated proteins (MAPs) known to promote tubulin assembly and microtubule stability during neuronal morphogenesis.

The results obtained indicate that estradiol 17-B enhances axonal growth by hypothalamic neurons; it also causes an acceleration in the time course of initial axonal elaboration, and hence may regulate the onset of neuronal polarization. In addition, estradiol 17-B promotes an increase in Tau, but not in tubulin, MAP-1a, or MAP-2 protein levels. This response precedes and accompanies an increase in stable microtubule polymer within axonal shafts. Taken collectively, our results suggest that estrogen-enhanced axonal growth is mediated by a selective induction of microtubule stabilizing factors, namely the Tau proteins.
Supported by grants from CONICET and CONICOR.

S3.SC1

ESTRADIOL INDUCED NEUROPLASTIC CHANGES IN THE HYPOTHALAMUS IS ACCOMPANIED BY INCREASED ENDO-EXOCYTOTIC ACTIVITY OF NEURONAL MEMBRANES. A. Parducz, T. Szilagyi, S. Hoyk and L.M. Garcia-Segura. Institute of Biophysics, Biological Research Center, Szeged, Hungary; Instituto Cajal, CSIC, Madrid, Spain.

The organizational effects of gonadal steroids on neuronal connectivity is well documented and recent studies have shown that this influence is not limited to developmental stages. In the hypothalamic arcuate nucleus the number of axo-somatic synapses fluctuates during the ovarian cycle and experiments on ovariectomized animals clearly show that estradiol plays a decisive role in this phenomenon. It was found that 24 hours after estrogen treatment there is a transient and significant decrease in the number of GABAergic axo-somatic synapses and simultaneous increase in glial covering of perikaryal membranes. The synaptic changes in arcuate nucleus are accompanied by dramatic modifications in the ultrastructure of neuronal plasma membrane as well, and our hypothesis is that the hormonal induction of synaptic plasticity may be, at least in part, the result of an effect of estradiol on the distribution/internalization of adhesion or recognition molecules in neuronal membranes. The coated vesicles are thought to be the cell organelles which may transport these molecules to and from the membranes, therefore we performed experiments to determine if there is a change in the number of coated vesicles and coated pits following estrogen treatment i.e. during the synaptic remodelling.

The present results clearly show that in estradiol treated animals the number of coated pits and vesicles is increased and in freeze-fracture replicas the increased number of exo-endocytotic pits are also signalling a more active transport or turnover of perikaryal membrane constituents.

S3.SC2

GONADAL HORMONE REGULATION OF NEURO-GLIAL PLASTICITY IN THE ADULT RAT HYPOTHALAMUS. L.M. Garcia-Segura, J.A. Chowen, S. Busiguina, F. Naftolin and A. Párducz. Instituto Cajal, C.S.I.C., 28002 Madrid, Spain, Dept. OB/GYN, Yale Univ. School of Medicine, New Haven, CT, USA and Institute of Biophysics, Biological Research Center, H-6701 Szeged, Hungary

The influence of gonadal steroids on the ultrastructure of glial cells, the surface density of glial fibrillary acidic protein (SvGFAP) and the number of axo-somatic synapses was assessed in the arcuate nucleus of adult female rats. SvGFAP, the number of astroglial profiles in the arcuate neuropil and the proportion of neuronal perikaryal membrane covered by glia showed a rapid and reversible increase after the rise of estradiol levels in plasma during the estrous cycle. In contrast, the number of GABAergic axo-somatic synapses was decreased by estradiol. These results suggest that coordinated changes in glial cells and GABAergic synapses may be actively involved in the modulation of neuroendocrine events by the hypothalamus.

S4.1

CONTROL OF PROLACTIN SECRETION IN SHEEP. I.J. Clarke and G. A. Lincoln*, Prince Henry's Institute of Medical Research, P.O. Box 152, Clayton, 3168, Australia and *MRC Unit of Reproductive Biology, 37 Chalmers Street, Edinburgh, Scotland.

In sheep, as in other species, the secretion of prolactin from the pituitary gland is under tonic inhibitory control by hypothalamic factors. Thus, hypothalamo-pituitary disconnection (HPD) causes an increase in prolactin secretion. However, the levels of dopamine in hypophyseal portal blood were not higher than those in peripheral blood; noradrenalin levels were 3-fold higher in portal blood. Noradrenalin inhibits prolactin secretion in sheep. suggesting that this amine may act as a prolactin inhibitory factor in this species. On the other hand dopamine may reach the anterior pituitary through the short portal vessels via the posterior pituitary.

With the exception of thyrotrophin releasing hormone (TRH), we have not identified any factor that will cause prolactin release from the isolated pituitary gland. TRH is unlikely to be the physiological releasing factor because it's pulsatile release into hypophyseal portal blood do not correlate with prolactin secretion

Prolactin secretion shows a circannual rhythm in sheep with levels in plasma being elevated during long days. Surprisingly, this rhythm persists following HPD. This could be manipulated by artificial lighting regimens and by melatonin treatment. Since the pars tuberalis of the pituitary gland contains a high concentration of melatonin receptors, we propose that seasonal regulation of prolactin is by direct action of melatonin on the pituitary gland.

S4.2

A PHYSIOLOGICAL ROLE FOR DOPAMINE AS A HYPOTHALAMIC PROLACTIN RELEASING HORMONE. Marc E. Freeman, Department of Biological Science, Florida State University, Tallahassee, FL 32306-4075 USA

Stimuli inducing prolactin (PRL) secretion must act by diminishing the release of hypothalamic dopamine (DA), the PRL-inhibiting hormone, into hypophysial portal blood. The secretion of PRL in physiologically significant quantities requires the added release of PRL-releasing hormones of hypothalamic origin into portal blood superimposed upon this diminution of PRL-inhibitory activity. We have found that DA is actually a candidate for a PRL-*releasing* hormone. In perifused pituitary cells, lowering the DA concentration caused a greater release of PRL than complete withdrawal of DA. This phenomenon could be reproduced in cultured pituitary cells in which PRL secretion was measured by RIA or reverse hemolytic plaque assay (RHPA). Moreover, low doses of DA stimulated PRL secretion *in vivo*. Distinct signal transduction mechanisms were responsible for stimulation and inhibition of PRL secretion: pertussis toxin, an inhibitor of G_i, blocked inhibition but not stimulation of PRL secretion by DA while cholera toxin, an activator of G_s, enhanced stimulation but had no effect on inhibition of PRL secretion. Enriched lactotrophs responded to 10 μM DA with an 80% inhibition of PRL secretion while 100 pM DA stimulated PRL secretion by 40%. DA over a wide range of doses failed to affect phosphatidylinositol turnover while intracellular cAMP formation was only inhibited by DA. PRL-inhibitory doses of DA decreased intracellular calcium ([Ca]i) in 83% of lactotrophs while PRL-stimulatory doses of DA enhanced [Ca]i in 44% of the lactotrophs. Nifedipine, an inhibitor of L-type calcium channels, prevented the stimulatory effect of DA on PRL secretion. These studies suggest that the cascade mediating DAergic *inhibition* of PRL secretion involves activation of a G_i after binding to a D2 receptor leading to inhibition of cAMP-dependent [Ca]i and PRL secretion. *Stimulation* of PRL by lowering (but not withdrawing) DA involves binding to a D2 receptor leading to activation of a G_s, directly enhancing [Ca]i and PRL secretion. (Support: NIH, DK43200).

S4.3

IMPLICATION OF CALCIUM IN STIMULUS SECRETION COUPLING AND ITS REGULATION IN ANTERIOR PITUITARY CELLS. P.-M. Lledo, P. Vernier & J.-D. Vincent, C.N.R.S., Inst. A. Fessard, 91198 Gif-sur-Yvette, France.

Our work is centered in the study of the cellular mechanisms which control hormone secretion in anterior pituitary cells, with special interest on Ca^{2+} and second messengers. Single cell recording and intracellular perfusion were used to measure plasma membrane conductances and to assess directly the rapid changes in membrane surface area associated with secretory granule fusion and exocytosis. This has been combined with photometry for measuring the free intracellular [Ca^{2+}].

We have demonstrated that secretory events, known to involve intracellular Ca^{2+} as a key facilitator of exocytosis, were modulated by other intracellular signals which may act in concert to regulate secretion. Calcium elevation within the cell arise from both extracellular space via voltage- and agonist-gated ion channels and intracellular store release. Calcium influx may be very specifically modulated by signaling systems using receptors coupled to GTPases. The signal transduction mechanism that links D_2 receptor activation to a specific modulation of four different types of ionic channels will be briefly presented. The presence of Ca^{2+}-binding proteins also contributes to regulate the free intracellular Ca^{2+} level. We will describe the effect of calbindin on intracellular Ca^{2+} signals. Finally, experiments with patch-clamp measurements of Ca^{2+}-triggered exocytosis, were performed on injected pituitary cells with antisense directed at a small G-protein (rab3 protein). This provided the intriguing result that Ca^{2+} itself is not a sufficient stimulus for secretion: a component of Ca^{2+}-dependent exocytosis is regulated by this small G-protein and these two factors must act in concert to facilitate secretion in pituitary cells.

S4.SC1

DOPAMINE AND ENDOTHELIN SYNERGISTICALLY REGULATE PROLACTIN SECRETION. Béla Kanyicska* and Marc E. Freeman, Department of Biological Science, Florida State University, Tallahassee, FL 32306-4075 USA

The discovery of the PRL release-inhibiting potential of endothelins (ET) and their presence in the hypothalamic magnocellular neurons suggested that ET and dopamine (DA) may act in concert to modulate PRL secretion. To evaluate this possibility, a perifusion method was applied to follow the temporal pattern of PRL secretion as affected by ET and/or DA. Enzymatically dispersed anterior pituitary cells obtained from random cycling female rats were perifused with Dulbecco's Modified Eagle's Medium supplemented with 0.2 % BSA and 100 μM ascorbic acid. Six 0.5 ml perifusion chambers loaded with 10^6 cells were run in parallel and 3 minute fractions were collected at the rate of 0.2 ml/min. ET-1 (20 nM; 12 min/pulse) alone elicited a rapid and transient (<3 min) elevation of PRL release followed by an inhibitory phase which lasted for about 60 min. Extended exposure to 500 nM DA (≥48 h) dramatically shifted the responsiveness of the lactotrophs: the fast stimulatory response was robustly enhanced and the inhibitory phase was replaced by a modest but long lasting elevation of basal PRL secretion. Pharmacological desensitization (200 nM phorbol 12-myristate 13-acetate, PMA) or inhibition (200 nM staurosporine) of protein kinase C (PKC) mimicked the effects of DA. Taken together, long exposure to DA, a condition most closely resembling the *in vivo* environment of the lactotrophs, can synergistically affect some signal transduction processes mediating ET-induced stimulation of PRL secretion. The mechanism of this phenomenon likely involves specific phosphorylation events in which PKC plays an important role. Supported by NIH, DK43200.

S4.SC2

EFFECT OF NON SUCKLING INTERVAL UPON REGIONALIZATION OF PROLACTIN (PRL) SECRETION BY THE LACTATING RAT ANTERIOR PITUITARY (AP). Mena, F*, Aguayo, D and Morales, MT. Center of Neurobiology, National University of México, México, D.F. México 04510.

Previous studies showed that both transformation and suckling-induced release of PRL by the lactating rat AP are critically influenced by the length of the previous non-suckling interval. On the other hand, it has recently been shown that regional differences in transformation and release of PRL exist between the central, i.e., the inner region of the AP surrounding the intermediate lobe of the pituitary gland, and the peripheral region of the gland; and it was suggested that such differences could account for increased PRL secretion during lactation. In the present study we analyzed whether the length of non suckling may influence the occurrence of regionalization within the lactating rat AP. Methods: Lactating rats were isolated from their pups for either 0, 2, 4, 8, 12, 16 or 24h and then they were either killed or suckled by their pups for 15 min and then sacrified. AP fragments from each region were incubated for 30-120 min. Changes in PRL concentration and release were determined by polyacrylamide-disc-gel electrophoresis and densitometry. Results: *In vitro* transformation and release of PRL were significantly higher in AP fragments from the central than from the peripheral regions of the AP of non suckled rats. However, such differences were observed only in tissue fragments from 4-12h but not on either 0-2 or 16-24h non suckled rats. On the other hand, acute suckling to 4-12h non suckled rats abolished differences in release between the two regions of the gland. Conclusions: These results suggest that regionalization of PRL secretion develops as a function of time in which the mother is deprived of suckling by the litter and, that this stimulus prevents the occurrence of such phenomenon.

S5.1

Abstract not received

S5.2

MINERALOCORTICOIDS AS STABILIZING FACTOR FOR NEURONAL EXCITABILITY. M. Joëls. Inst. for Neurobiology, Univ. of Amsterdam, 1098 SM Amsterdam, The Netherlands.

The mineralocorticoid receptor (MR) in rat brain is structurally similar to the MR in peripheral tissue but, in contrast to the latter, binds corticosterone effectively: The affinity of the MR in rat brain for corticosterone is even higher (Kd~0.5nM) than of the glucocorticoid receptor (GR; Kd~5nM). With electrophysiological methods in vitro we examined the electrical properties of CA1 hippocampal neurons under conditions 1. that MRs (and GRs) are unoccupied (i.e. in untreated tissue from adrenalectomized rats), 2. that there is a predominant MR activation and 3. that GRs are occupied in addition to MRs. In particular, the transition from 2 to 3 is physiologically interesting, since it probably occurs daily, due to fluctuations in endogenous corticosterone levels.

In the absence of corticosterone (MRs unoccupied), amino acid carried input to CA1 neurons was found to attenuate with repeated stimulation; low-threshold Ca-currents were large. Low levels of corticosterone (predominant MR occupation) resulted in stable amino acid transmission, small Ca-currents and small responses to modulatory aminergic input. Further increase of the steroid level (GRs also activated) again induced less optimal responses, with attenuation of the amino acid input and large Ca-influxes. We conclude that the CA1 neuronal circuit may be most stable under conditions of predominant MR activation, that is with low to moderate levels of corticosterone.

S5.3

CENTRAL MEDIATORS IN MINERALOCORTICOID INDUCTION OF SALT APPETITE. A.F. De Nicola. Lab. Neuroendocrine Biochemistry, Instituto de Biologia y Medicina Experimental-CONICET, Obligado 2490, 1428 Buenos Aires, Argentina.

High doses of deoxycorticosterone acetate (DOCA) incited a salt appetite in rats due, at least in part, to a direct action in the central nervous system. Natriogenesis was partly delayed by administration of the mineralocorticoid (MC) antagonist ZK 91587 whereas the antiglucocorticoid RU 486 was ineffective, suggesting involvement of MC receptors (MR). In DOCA-treated rats, binding of (^{3}H)-corticosterone to MR was reduced in hippocampus, unchanged in amygdala but highly stimulated in the hypothalamus. Binding to glucocorticoid receptors (GR) was reduced in all regions. However, GR were not activated because the glucocorticoid-dependent enzyme ornithine decarboxylase was not stimulated by DOCA. At the time of maximum salt ingestion, DOCA-treated rats presented reduction of the activity of Na,K-ATPase in two amygdaloid nuclei and lateral hypothalamus. This was accompanied by a reduction in the biosynthesis of the ß-subunit of the enzyme in some amygdaloid and hypothalamic nuclei, according to in situ hybridization data. Therefore, modulation of the enzyme Na,K-ATPase as well as MR in specialized neuroendocrine areas may be part of the mechanisms for DOCA effects on salt appetite .

S5.SC1

TRANSCRIPTIONAL INDUCTION OF THE RAT MINERALOCORTICOID RECEPTOR GENE BY CORTICOSTEROIDS. Maija Castrén*, Benedikt Berninger, Thorsten Trapp, Eero Castrén and Florian Holsboer. Dept. of Neuroendocrinology and Neurochemistry, Max-Planck-Institute of Psychiatry, Munich, Germany

We have investigated the regulation of the mineralocorticoid receptor (MR) gene expression by corticosteroids in primary hippocampal neurons, the primary target of glucocorticoids in the brain. By using quantitative reverse transcriptase-PCR, 4.0 fold induction by aldosterone and 4.5 fold induction by dexamethasone was detected in MR mRNA levels. We used transient transfections into neuroblastoma cells to show that aldosterone and dexamethasone can directly activate the rat MR promoter demonstrating that the steroid-induced increase in the MR mRNA concentration is transcriptional. The induction of the promoter activity by aldosterone and dexamethasone was significantly reduced by competitive receptor agonists indicating that the induction was mediated predominantly by glucocorticoid receptor and MR, respectively. Progressive 5'-deletions of the MR promoter sequences defined a glucocorticoid responsive region between -520 and 297 base pairs (bp). A consensus half-glucocorticoid responsive element (half-GRE) is located at -319 bp and the oligonucleotide comprising the putative MR GRE (-298/-315) in front of Simian virus promoter responded to aldosterone and dexamethasone. The identified MR GRE is a weak enhancer as a single element, but cloning three of these enhancers in tandem greatly potentiated the response to corticosteroids.

S5.SC2

THE NON-GENOMIC MECHANISM OF GLUCOCORTICOID ACTION ON NEURONS. Y.Z. Chen, X.Liu, C.A.Wang, A.L.Ye, H.Fu, Z.Guo. Dept. of Physiology, Second Military Medical University, Shanghai, P.R.China, 200433.

Since 1987 we have provided electrophysiological evidences that GC could act non-genomically. Further biochemical data revealed that GC could bind to the purified neuronal membrane preparation specifically with a reasonably high affinity. With an antibody, which recognizes the N-terminal of the traditional GC receptor, it has been shown that GC membrane receptor could be visualized with the immunogold technique under electron microscope. Recently the influences of GC and other drugs on the release of arginine vasopressin(AVP) from superfused hypothalamic slices containing paraventricular and supraoptic nuclei were observed. The AVP released from the slice were determined by radioimmunoassay. The results showed that, the steady release rate of AVP was 9.06±1.23pg/min, which lasted as long as 6 hours. The release of AVP was inhibited within 20min by corticosterone(B) in a dose-dependent manner from 10^{-7}-10^{-4}mol/L. The inhibitory effect of B persisted in the presence of actinomycinD(4×10^{-4}mol/L) or puromycin(4×10^{-4}mol/L). Furthermore, the inhibitory effect of GC could be antagonized by RU38486, and corticosterone-bovine serum albumin was also inhibitory to the releasing process. So the results depicted the non-genomic action of GC on neurosecretory process. Because GC manifested its effect on neurons at or close to its physiological concentration, it might finally be proved to be a new class of neuromodulators.

Acknowledgements: This work was supported by NSFC.

S6.1

CELL BIOLOGY OF GT1 GnRH NEURONAL CELL LINES. R.I. Weiner, E.A. Vitalis, P.-S. Tsai, L. Milenkovic, A.L.H. Choi, G. Martinez de la Escalera. Reproductive Endocrinology Center, University of California, San Francisco, USA, 94143.

GT1 GnRH cell lines were established by genetically targeted tumorigenesis in transgenic mice. The cell lines are both morphologically and genetically highly differentiated neurons which express the GnRH gene at high levels. The secretion of GnRH is coupled to depolarization. Basal release from cultures of cells is pulsatile with a pulse frequency identical to that seen in castrated mice. Therefore, pulsatile release is an intrinsic property of GT1 cells demonstrating that cultures of the cells have the ability to time and synchronize GnRH release. The secretion of GnRH is regulated by a variety of receptors expressed by the cells including excitatory: ß1 adrenergic, D1 dopaminergic, and $GABA_A$ receptors; and inhibitory: $GABA_B$ and the short and long forms of the prolactin receptor. The receptors stimulate signaling pathways involving the activation or inhibition of protein kinases and phosphatases which may comprise a timing mechanism for pulsatile release. The cells also express functional FGF receptors which appear to mediate the neurotropic action of basic FGF. These observations begin to explain the complexity of GnRH regulation observed in animals.

S6.2

UNCONVENTIONAL SIGNALLING BY THE LHRH RECEPTOR. R. Mitchell, M.S. Johnson, J. Simpson, P.J. Sim, W.B. Wolbers, M. Fennell and A.J. Ison. MRC Brain Metabolism Unit. University Department of Pharmacology, 1 George Square, Edinburgh EH8 9JZ, Scotland

The LHRH receptor is a member of the family of G protein-linked receptors coupled to hydrolysis of phosphoinositides. The dependence of LHRH-induced gonadotropin secretion upon phospholipase C activity has however been questioned. In view of the unique ability of the LHRH receptor to elicit the phenomenon of self-priming, we have sought to define unconventional signals emanating from this receptor that may not be generated by other members of the receptor family. The phenomenon of LHRH self-priming is dependent upon an apparently novel species of PKC (with a pituitary-selective distribution) that we have partially purified and characterised. Amongst the cellular targets of a PKC with these properties are PLA_2 and PLD.
Signalling by means of tyrosine kinase and MAP kinase cascades is classically associated with growth factor receptors. Nevertheless we have shown that each of these is strongly activated by LHRH both in normal pituitary tissue and in the αT3-1 gonadotropin cell line. LHRH-induced production of phosphotyrosine-immunoreactive proteins is mimicked in part by phorbol esters but not by ionomycin and is essential for LHRH-induced PLD activation and LH secretion. LHRH-induced MAP kinase activation correlates strongly with the ability of gonadotrophs to demonstrate self-priming and occurs through a PKC-dependent rather than Ca^{2+}-dependent or tyrosine kinase-dependent mechanism. Since MAP kinase is involved in the regulation of transcription, translation and cytoskeletal organisation, it is a strong candidate for a central role in the self-priming phenomenon which is reliant on the rapid induction of protein synthesis and cytoskeletal changes.

S6.3

LIGAND-RECEPTOR INTERACTIONS AND SIGNAL PROPAGATION IN THE GnRH RECEPTOR: INSIGHTS FROM MUTAGENESIS. *N. Illing[1,2], I. Becker[2], C. Flanagan[2], J.S. Davidson[2], W. Zhou[3], S. Sealfon[3], and R.P. Millar[2]. [1]Dept of Biochemistry and [2]MRC Regulatory Peptides Research Group, University of Cape Town Medical School, Observatory 7925, South Africa; [3]Fishberg Center in Neurobiology and Dept of Neurology, Mount Sinai School of Medicine, New York.

Our recent cloning of GnRH receptors (GnRHR) from different vertebrate species paves the way for the molecular dissection of the functioning of the GnRHR. The GnRHR is a G-protein-coupled receptor (GPCR) with seven transmembrane (TM) α-helical domains connected by intracellular (IC) and extracellular (EC) loops. A unique feature of the receptor is the absence of an intracellular C-terminal tail which is the target for phosphorylation-induced desensitization of a number of GPCRs. We have shown that there is no homologous desensitization of phospholipase C activity by GnRH. Our research focuses on the following areas of investigation: 1) interhelical interactions 2) ligand-receptor interactions 3) the nature of the molecular switch that propagates ligand activation of the receptor and 4) coupling of IC loops to signal transduction pathways. We have exploited the putative reciprocal mutation of interacting residues of the TMs, and this has allowed the assignment of relative positions of helices TM2 and TM7. In addition to testing and refining our model of interhelical interactions, this provides insight into the orientation of side chains of TM amino acids which may be candidates for ligand binding. While all of the vertebrate GnRHs are able to stimulate the release of gonadotropins, the specificity of the receptor differs among vertebrate species. We have identified an acidic residue in the EC domain that determines the specificity of the mammalian GnRHR for mammalian GnRH. Two consensus sequences (N-X-S/T) for N-glycosylation are located in the EC domains and are conserved in all the cloned GnRHRs. Mutagenesis studies have shown that these sites are important for normal GnRHR localization to the cell surface, but do not participate in ligand binding or signal transduction of the GnRHR.

S6.SC1

CROSS-TALK BETWEEN Ca^{2+} AND PROTEIN KINASE C IN GnRH ACTION UPON GONADOTROPIN SUBUNITS GENE EXPRESSION IN CULTURED RAT PITUITARY CELLS.

Z. Naor* and D. Ben-Menahem. Department of Biochemistry, Tel Aviv University, Ramat Aviv 69978, Israel.

Incubation of cultured rat pituitary cells with GnRH resulted in a biphasic (60 min and 24 h) elevation of gonadotropin subunit α, LHβ and FSHβ mRNA levels. Addition of the PKC activator TPA or the Ca^{2+} ionophore, ionomycin, mimicked the profile of GnRH-induced α- and LHβ mRNA elevation. The two phases of FSHβ mRNA elevation induced by GnRH could be mimicked by TPA. The rapid effect of GnRH was abolished by the PKC inhibitors staurosporine and GF 109203X, while the effect of GnRH on α- and LHβ, but not FSHβ, was abolished in Ca^{2+}-free medium. While additivity in LH release is elicited by combination of TPA and ionomycin for 30 min, LHβ and FSHβ gene expression is inhibited. Thus sequential and differential signalling by Ca^{2+} and PKC is responsible for GnRH-induced gonadotropin gene expression.

S6.SC2

GLUTAMATE, GABA, AND GNRH NEUROINTERACTIONS IN THE PRIMATE HYPOTHALAMUS. **P.C. Goldsmith*, K.K. Thind. Reproductive Endocrinology Center, University of California, San Francisco, CA 94143-0556.**

We have analyzed interactions between Glutamate (Glu) and GnRH neurons in the hypothalamus of adult, juvenile and fetal *M. fascicularis* and *M. macaca* using double-label immunostaining. Axo-dendritic Glu/GnRH interactions seen in the OVLT, medial septum (MS), and VHT1 by light microscopy were verified as classical asymmetrical synapses by EM. Reverse GnRH/Glu interactions including axo-dendritic (AXO/DEN) synapses and poorly specialized dendro-dendritic (DEN/DEN) contacts were also present. These results are the first anatomical evidence in any species that GnRH neurons are under direct Glu control. In a related study, we examined Glu and GABA interactions in the adult female *M. fascicularis* by immunostaining for Glu and glutamic acid decarboxylase (GAD). Immunoreactive (-ir) profiles (*n=785)* were 63% Glu-ir, 28% GAD-ir, and 9% Glu+GAD-ir. Glu-ir afferents were seen in 59% *(n=177)* of labeled synapses (36%) and contacts (64%), and in 69% of all AXO/DEN and 80% of all DEN/DEN interactions. AXO/DEN's were 29% Glu/GAD, 22% Glu/Glu, and 18% Glu/Glu+GAD, while DEN/DEN's were 50% Glu/GAD, 12% Glu/Glu, and 18% Glu/Glu+GAD. Asymmetrical synapses were found only in the MS, VHT1, and SON (40-49%), where GnRH-ir neurons occur in primates. Only symmetrical synapses occurred in the PVN (13%), where GnRH-ir neurons are rare. In summary, predominant Glu-ir in hypothalamic afferents attests to its powerful influence on neuroendocrine activity. However, GAD-ir also exists in 47% of Glu's AXO/DEN and 68% of Glu's DEN/DEN efferents. Since GnRH-ir neurons express excitatory Glu, excitatory $GABA_A$ and inhibitory $GABA_B$ receptors, the integrated output of Glu-GABA interactions may contribute significantly to the membrane potential of GnRH neurons in primates. (Supported by NIH grants HD10907 and HD11979.)

S7.1

THE SUPRACHIASMATIC NUCLEUS DRIVING NEUROENDOCRINE RHYTHMS.

R.M. Buijs, A. Kalsbeek. Netherlands Institute for Brain Research, Meibergdreef 33, 1105 AZ Amsterdam, The Netherlands.

The suprachiasmatic nucleus (SCN) synchronizes the daily or nightly activity and steroid hormone secretion of most mammals, with the day/night cycle. The SCN has an endogenous rhythm in electrical activity and neurotransmitter synthesis. We have hypothesized that this circadian rhythm in neurotransmitter synthesis and release is the physiological basis of the entrainment properties of the SCN.

We have investigated by which anatomical connections the SCN may impose its endogenous rhythm onto the hypothalamo-adrenal axis. Thus we found no evidence for direct contacts between the SCN and CRH producing neurons, but for an indirect route, probably containing vasopressin as a neurotransmitter, via the dorsomedial hypothalamus (DMH). Furthermore, it was demonstrated that GABA is present in approximately 30% of the SCN terminals and that it is colocalized with several SCN peptides.

Microinfusion of vasopressin and vasopressin antagonists in DMH inhibited respectively stimulated ACTH (corticosterone) release. Thus we propose specifically that vasopressin released as a neurotransmitter from the SCN terminals in the DMH area serves as a corticotrophin inhibiting factor and in general that vasopressin of SCN origin regulates as a neurotransmitter those physiological processes that serve to maintain the nocturnal animal in its rest state. Whether the opposite mechanism holds in day-active animals still has to be investigated.

S7.2

EFFECT OF LIGHT ON NEUROTRANSMITTER CONTENTS AND NEUROPEPTIDE SYNTHESIS IN THE SUPRACHIASMATIC NUCLEI.

Shin-Ichi T. Inouye, Mitsubishi Kasei Institute of Life Sciences, Machida, Tokyo 194 Japan

The suprachiasmatic nucleus (SCN) of the hypothalamus contains a circadian pacemaker that drives many behavioral and humoral rhythms in mammals. These rhythms are synchronized to the external light-dark cycle. To explore neurochemical mechanisms through which light regulate the phase of the circadian rhythms, we investigated the change in neurotransmitter contents in the SCN induced by environmental light-dark cycles or by short light exposure. While vasopressin and somatostatin contents were unaffected by the presence or absence of the light-dark cycle, vasoactive intestinal polypeptide (VIP), gastrin releasing peptide (GRP) and neuropeptide Y (NPY) levels in the SCN distinctively responded to change in ambient light . Light reduced VIP and enhanced GRP level, and constant darkness kept the levels stable. Phase dependence was also found in VIP and NPY responses to light pulses. VIP response to light was strongest during the late subjective night and weakest during the early subjective night. NPY level responded transitorily to light to dark and dark to light transitions. Messenger RNA abundance encoding VIP showed a similar change to VIP peptide in response to light exposure, but with faster time course. Moreover, serotonin and norepinephrine levels in the SCN were also dependent on lighting conditions. These observations suggest that light information is transduced in the SCN into activity of transmitters and processed to determine the phase of the circadian pacemaker.

S7.3

MELATONIN RECEPTORS IN CIRCADIAN AND SEASONAL RHYTHMS. M. Masson-Pévet. URA-CNRS 1332, Université Louis Pasteur, 12 rue de l'Université, 67000 Strasbourg, France.

Suprachiasmatic nuclei (SCN) and pars tuberalis (PT) are two structures exhibiting high affinity receptors for melatonin. The regulation of these receptors has been studied at the daily and the seasonal level. Melatonin receptor density in the two structures is elevated at day-time and low at night-time. In the PT, variations persist in constant darkness and can only be blocked by pinealectomy ; thus these daily variations are directly induced by the circadian rhythm of plasma melatonin concentrations. In contrast, this process of desensitization does not determine the daily variations in SCN melatonin receptor density. Indeed, in the SCN, the light/dark cycle is the regulatory factor : melatonin receptor density is specifically reduced during the night, even in absence of melatonin, while one hour light reverses this nocturnal decrease in the SCN. This light effect on melatonin receptor density in the SCN is mediated by activation of NMDA-type receptors. At the seasonal level, short photoperiod which induces gonadal regression, also induces a decrease in the density of melatonin receptors of the PT. In constrast no change is observed in SCN melatonin receptors with photoperiod.
The regulation of melatonin receptors is thus totally different in the PT and SCN at the daily as well as at the seasonal level.

S7.SC1

SUPRACHIASMATIC (SCN) AND SUBPARAVENTRICULAR (SPV) EFFERENTS TARGET MEDIAN EMINENCE PROJECTIVE NEURONS CONTAINING CALBINDIN (CB), TYROSINE HYDROXYLASE (TH), GALANIN (GAL) AND β-ENDORPHIN (β-END). T.L. Horváth*, C. Leranth, F. Naftolin. Dept. of OB/Gyn, Yale Univ. School of Med., New Haven , CT., 06510, U.S.A.

This study aims to describe connections between the circadian pacemaker SCN and neuroendocrine cells of the hypothalamus using the combination of anterograde and retrograde tracer techniques and immunocytochemistry. Experimental: *Phaseolus vulgaris* leucoagglutinin (PHA-L) was injected into either the bilateral SCN or the SPV of 8 female rats to label their efferents. Two days later, the retrograde tracer fluorogold (FG) was administered intraperitoneally, to identify neurons projecting to the median eminence. After visualization of PHA-L with a nickel-diaminobenzidine reaction (dark blue reaction product), sections were immunostained for FG (granular cytoplasmic staining), followed by CB, TH, GAL and β-END immunostaining. PHA-L immunopositive SCN efferents were most abundant in the SPV zone; fewer fibers were observed in the medial preoptic area and paraventricular nucleus, and only a very limited number of axons were detected in the arcuate nucleus. These regions contained a high number of cells immunoreactive for FG. Some of these neurons were observed to be targets of SCN axon terminals while containing either CB, TH, GAL or β-END. The efferents of the SPV zone were abundant in the same areas, and the instances of connections between these fibers and median eminence projective, chemically identified neurons were frequent. Electron microscopic examination confirmed the putative connections to be synaptic. Conclusions: This experiment provides the first evidence that the SCN has limited, but direct efferents to neuroendocrine cells containing CB, TH, GAL and β-END. These neurons may also be indirectly regulated by the SCN via interneurons located in the SPV region.

S7.SC2

ACUTE AND CHRONIC ADMINISTRATION OF GLUCOCORTICOIDS CHANGE LEVELS OF PEPTIDE GENE EXPRESSION IN THE RAT SUPRACHIASMATIC NUCLEUS.

Jens D. Mikkelsen, Niels Vrang, Morten Møller, Philip J. Larsen. Department of Anatomy, The Panum Institute, University of Copenhagen, Denmark

In this study we have investigated the effects of chronic and acute administration of glucocorticoids upon the the diurnal expression of vasopressin and vasoactive intestinal peptide (VIP) mRNA in the SCN by semiquantitative in situ hybridization histochemistry. Male rats entrained to a 12:12 photoperiod were either adrenalectomized (ADX) or sham-operated. The adrenalectomized rats were either treated with corticosterone, dexamethasone or saline for 14 days. The animals were seperated in groups of 6, which were decapitated at various *zeitgeber* times (ZT). The chronic administration of exogenous glucocorticoids significantly enhanced vasopression gene expression to higher levels only at ZT5, while at other ZTs (ZT11, ZT17, and ZT23), no change was detected. The same treatment abolished the rhythmic expression of VIPmRNA resulting in constantly elevated levels. These data show that the internal clock located within the vasopressin neurons of the SCN can be regulated only at times, where non-photic phase-shifts can also be achieved. Furthermore, in ADX rats given a supplement of dexamethasone in their drinking water, the expression of both vasopressin and VIP mRNA was elevated the following morning at ZT6 when compared to vehicle. These data suggest that glucocorticoids could play a role as a hormone with phase-shifting (non-photic) effects on the circadian clock.

S8.1

NEURAL CONTROL OF ADRENOCORTICAL FUNCTION. TJH. Tilders & I. Dijkstra. Res Inst Neurosci Free University, Fac Med, Dept Pharmacol, 1081 BT Amsterdam, The Netherlands.

The production of gluccorticoids (CORT) in the adrenal gland is primarily controlled by circulating ACTH. Nonetheless, in many (patho)physiological conditions, deviant plasma CORT levels are not sufficiently explained by changes in circulating ACTH. Several neuro-transmitters, neuropeptides including CRH, cytokines, NO e.a. stimulate CORT production by adrenal(cell)s in vitro. Most of these substances, including NO, are produced in the adrenal gland and are present in chromaffin and/or ganglion cells and (varicose) fibres in the medulla and/or cortical zones. We hypothesize that the activity of these cells is CNS controlled (splanchnic nerve) and exert their action at the CORT producing cells directly or by affecting the adrenal blood flow that correlates with adrenal CORT production. Diurnal variations in resting CORT levels are partly due to diurnal changes in the sensitivity to ACTH. In perfused adrenal glands, CRH increases the CORT response to ACTH. Conversely, blockade of CRH reduces adrenal sensitivity and abolishes the nocturnal rise in ACTH sensitivity. The adrenal ACTH hyperresponsiveness found during chronic stress, depression and other psychopathologies may be determined by similar mechanisms.

S8.2

NEURAL MODULATION OF LOCAL PEPTIDE ACTION IN THE TESTIS.

I. Gerendai. 2nd Department of Anatomy, Semmelweis University Medical School, Budapest, Hungary, H-1094.

Our previous studies indicated that in immature rats intratesticular administration of opiate receptor antagonists or enkephalin decrease, while oxytocin stimulates testicular steroidogenesis. It has also been demonstrated that testicular nerves are also involved in the control of testicular functions. Therefore, we investigated whether testicular nerves might exert modulatory effect on local peptide actions. Partial denervation of the testis was performed surgically (vasectomy, i.e. transection of the inf. testicular n.) or pharmacologically [testicular injection of 6-hydroxydopamine (6-OHDA) or 5,6 dihydroxytryptamine (5,6-DHT)]. Hemivasectomy and treatment of the testis with naloxone or enkephalin analog, in spite of the suppressive effect of these interventions, resulted in a paradoxical effect, i.e. increased steroidogenesis in the case of naloxone administration, and normalization of basal testosterone secretion in vitro after enkephalin treatment. Effect of oxytocin (stimulatory) observed in rats with intact testis was reversed following pharmacological sympathectomy. Pretreatment of the testis with 5,6-DHT prevented the oxytocin-induced rise in steroidogenesis. Results indicate that testicular nerves are involved in the control of local peptide effects. (These studies were supported by OTKA 1007 and ETT 10-201 grants.)

S8.3

NEURAL CONTROL OF IMMUNE FUNCTION.

K. Bulloch. The Rockefeller University, Lab. of Neuroendocrinology, New York, N. Y. 10021 and UCSD, Dept. of Psych, San Diego, Ca. 92161.

Some of the most compelling evidence for the existence of interaction between the immune and nervous systems has come from studies which describe the distribution and function of autonomic and neuroendocrine molecules within the organs and tissues of the immune system. Calcitonin gene related peptide (CGRP) is a prime example of such a molecule. CGRP has been identified by ICC in nerves and a discrete cell population within the thymus, and pharmacological studies demonstrate the presence of specific receptors for CGRP on thymocytes. Functional studies indicate that CGRP is a potent inhibitor of mitogen and antigen stimulated T cells proliferation and is involved in apoptosis within this gland. These data suggest that endogenous CGRP may serve as a natural inhibitor of inappropriate induction of antigen sensitive mature T cells within the thymus as well as play a role in T cell education and the positive and negative selection of the T cell repertoire.

S8.SC1

LOCALIZATION OF CATECHOLAMINERGIC NEURONAL ELEMENTS IN RAT ADRENOCORTICAL ZONA GLOMERULOSA AND JUVENILE THYMUS: SIMILARITIES AND DIFFERENCES.

E. Orsó, I.E. Tóth, I.J. Elenkov, E.S. Vizi. Institute of Experimental Medicine, Hungarian Academy of Sciences, H-1450 Budapest, P.O.Box 67. Hungary.

An extensive peripheral noradrenergic neuronal meshwork was demonstrated both in adrenocortical zona glomerulosa and juvenile rat thymus by light and electron microscopic immunocytochemistry. About 20% of noradrenergic varicosities lies in close proximity of zona glomerulosa cells making non synaptic interaction which forms the possibility for the fine tuning of zona glomerulosa function by a paracrine way. Thymic noradrenergic varicosities were localized in the extraparenchymal compartment, in trabecules and septa. These extraparenchymal spaces form a closed channel-network, where catecholamines, released from local varicose axon terminals, are able to diffuse along collagen fibrills (helped with contractile elements of epithelial cells) for a relatively long distance and get to the thymic parenchymal cells. Large number of mast cells could be shown in close association with tyrosine-hydroxylase and/or dopamine-ß-hydroxylase-immunoreactive nerve fibres in the thymus. This close apposition of mast cells and autonomic nerve fibres may be of crucial significance for indirect neuroimmunomodulatory mechanism in the thymus. We have confirmed, that while in adrenocortical zona glomerulosa there is a close contact between catecholaminergic nerve terminals and parenchymal cells, thymic parenchyma has no direct innervation, but the morphological structure makes possible the diffusion of catecholamines from the nerve endings to the parenchymal cells.

S8.SC2

DIFFERENT REGULATION OF ADRENAL TYROSINE HYDROXYLASE GENE EXPRESSION IN RATS AFTER INSULIN HYPOGLYCEMIA AND IMMOBILIZATION STRESS.

R. Kvetnansky, I. Vietor, M. Rusnak, E. Viskupic, S. Zorad, E.L. Sabban*[1] Institute Exp. Endocrinology, Slovak Acad. Sci., Bratislava, Slovakia, and [1]Dept. Biochem. Mol. Biol., New York Medical College, Valhalla, N.Y., USA.

Both immobilization (IMO) of rats for 2 hours and administration of insulin (5 IU/kg, i.p., 5 hours) have been shown to elevate adrenal tyrosine hydroxylase (TH) mRNA levels about 4 - 6-fold. The aim of this study was to examine the mechanism(s) responsible for these changes. The innervation of the adrenal medulla is cholinergic and is predominantly mediated via splanchnic nerve. The IMO-induced rise in TH mRNA levels was not reduced by antagonists of both nicotinic and muscarinic receptors. Denervation of the adrenals by unilateral or bilateral splanchnicotomy, surprisingly, did not block the IMO induced rise in TH mRNA found in innervated adrenals. In contrast, adrenal denervation completely prevented the rise in TH mRNA levels induced by insulin administration. Nitric oxide (NO) is a newly discovered second messenger which might affect TH. Inhibition of NO synthesis by administration of L-nitroarginine (40 mg/kg, i.p.) significantly reduced the IMO induced rise in the adrenal TH mRNA levels. These data suggest that mechanisms regulating the expression of the gene coding for TH differ depending on the stress model used: insulin-mediated induction depends on splanchnic innervation, whereas IMO-mediated induction is non-neuronal and occurs even in the absence of splanchnic innervation. Nitric oxide appears to be involved in IMO stress induced elevation of TH mRNA levels in rat adrenals.

Supported by Fogarty Award FIRCA (TW-00108) and Slovak Grant Agency for Science (2-543/93).

S9.1

GLUCOCORTICOID REGULATION OF TGF-$\beta 1$ mRNA IN HIPPOCAMPUS AND EFFECTS OF AGING. N.R. Nichols, Morgan, T.E., Laping, N.J., Finch, C.E. Andrus Gerontology Center and Dept. of Biological Sciences, Univ. of Southern California, Los Angeles, CA, USA, 90089-0191.

The anti-inflammatory and immunosuppressive actions of glucocorticoids are often mediated by their interactions with cytokines. Recently, we cloned TGF-$\beta 1$ from hippocampus of adult male F344 rats as a mRNA that was decreased in response to corticosterone (CORT) treatment. This response exhibited glucocorticoid receptor (GR) specificity and was elicited by CORT in the drinking water. TGF-$\beta 1$ mRNA increased early in the response to deafferenting and neurotoxic lesions and was expressed in microglia. Adrenalectomy (ADX) promotes neurodegeneration in the hippocampal dentate gyrus, an area still undergoing development in the adult rat brain. By in situ hybridization, TGF-$\beta 1$ mRNA was dramatically increased in the dentate granule cell layer after ADX, coincident with the appearance of both pyknotic cells and OX-42 immunoreactive microglia with an activated morphology. This expression disappeared within 2 h CORT treatment. In a study of aging, hippocampal TGF-$\beta 1$ mRNA increased by 24 mo of age in two cohorts of rats by RNA blot hybridization. This change was of the same magnitude (30%), but in the opposite direction to the response to CORT in young rats. In human post-mortem brain, TGF-$\beta 1$ mRNA increased ($P < 0.05$) in the cortex of old (60-89 y) compared with middle-aged (25-59 y) individuals; a similar trend was observed in the hippocampus. If the decrease in TGF-$\beta 1$ mRNA in response to glucocorticoids is an adaptive response (i.e. anti-inflammation), then the increase during aging may represent a failure in homeostatic mechanisms due to altered neuroendocrine regulation at the level of target responsiveness. New roles for TGF-$\beta 1$ in brain development and aging are proposed, that suggest interaction between neuroendocrine and neuroimmune circuits. Supported by PHS AG-07909.

S9.2

HORMONAL REGULATION OF NEUROTROPHIC FACTORS IN BRAIN. D. Lindholm, Dept. Neurochemistry, Max Planck Institute for Psychiatry, Munich, Germany, D-82152

Hormones produced by the adrenal and thyroid glands have important effects on normal brain function. Glucocorticoid hormones mediate the stress response in brain but have also essential neurophysiological and cell survival effects in eg hippocampus. We have studied whether some of the effects of glucoccorticoids involve changes in expression of neurotrophic factors such as nerve growth factor (NGF), brain-derived growth factor (BDNF) and neurotrophin-3 (NT-3). In the rat hippocampus corticosterone and the synthetic glucocorticoid, dexamethsone influenced the expression of NGF and NT-3 whereas at early time points BDNF remained constant. There is also an important interaction between the hormones and the neurotransmitter-dependent regulation of NGF and BDNF in the hippocampus suggesting a complex set of regulatory mechanisms for these genes within neurons. Tri-iodothyronine enhanced NT-3 expression particularly in the rat cerebellum whereas experimental hypothyroidism decreased the levels of NT-3 mRNA. T3 had only minor effects on NGF and BDNF mRNA expression. T3 also increased survival of both cerebellar granule and hippocampal neurons in culture. The interplay between the various hormones and the neurotrophic factors in regulating neuronal survival and differentiation in brain will be further discussed.

S9.3

LOCALLY PRODUCED GnRH AS AN INHIBITING GROWTH FACTOR IN ENDOCRINE-DEPENDENT TUMORS. P. Limonta*, D. Dondi, M. Montagnani Marelli, R.M. Moretti. Dept. of Endocrinology, University of Milano, 20133 Milano, Italy.

The tumor of the prostate is a hormone-dependent pathology, at least in its early stages. Locally produced growth modulating factors have been proposed to play a crucial role as mediators of steroid action in the proliferation of this type of tumor. In the authors' laboratory, it has been shown that GnRH agonists exert a direct antiproliferative action on the human androgen-responsive prostate cancer cell line LNCaP. The specificity of this action has been confirmed by the observation that low affinity high-capacity binding sites for GnRH analogs are present on LNCaP cells, particularly when cultured in a steroid-free medium. These data suggested that GnRH itself, or a GnRH-like peptide, might be produced by prostatic tumor cells to act as a paracrine/autocrine growth modulating factor. By means of the reverse transcription-polymerase chain reaction (RT-PCR) technique, it has been demonstrated that a mRNA for GnRH is expressed in LNCaP cells. To clarify the possible role played by this factor in the local control of tumor growth, LNCaP cells, grown in steroid-free conditions, have been treated with a potent GnRH antagonist; the treatment resulted in a significant increase of cell proliferation.Taken together, these data point to GnRH as a locally produced inhibiting growth factor in the endocrine-dependent tumor of the prostate. Additional observations seem to indicate that GnRH might act by antagonizing the EGF/TGFα growth stimulating system. These data underline the multiple relationships among different growth factors in the local regulation of prostatic tumor cell proliferation. *(Supported by AIRC, by CNR through the special projects "ACRO", "FATMA", "BTBS", and by MURST).*

S9.SC1

SYNAPTIC REMODELLING INDUCED BY TROPHIC FACTORS. A. Claudio Cuello. Depart. of Pharmacology & Therapeutics, McGill University, Montreal, Quebec, Canada, H3G 1Y6

Neurotrophins and other trophic factors have been shown to preserve cholinergic injured neurons of the nucleus basalis (nbm) and medial septum of adult animals. Experimental evidence gathered in our laboratory indicates that the action of neurotrophic factors can go beyond the maintenance of neural phenotypic characteristics. Thus, NGF provokes a dose-dependent up-regulation of choline acetyltransferase enzymatic activity and high affinity choline uptake in the remaining cortex of rats bearing unilateral cortical infarctions. These effects are not observed in naive, non-lesioned animals. After intracerebroventricular administration of NGF, rats with limited cortical infarction experience retraction of the cholinergic terminal fibre network and loss of varicosities in the remaining neocortex. This parallels the cell body shrinkage observed in the nbm. NGF treatment compensates for these cholinergic deficits in CNS-lesioned rats by expanding the fibre network and increasing the number of varicosities. Furthermore, ultrastructural studies combined with image analysis reveal a hypertrophy of cholinergic presynaptic sites and an increase in synaptic differentiations. This cortical "synaptic modelling" could explain the remarkable functional and behavioural changes observed in cortically injured animals treated with NGF.

References: Cuello, A.C., (1993) Progr. Br. Res., 98: 265-277; Garofalo, L. et. al., (1992) Proc. Natl. Acad. Sci., USA., 89: 2639-2643; Garofalo, L. et.al., (1993) Neuroscience, 57(1): 21-40; Garofalo, L. and Cuello, A.C., (1994) Expl. Neurol., 125: 195-217.

Acknowledgements: Medical Research Council of Canada (MRC)

S9.SC2

ROLE OF NERVE GROWTH FACTOR IN THE DIFFERENTIATION AND PROLIFERATION OF PITUITARY CELLS. C. Missale, F. Boroni, M. Losa*, M. Giovanelli*, P.F. Spano. Div. of Pharmacology, Dept. of Biomedical Sciences and Biotechnology, University of Brescia, Brescia, Italy and * Div. of Neurosurgery, Scientific Institute S. Raffaele, University of Milano, Italy.

The phenotypical characteristics of 13 human prolactinomas (5 sensitive to dopamina (DA) D-2 receptor agonists and 8 refractory to this therapy) were studied. Cells from DA-sensitive tumors are very similar to lactotroph cells as shown by their very low degree of malignancy and the expression of DA D-2 receptors. By contrast, cells from totally resistant patients have a very high malignancy potential and lack D-2 receptors. Both prolactinoma phenotypes express receptors for nerve growth factor (NGF). Exposure of the most malignant DA-resistant prolactinoma cells to NGF for 4 days results in their permanent differentiation into lactotroph-like cells characterized by a marked decrease of the proliferation rate, the loss of capability to grow in soft agar and to form tumors in nude mice and the expression of DA D-2 receptors. Measurement of NGF production revealed that DA-sensitive cells produce and secrete NGF, while DA-resistant cells lack this autocrine loop. Exposure of DA-resistant cells to NGF restores the autocrine loop mediated by NGF. Inactivation of this loop in DA-sensitive cells by an antisense oligonucleotide targeted to NGF cDNA results in their transformation into highly malignant DA-resistant cells. NGF is thus an autocrine factor produced by PRL-secreting adenomas which plays a central role in maintaining their differentiated characteristics.

S10.1

HYPOTHALAMIC CONTROL OF ACTH SECRETION IN THE SHEEP. C. Oliver, V. Guillaume, M. Grino, B. Conte-Devolx, INSERM U 297, Fac. Med. Nord, 13916 Marseille, France.

The respective roles of CRH and AVP in the regulation of ACTH secretion in the sheep were investigated using two experimental approaches : measurement of both neurohormones into hypophysial portal blood (HPB) and active immunization against CRH or AVP. Both peptides are present in HPB and their secretion increases during stress exposure. When intensity of stress is more pronounced, AVP release into HPB predominates over that of CRH. Both neurohormones appear to play a physiological role in the corticotropic response to stress since ACTH increase is significantly reduced in animals actively immunized against CRH or AVP. During and after metyrapone administration, CRH and AVP secretion into HPB increases with a clear predominance of AVP stimulation. CRH appears to play a major role in basal and circadian variations of the HPA axis as shown by the diminution of circulating ACTH and cortisol levels in animals actively immunized against CRH ; the reduction of cortisol is strikingly reduced in comparison to that of ACTH, suggesting a physiological role for endogenous adrenal CRH. In contrast, AVP does not appear to play a role in basal and circadian variations of ACTH secretion since ACTH and cortisol are unaltered after active immunization anti-AVP.

S10.2

ROLE OF ION CHANNELS IN HORMONE SECRETION BY ANTERIOR PITUITARY CORTICOTROPHS. F. A. Antoni*. MRC Brain Metabolism Unit, Department of Pharmacology, University of Edinburgh, Edinburgh, EH8 9JZ, Scotland, U.K.

Anterior pituitary corticotroph cells fire action potentials and display marked voltage-dependent fluctuations of intracellular free Ca^{2+} concentration. Various lines of evidence show that L- and possibly T-type voltage-operated Ca^{2+} channels play a pivotal role in the secretion of adrenocorticotrophic hormone (ACTH). The membrane potential is regulated by at least four distinct potassium currents (A-type, BK, SK, inward rectifyer). K^+ currents appear essential for glucocorticoid and atrial natriuretic peptide (ANP) mediated inhibition of ACTH secretion. Glucocorticoid treatment enhances an A-type K^+ current in AtT20 mouse corticotroph tumour cells. Several K^+ channel blockers with distinct pharmacological specificities reverse the inhibition of stimulated ACTH release by ANP. The latter finding indicates that an intricate functional interplay between K^+ currents is required for the physiological responsiveness of corticotroph cells. Although present, tetrodotoxin sensitive Na currents do not appear to be important for the actions of either stimulatory or inhibitory regulators. A further important area of regulation is the interaction between the electrical and chemical messenger systems of corticotroph cells. Recent studies show that CRF-evoked cAMP production in normal rat anterior pituitary cells as well as AtT20 cells is inhibited by Ca^{2+}. In AtT20 cells the Ca^{2+} is derived from the extracellular space by entry through L-type channels, whereas in normal corticotrophs a significant portion is also mobilised from the ryanodine/caffeine sensitive intracellular pool. In AtT20 cells the inhibitory effect of Ca^{2+} on cAMP accumulation is apparently mediated by the protein phosphatase calcineurin as deduced from studies with immunosuppressant blockers of this enzyme. In sum, voltage-operated ion channels are integral elements of signal processing in anterior pituitary corticotroph cells.

S10.3

RAPID INDUCTION OF c-*fos* AND AP-1 MODULATE CORTICOTROPH RESPONSIVENESS TO GLUCOCORTICOIDS. D.J. Autelitano. Baker Medical Research Institute, Prahran, Vic.3181 Australia.

It is well established that stress leads to facilitation of hypothalamic-pituitary-adrenal (HPA) axis activity and blunting of the inhibitory feedback effects of glucocorticoid (GC) hormone. We have examined whether a component of this facilitation occurs at the level of the pituitary corticotroph. *In vitro* studies on rat anterior pituitary (AP) cultures or the corticotroph cell line AtT-20 have shown that prior exposure to corticotropin releasing factor (CRF) abolishes subsequent inhibitory actions of GC on POMC gene transcription and peptide release. Given the recent reports of mutual antagonism between AP-1 and the glucocorticoid receptor (GR), we have examined whether rapid induction of AP-1 related proteins may be involved in the CRF-mediated antagonism of GC responses. CRF-mediated blockade of GC function is dependent upon rapid *de novo* protein synthesis. Both pulsatile and chronic administration of CRF to AtT-20 cultures results in a rapid but transient stimulation of c-*fos* mRNA with a concurrent decrease in c-*jun* mRNA levels, associated with a prolonged enhancement of AP-1 DNA binding. The introduction of c-*fos* antisense oligonucleotides reduced the CRF-mediated increase in AP-1 DNA binding and blocked the ability of CRF to antagonize subsequent GC effects. In vitro gel shift analysis using nuclear extracts derived from CRF-treated and GC-treated AtT-20 cells suggests that there is a mutual repression between AP-1 and GR in the corticotroph cell. In addition, subjecting rats to acute restraint stress was shown to activate expression of c-*fos* in AP, hypothalamus and hippocampus, suggesting that the CRF-mediated effects demonstrated in vitro occur in the intact animal in reponse to stress. These data show that the rapid induction of c-*fos* in the corticotroph cell in response to CRF stimulation antagonizes GC action and suggests that this may be part of a physiological mechanism to facilitate HPA function during stress.

S10.SC1

THE MODULATORY EFFECTS OF THE HIPPOCAMPUS (HIPP) AND AMYGDALA (AMG) ON ACTH AND CORTICOSTERONE (CS) RESPONSES ARE MEDIATED BY MEDIAN EMINENCE (ME) CRF-41. S. Feldman, J. Weidenfeld. Dept. Neurology,Hadassah Univ.Hosp. Jerusalem. Israel.

The HIPP and AMG have mainly inhibitory and facilitatory effects respectively, on the hypothalamo-pituitary-arenocortical (HPA) axis. In intact rats photic or acoustic stimuli cause CRF-41 release from the ME, which stimulates ACTH and subsequently CS secretion. This response is blocked by the negative feedback effects exerted by local CS paraventricular nucleus implants. The blockage is reversed in rats with bilateral hippocampectomy, suggesting the removal of a tonic inhibitory input to the hypothalamus, which acted synergistically with the negative feedback effect, and modulated ME CRF-41 secretion. Lesions in the medial or central AMG nuclei prevented the release of ME CRF-41 and the rise in plasma ACTH and CS following photic or acoustic stimul. Lateral AMG lesions were not effective. These results indicate a differential effect of AMG nuclei on the HPA axis and that a tonic facilitatory input from the AMG to the hypothalsmus is essential for the release of CRF-41 in response to neural stimuli.

S10.SC2

ANTAGONIST SUPPRESSION OF THE ACTH-RELEASING ACTIVITY OF CRH, AVP AND HYPOTHALAMIC-CONDITIONED MEDIA IN VITRO. M.J.Ellis,* R.S.Mulligan, M.J.Evans, R.A.Donald. Dept.Endocrinology, Christchurch Hospital, Christchurch, New Zealand.

Receptor antagonists were studied for their effects on pituitary cell ACTH release stimulated by (1) CRH plus AVP (to define antagonist efficacy) and (2) stalk median eminence (SME) or hypothalamic-conditioned media (to investigate possible non-CRH/AVP bioactivity). ACTH was measured in the effluent from perifused horse anterior pituitary cells stimulated (5min pulses) alternately with secretagogue ± antagonists. Bioactivity was expressed as percent expected ACTH for a given pulse. Tissue-conditioned media were prepared by incubating fragments of SME and hypothalamic tissue in the pituitary bioassay medium. Chromatography (FPLC) indicated CRH-binding activity in the hypothalamic but not SME-conditioned medium. The bioactivity of CRH plus AVP at levels comparable to SME and hypothalamic media, CRH(0.3nM) plus AVP(12.5nM) and CRH(0.03nM) plus AVP(2.5nM), was inhibited reversibly by antagonists to -0.5 ± 1.3% and 0.8 ± 1.5% expected ACTH (n = 9) respectively. The same antagonists, αhelical CRH(12-41) (5μM) plus $d(CH_2)_5$[Tyr(Me)]AVP (25μM), suppressed the bioactivity of SME and hypothalamic media to -4.4 ± 3.3% and 13.5 ± 1.8% (n = 6) respectively (ACTH rise 2-fold over basal for the latter). Specificity of ACTH blockade was confirmed by measuring FSH release. We conclude that (1) combined CRH and AVP antagonists can block the ACTH response to CRH plus AVP and (2) while CRH and AVP are the predominant ACTH secretagogues released by the unstimulated equine SME and hypothalamus, the latter possesses additional ACTH-releasing activity.

S11.1

GENE REGULATION IN THE PVN. S.L. Lightman, Department of Medicine, University of Bristol, Bristol Royal Infirmary, Marlborough Street. Bristol BS2 8HW, UK.

The paraventricular nucleus acts as a major relay for the neuroendocrine responses to multiple environmental stimuli. At the level of the magnocellular cells within the nucleus, stimuli of increased plasma osmolality result in increased expression of vasopressin and dynorphin mRNA in the vasopressin cells, and an increase in oxytocin and CRH mRNA's in the oxytocin cells. Interestingly the same stimulus that increases magnocellular CRH mRNA also decreases parvocellular CRH mRNA. In addition to changes in gene expression in response to altered fluid balance, changes in food intake also affect the PVN. Food deprivation causes a marked diminution of TRH mRNA, an effect which can be reproduced by equicaloric protein free diet. Thyroid status also affects the HPA axis and experimentally induced hypothyroidism results not only in the expected increase in TRH mRNA, but also in a marked decrease in CRH transcripts in the parvocellular paraventricular nucleus. A similar reduction in CRH mRNA is found in hypothyroid animals whose plasma levels of corticosterone have been clamped. CRH mRNA itself is, of course, clearly regulated by feedback from circulating corticosteroids and by afferent pathways responding to stressful stimuli. Multiple pathways are undoubtedly involved in the complex regulation of PVN TRH and CRH mRNA's and studies will be described in which we have demonstrated a role for hippocampal inputs in setting the basal activity of the hypothalamo-pituitary-thyroid axis in addition to their previously described effects on the hypothalamic pituitary adrenal axis.

S11.2

PITUITARY-ADRENAL REGULATION OF THE IMMUNE SYSTEM AND SUSCEPTIBILITY TO INFLAMMATORY DISEASE. **Esther M. Sternberg, Natl. Inst. Mental Health, NIH, Bethesda, MD. USA**

Communication between the central nervous and immune systems plays an important role in susceptibility to inflammatory and infectious disease, and also influences behavior. This communication involves activation of the central nervous system by immune cytokines, such as interleukin-1 and conversely regulation of immune responses through hormonal as well as direct neuronal mechanisms. Cytokine activation of the hypothalamic-pituitary-adrenal axis and the resultant suppression of immune and inflammatory responses through the action of the corticosteroids, represents an important mechanism through which the central stress response modulates peripheral inflammation. Interruption of this communication on a genetic basis, as in inflammatory diseases susceptible Lewis rats, on a pharmacologic basis, with drugs such as the glucocorticoid receptor antagonist RU 486, on a surgical basis through adrenalectomy or on a toxic basis, is associated with exacerbation of inflammatory disease.

S11.3

FOOD INTAKE IS A MAJOR REGULATOR OF ACTIVITY IN THE HPA AXIS. M.F. Dallman*, S.F. Akana, E.S. Hanson, A.M. Strack, M.J. Bradbury. Dept. Physiology, University of California San Francisco, CA USA 94143-0444

Ad lib food intake occurs primarily during the hrs of dark; thus when rats are stressed in the PM, before lights off, they are relatively fasted. We have previously reported greater responsivity of ACTH to stressors, B feedback, and facilitation (induced by prior stress) of ACTH responses to novel stress in the AM (after lights on) when rats are relatively fed, than in the PM (before lights off) when they are relatively fasted. When ADX rats are exposed to an overnight fast (ONF), the magnitude of the ACTH response to restraint is markedly reduced, although basal ACTH is not elevated compared to fed controls gavage with calories during the ONF increases ACTH responses to stress. Thus, with a short-term fast, the basal rhythm in the HPA axis is not affected but the diurnal rhythm in stress responsivity is determined by food intake. Next we studied intact rats during ONF. ACTH and B in fasted rats reflected the pattern of feeding in fed rats but was lagged by 3 hr. ACTH and B in fasted rats decreased to control at lights on. Thus, activity in the HPA axis in fasted rats serves as a default pathway for the stimulus to feeding in rats with access to food. In the AM, fasted rats had smaller ACTH responses to stress, were resistant to exogenous B feedback and did not exhibit facilitation to restraint despite the enhanced ACTH and B that occurred during ONF. Thus, food intake determines all diurnal rhythms in stress responsivity. We conclude that the HPA axis functions as an integral part of the larger hypothalamic system that regulates energy flow. (DK28172)

S11.SC1

ANTISENSE TARGETING OF HYPOTHALAMIC NEUROPEPTIDES IN VIVO: BIOCHEMICAL; NEUROENDOCRINOLOGICAL AND BEHAVIORAL ASPECTS. T. Skutella, J.C. Probst, G.F. Jirikowski.
Max Planck Institute of Psychiatry, Clinical Institute, Dept. of Neuroendocrinology, Munich, Germany

The effectiveness of centrally applied antisense oligodeoxynucleotide (ODN) designed to target the untranslated 5'region and the initiation codon of vasopressin (VP), oxytocin (OT) and corticotropin-releasing hormone (CRH) mRNA were tested in vivo biochemically, morphologically and on a behavioral level. Probes were protected against degradation by inversion-capping or by phosphorothioate modification. VP antisense reduced VP mRNA, peptide content and induced a temporary diabitis insipidus. Intracerebroventricular injection of OT antisense probe into lactating females caused reduction of OT levels and inhibition of milk-ejection, whereas maternal behavior was not affected in these rats. Antisense blockade of CRH transcripts resulted in a clearcut anxiolytic effect in a shuttle-box and social-defeat/elevated plus maze task. The reduced acute stress response were paralleled by a reduction of CRH, ACTH and corticosterone.
Our studies indicate that antisense targeting with inverted and phosphorothioate modified ODN facilitates reversible specific inhibition of hypothalamic neuropeptides in neuroendocrinological and behavioral settings. This technique may also allow for new therapeutic approaches in human psychiatric disorders.

S11.SC2

REGULATION OF IMMEDIATE-EARLY GENES (NGFI-B AND c-FOS) IN STRESS-RELATED NEUROSECRETORY NEURONS. K.J. Kovács and Paul E. Sawchenko. Laboratory of Neuroendocrinology, Institute of Experimental Medicine Budapest, Hungary H-1083 and LNSF, The Salk Institute, La Jolla, CA 92037 USA

The promoter regions of corticotropin releasing-factor (CRF) and vasopressin (AVP) genes contain sequences similar to NGFI-B and glucocorticoid response elements (NBRE and GRE respectively). NGFI-B is also a member of steroid receptor superfamily and its expression is induced by various stimuli. c-fos, another immediate-early gene and its protein product, c-Fos have been widely used as a marker for activated neurons.
Ether stress results elevation of ACTH and corticosterone plasma levels, as well as rapid and transient induction of NGFI-B gene and Fos immunoreactivity in the parvocellular neurons of the paraventricular nucleus. The effect of steroid hormones on the stress-induced induction of immediate-early genes was studied in adrenalectomized (ADX) rats and rats with subcutaneous implants of 25 mg (LOW CORT) or 200 mg (HIGH CORT) corticosterone pellets and compared to that of intact rats. The pattern of induction of immediate-early genes in ADX and LOW CORT animals was similar to intact rats, although the Fos expression was longer lasting (1-3 hours) after adrenalectomy without steroid replacement. In contrast, in HIGH CORT rats the expression of both immediate-early genes was totally supressed in neurosecretory neurons of the hypothalamus.
These results suggest that feedback effects of steroids on stress-induced activation of hypophyseotropic neurons involves not only direct inhibition of the CRF and AVP genes but also inhibition of immediate-early genes.

S12.1

GENE REGULATION OF THE VIP SYSTEM. I. Gozes*, R. Glazer, A. Davidson, I. Ashkenazi, A. Ticher, W. Rostene, B.S. McEwen and D.E. Brenneman. Chemical Pathology, Sackler Medical School, Tel Aviv University, Israel; INSERM U339, Paris, France; SDMP, NICHD, NIH, Bethesda MD, Neuroendocrinol. Rockefeller University, NY, U.S.A.

Vasoactive intestinal peptide (VIP) is a 28 amino acid peptide widely distributed among neurons of the central and peripheral nervous tissue. Sex steroids as well as physiological inputs (lactation, blood pressure) differentially regulate VIP gene expression [Molec. Neurobiol. 3,1 (1989); J. Molecular Neurosci. 4, 1 (1993)]. Anatomical, as well as physiological data suggest a neuro-endocrine role of VIP, modulating the secretion of various pituitary hormones. Since the secretion of pituitary hormones can be under control of adrenal steroids, VIP levels may be regulated by adrenal steroids as well. Adrenalectomy performed on adult male rats resulted in a significant decrease in VIP-mRNA in the hypothalamus (from 10.6 $\pm$ 0.3 to 3.5 $\pm$ 0.2 arbitrary units). In situ hybridization experiments revealed that a major site of VIP-mRNA expression in the hypothalamus is the suprachiasmatic nucleus (SCN). Indeed, adrenalectomy resulted in a two fold decrease in VIP transcripts in this nucleus. However, this decrease was not reversed by replacement treatment with corticosterone or the glucocorticoid agonist, RU28362 (Neurosci. Lett, in press). Thus, VIP-mRNA may be regulated by indirect mechanisms, influenced by the adrenal gland. Also, in the SCN, in which the circadian clock resides, day-night cycles are paralleled by rhythmical alteration in the levels of the mRNA encoding VIP. By Northern blot hybridizations we now show that diurnal oscillation in VIP-mRNA preceded eye opening. In addition, more pronounced day-night oscillations in VIP-mRNA were observed in animals reared in the dark, suggesting an endogenous (perhaps autocrine) as well as an exogenous (environmental-light associated) control. Blockade of VIP activity resulted in blockade of diurnal rhythms, including rhythms of adrenal hormones [Neuroscience Soc. Abs. 18, 2 (1992)] and of motor activity.

S12.2

IDENTIFICATION AND FUNCTION OF PACAP. *Y. Masuo, T. Ohtaki, N. Suzuki, H. Matsumoto, Y. Masuda, Y. Matsumoto, F. Tokito, M. Fujino. Discovery Research Laboratories I, Takeda Chemical Ind., Ltd., 10 Wadai, Tsukuba, Ibaraki, 300–42 Japan.

We investigated the regional distribution and ontogeny of endogenous PACAP and its binding site densities in the rat brain using a sandwich–enzyme immunoassay and binding autoradiography. Marked regional variation in the levels of PACAP was found in adult animals. High levels were observed in the lateral septal nucleus intermediate, diagonal band, central amygdaloid nucleus, several parts of the hypothalamus, central gray, interpeduncular nucleus and dorsal raphe. In most regions the peptide levels were low at 2 days of age, peaked within 30–60 days, and then remained constant. The distribution of PACAP differed from that of VIP, although the age-related variation was similar to that for both VIP and classical neurotransmitters. These results suggest the existence of PACAP–containing neurons that are independent of VIP. The densities of PACAP binding sites were higher than those for VIP, and their localization was relatively homogeneous in adult rats. However, the site density was notably higher than that for VIP in the hippocampal formation, lateral hypothalamic area, substantia nigra pars compacta, pontine reticular nucleus, and cerebellum. The density of PACAP binding sites was already high at day 2 and varied only slightly up to day 240, in most regions. These variations in distribution and ontogenesis differed from those of VIP. PACAP binding sites may be expressed in both neurons and glial cells. Previous studies suggested that VIP has presynaptic effects on cholinergic terminals in the hippocampus. Since PACAP binding sites markedly predominated over those for VIP in this structure, we further studied the effects of PACAP and VIP on the spontaneous release of acetylcholine (ACh) from the hippocampus using brain microdialysis. Intrahippocampal injections of these peptides caused dose–related increases in ACh release, which were highly calcium– and tetrodotoxin–dependent. Therefore, PACAP and VIP could presynaptically stimulate cholinergic activity in the hippocampus. However, the ability to enhance ACh release was determined to be as follows: VIP > PACAP38 > PACAP27. The present results suggest that PACAP plays an important role in regulating the central nervous system and in the modulation of brain development.

S12.3

MOLECULAR BIOLOGY OF RECEPTORS FOR PACAP AND VIP. E.M. Lutz, W.J. Sheward, K.M. West, J.A. Morrow, *A.J. Harmar. MRC Brain Metabolism Unit, University Department of Pharmacology, Edinburgh, Scotland EH8 9JZ.

In order to identify novel neuropeptide receptors which may play a role in neuroendocrine function, we amplified pituitary cDNA by PCR using primers corresponding to conserved regions in the 3rd and 7th transmembrane domains of the calcitonin/secretin/parathyroid hormone receptor family. Several classes of PCR product were obtained, subcloned and sequenced. Partial cDNAs encoding two novel receptors were identified and cDNAs encoding the full-length receptor proteins were isolated from a rat olfactory bulb cDNA library. The most abundant clone (RPR7) was very similar in sequence to the VIP receptor, but distinct from all the known members of the family. We concluded from the order of potency of ligands in stimulating cyclic AMP formation in COS cells transfected with RPR7 cDNA that RPR7 encodes a receptor for pituitary adenylate cyclase activating polypeptide (PACAP). The pharmacology of the second novel receptor cDNA (RPR4) is that of a VIP receptor (the VIP_2 receptor) which is distinct from the VIP receptor recently cloned from rat lung (the VIP_1 receptor). VIP_1 and VIP_2 receptors have distinct distributions in the CNS, with high levels of VIP_1 receptor mRNA in cortex, hippocampus, hypothalamus and cerebellum and VIP_2 receptors in hippocampus, thalamus and suprachiasmatic nucleus. The distribution of VIP binding sites in the CNS, determined by autoradiography, is consistent with the combined distributions of the VIP_1 and VIP_2 receptor mRNAs. The cloning of receptors for PACAP and VIP is an important step towards an understanding of the physiological roles of the two peptides. Our work has provided the first evidence for VIP receptor heterogeneity at the molecular level and will enable drugs which act selectively as agonists or antagonists of VIP_1 or VIP_2 receptors to be identified. Such agents will be powerful tools in the analysis of the hormonal and neurotransmitter role of VIP and may have important therapeutic implications.

S12.SC1

EVIDENCE FOR A STEROID MODULATED EXPRESSION OF PITUITARY ADENYLATE CYCLASE ACTIVATING POLYPEPTIDE (PACAP) IN THE ANTERIOR PITUITARY OF RATS. W. Wuttke*, S. Benter, H. Jarry, Dept. Clin. & Exptl. Endocrinology, University of Göttingen, 37075 Göttingen, Germany

PACAP is believed to be a hypothalamic hypophysiotropic factor. However, the presence of PACAP immunoreactive material within the anterior pituitary (AP) has been demonstrated by RIA. This finding points to a local production of the peptide. To give direct evidence for local synthesis of PACAP we developed a RT-PCR assay based on a published rats PACAP cDNA. Using this approach we addressed the questions I) whether PACAP mRNA is detectable in the AP and II) mRNA levels change during the proestrous day. In the morning of proestrous rats were implanted with a jugular vein catheter and blood samples were collected at 30 min intervals beginning 1300 hrs. Rats were sacrificed at various time points of proestrus and pituitaries were rapidly removed. mRNA was isolated with magnetic oligo-(dT) coated beads. A PCR signal of predicted size was readily dectable after 35 amplification cycles. Sequence analysis of the cloned PCR product confirmed that PACAP mRNA was reverse transcribed and amplified. Animals were grouped according to their LH- and prolactin values prior to decapitation in groups of rats showing either constantly low, increasing or decreasing hormone values. The amount of PACAP transcript was determined by densitometry analysis of agarose gels of PCR products. During the preovulatory LH- and prolactin surge expression of PACAP significantly ($p<0.01$) increased. The presence of PACAP mRNA in the AP indicates local synthesis of PACAP. Since expression of PACAP in the AP changes during proestrous, it is likely that sex steroids modulate PACAP gene expression.

S12.SC2

EFFECT OF THYROID STATUS ON THE PROLACTIN-RELEASING ACTION OF VASOACTIVE INTESTINAL PEPTIDE(VIP) IN HUMANS : COMPARISON WITH THE ACTION OF TRH.
S. Sakihara*, H. Watanobe, S. Sasaki, K. Takebe. Third Department of Internal Medicine, Hirosaki University School of Medicine, Hirosaki, Japan, 036

Recent studies have shown that primary hypothyroidism induced in the rat was able to stimulate the biosynthesis of VIP in the anterior pituitary(AP). Since the AP VIP is known to stimulate PRL secretion through a paracrine and/or autocrine mechanism, it is interesting to hypothesize that hyperprolactinemia seen in hypothyroid patients may at least in part be due to a paracrine effect of elevated VIP on AP PRL secretion. Prompted by this information , we examined the effect of VIP load on PRL secretion in patients with primary hyperthyroidism or hypothyroidism, and compared the data with those from TRH load performed in the same patients. Eight female patients with Graves'disease and 8 females with chronic thyroiditis received iv bolus injections of VIP(100 μg) and TRH (500 μg) 2-3 days apart from each other, during both the dysthyroid and euthyroid (attained by medical treatment) states. Compared to the data in the euthyroid state of the respective group , hyperthyroidism was associated with a lower basal PRL level and a lower PRL responsiveness to TRH, whereas hypothyroidism was associated with higher values of these parameters. In contrast, PRL responsiveness to VIP was essentially the same regardless of thyroid status. These results suggest that PRL responsiveness to VIP may not be so sensitively regulated by thyroid hormones as that to TRH in humans.

S13.1

INTERLEUKINS, NITRIC OXIDE (NO) AND CORTICOTROPIN-RELEASING HORMONE (CRH) RELEASE. S.M. McCann*, S. Karanth, K. Lyson, N. Belova, W.H. Yu, V. Rettori. Dept of Physiology, UT Southwestern Medical Center, Dallas, TX 75235-8873.

Various cytokines (IL-1, IL-2, IL-6, γ-interferon and cachectin) stimulate ACTH release following their third ventricular (3V) injection via hypothalamic action. IL-2 stimulates CRH release *in vitro* by combination with its receptors on cholinergic interneurons which synapse with nitricoxidergic neurons. These neurons release NO which diffuses to the CRH neuron, activates cyclooxygenase to generate PGE_2 which produces CRH release by activating adenylate cyclase to generate cyclic AMP which activates protein kinase A. The evidence is that CRH release induced by IL-2 is blocked by atropine and inhibitors of NO synthase (NOS) and that releasers of NO, such as nitroprusside, induce CRH release from hypothalamic explants. Cyclosporin A, a potent immunosuppressive drug, acutely blocks the action of IL-2 to stimulate CRH release, probably by blocking NOS. Dexamethasone and α-MSH, the latter via blockade of protein kinase C, also block the action of cytokines to release CRH. Blockade of NOS by N^G-monomethyl-L-arginine (NMMA) injected into the 3V prevented IL-1α-induced stimulation of prolactin and suppressed LH and GH release, but had no effect on ACTH secretion which suggests that there are both inhibitory and stimulatory roles for NO in the control of CRH release. (Supported by NIH Grants DK43900 and DK10073.)

S13.2

THE ROLE OF CYTOKINES IN SICKNESS BEHAVIOUR. R. Dantzer. Integrative Neurobiology, INSERM U394, Rue Camille Saint-Saens, 33077 Bordeaux Cedex

Non specific symptoms of infection include fever and profound psychological and behavioural changes. Sick individuals experience fatigue, malaise, listlessness and inability to concentrate. They also show hypersomnia, anorexia, depressed activity and loss of interest in their environment. These non specific changes are collectively termed "sickness behaviour".
Using pharmacological tools in the form of recombinant cytokines and their antagonist, we have shown that sickness behaviour is mediated by proinflammatory cytokines released by activated accessory immune cells during infection and inflammation. Peripheral or central injections of IL-1α, IL-1β and TNFα induce sickness behaviour in mice and rats, in the form of reduced social interest and decreased food-motivated behaviour. Although these behavioural changes are functionally related to the pyrogenic effects of cytokines, their receptor mechanisms are different from those mediating fever. The mechanisms which mediate the induction of sickness behaviour in response to peripherally released cytokines involve several steps: (1) the peripheral immune message activates primary afferent nerve endings, as evidenced by the induction of expression of sensory neuropeptides in the spinal cord in response to peripheral immune stimuli; (2) this neural message is conveyed to the brain to exert its effects since section of afferent nerves abrogates centrally mediated behavioural effects of peripherally released cytokines; (3) the neural message transmitted to the brain by primary afferents is transduced back into an immune message, as evidenced by the induction of the expression of brain cytokines at the mRNA and protein levels in response to peripheral immune stimuli; (4) the cytokines which are synthesized in the central nervous system in response to peripheral immune stimuli are released, as evidenced by *in vitro* studies; (5) the centrally released cytokines act on neurons to induce sickness behaviour, as evidenced by the ability of centrally injected cytokine antagonists to block the behavioural effects of peripheral cytokines; (6) the centrally released cytokines activate a variety of hormonal factors and neuropeptides which limit the extent of changes in neural activity induced by cytokines and promote recovery.

S13.3

STRESS AND CYTOKINES IN THE BRAIN INFLUENCE IMMUNE RESPONSES AND EXPERIMENTAL METASTASES. J.M. Weiss, N. Quan, R. Kitson[2], S.K. Sundar[1], W.H. Chambers[2], R.H. Goldfarb[2], Emory University School of Medicine, Atlanta, GA, USA, 30322; [1]Duke University Medical Center, Durham, NC, USA, 27710; [2]Pittsburgh Cancer Institute, PA, USA, 15213.

Experiments from two converging areas of investigation are described. First, experiments exploring the action of cytokines in the brain, particularly interleukin-1 (IL-1), are described. These studies demonstrate that IL-1 acting in the brain suppresses peripheral cellular immune responses via activation of corticotrophin releasing factor (CRF) in the brain to stimulate both the pituitary-adrenal axis and the sympathetic nervous system. This sequence of events apparently utilizes the same pathways by which stressors influence immune responses. Second, studies are then described utilizing an experimental model of cancer metastases in rats -- the MADB106 tumor which metastasizes to lung of syngeneic Fisher 344 rat. Findings suggest that changes in lymphocytes migrating to lung are important in surveillance of these metastases-generating tumor cells. Research is described indicating that these events involved in tumor surveillance are stress-sensitive, and consequently are regulated by stress-responsive pathways in brain. (Supported by MH-5042 and J.D. and C.T. MacArthur Foundation Health Network.)

S13.SC1

Hypothalamic CRF as an indicator of immune-mediated disease in mice and rats.
Harbuz,*M.S., [1]Blackwell, J.M. & Lightman, S.L. Dept. of Medicine, University of Bristol, Bristol Royal Infirmary, Marlborough St, Bristol. BS2 8HW. [1]Dept. of Medicine, University of Cambridge Clinical School, Addenbrookes Hospital, Hills Road, Cambridge. CB2 2QQ.

We have investigated the activation of the HPA axis in response to the immune-mediated diseases adjuvant-arthritis (AA) and experimental allergic encephalopathy (EAE) We have confirmed increased activity of the pituitary-adrenal axis in these models with increased POMC mRNA in the anterior pitutary and increased secretion of ACTH and corticosterone. We have however been unable to demonstrate any increase in the mRNA for CRF (the principal corticotrophin-releasing factor). Indeed, we have found paradoxical decreases in CRF mRNA in the PVG strain of rat following induction of mycobacterial adjuvant- or synthetic adjuvant-induced arthritis, and also in the Wistar strain of rat with EAE. We have now investigated CRF mRNA in the PVN of both susceptible and resistant strains of congenic mice infected with *Leishmania donovani*. Control levels of CRF mRNA in the resistant strain were approximately 50% below those in the susceptible strain. Infection reduced CRF mRNA by about 50% in the susceptible strain but had no affect in the resistant strain. In response to acute restraint stress the stress-induced increases in corticosterone and CRF mRNA were similar in both resisant and susceptible strains. These data, demonstrating a reduction in CRF mRNA in *L. donovani* infection together with our earlier findings in AA and EAE suggest the possibility of a common mechanism acting at the hypothalamic level to reduce CRF mRNA in response to T-cell, immune-mediated disease.

S13.SC2

THE THYMIC REPERTOIRE OF NEUROENDOCRINE-RELATED SELF-PEPTIDES IN T CELL LIFE AND DEATH. V. Geenen*, Institute of Pathology CHU-B23, University of Liège-Sart Tilman, B-4000 Liège, Belgium.

Both during phylogeny and ontogeny, the thymus appears as the crucial nodal point between the two major systems of cell-to-cell signalling, the neuroendocrine (NE) and the immune systems. Thymic epithelial and "nurse" cells from different species are a site for synthesis of polypeptide precursors belonging to neurohypophysial (NHP), tachykinin and insulin families. Through the primitive model of cryptocrine communication, thymic NE-related precursors constitute a source of signals that are able to influence the early steps of the immune response. Our most recent studies have shown that NHP-like signals exert a mitogenic action on thymocytes (pre-T cells), and enhance the phosphorylation of pre-T cell proteins involved in focal adhesion. These biological actions could be important for the establishment of cryptocrine signalling as an accessory pathway of T cell ***positive selection.***
On the other hand, thymic NE-related precursors are also a source of self-peptides which could induce the ***negative selection*** of T cells bearing a randomly rearranged TCR with a self-reactivity against NE families. We have investigated the intrathymic presentation of NE-related self-antigens through the purification of class I proteins derived from the major histocompatibility complex (MHC). The thymic OT self-antigen is synthesized under the form of a large 55-kD precursor which represents about 1.5-2% of the total NHP-related ir material detected in the thymic epithelium. This precusor bears both a MHC class I-related domain (45 kD) which is probably involved in its membrane targetting, as well as a neurophysin domain (10 kD) which may bind thymic OT as the NHP self-antigen for its direct presentation to the differentiating T cell system. The coexistence of these two domains within a single thymic protein nicely illustrates the probably common ancestral origin of a classical NE family and the Ig/MHC superfamily. Moreover, to our knowledge, this finding provides the first experimental evidence that the central T cell tolerance of NE self-antigens is not tightly MHC-restricted like the peripheral T cell response to allo- or auto-antigens.
(Supported by the Liège University Medical School, by the National Fund for Scientific Research of Belgium and by the European Science Foundation.)

S14.1

TRH METABOLISM AND ITS REGULATION.
P. Joseph-Bravo. Instituto de Biotecnologìa, Universidad Nacional Autònoma de Mèxico, A.P. 510-3, Cuernavaca Mor., Mexico, 62271.

The level of an active neuropeptide effective at its target is the resultant of multiple steps (biosynthesis, release and inactivation). We have attempted to study how are these events regulated studying different in vitro and in vivo paradigms and measuring the levels of TRH-mRNA and TRH as well as the activity of its degrading enzyme, pyroglutamyl peptidase II (PPII, EC 3.4.19.6). TRH-mRNA increases in a fast and transient manner in the paraventricular nucleus of male rats exposed to cold stress or in suckled female rats; stimulation is also observed in hypothalamic cell cultures incubated with dibutiryl-cAMP or phorbol ester suggesting a transynaptic regulation of TRH biosynthesis. Changes in TRHmRNA do not coincide in all circumstances with TRH levels or release activity, suggesting a possible regulation at the level of precursor processing.
Inactivation of TRH can be modulated at its target cell. In adenohypophysis, pyroglutamate peptidase II activity fluctuates during estrous cycle and is positively regulated by thyroid hormones; in cultured cells a down regulation occurs upon TRH or PKC-activators incubation. In the central nervous system, PPII is localized in neurons probably at the postsynaptic membrane. During electrical estimulation ("Kindling"), PPII shows opposite changes to TRH levels. These results suggest that the ectopeptidase responsible for TRH inactivation can be regulated to modify the levels of active substance attaining its target. Financed by DGAPA-UNAM and CONACYT.

S14.2

MECHANISM OF TRH ACTION: RECEPTOR LOCALIZATION AND CALCIUM RESPONSES IN PITUITARY CELLS AND CELLS TRANSFECTED WITH TRH RECEPTOR cDNA. P. M. Hinkle, E. J. Nelson, and R. Ashworth. Department of Pharmacology, Univ. of Rochester Medical Center, Rochester, NY, USA 14642
The cellular localization of receptor-bound TRH and the Ca^{2+} response to TRH were characterized in individual pituitary cells and cells of non-pituitary origin transfected with TRH receptor cDNA. Localization of the TRH peptide was monitored using a fluorescently labeled peptide, Rhod-TRH. Rhod-TRH binding was initially limited to the plasma membrane, but after 15 min at 37°C Rhod-TRH was concentrated in punctate endocytic vesicles. Calcium responses to TRH were measured in individual Fura-2-loaded pituitary cells and in nonexcitable cells transfected with receptor cDNA using digital fluorescence imaging. TRH stimulated an immediate spike in intracellular free Ca^{2+} ion, $[Ca^{2+}]i$, in all cell types. The amplitude of the initial $[[Ca^{2+}]i$ spike increased with the dose of TRH but the duration of the $[Ca^{2+}]i$ transient decreased. This was due to the dual action of TRH to stimulate release of Ca^{2+} from IP3-sensitive intracellular stores and to stimulate efflux of Ca^{2+} from the cytoplasm. Agonist-induced Ca^{2+} clearing was seen following activation of several Ca^{2+}-mobilizing receptors and in different cell types. The ability of agonists to stimulate efflux of cytoplasmic Ca^{2+} may provide a general mechanism limiting the duration of the $[Ca^{2+}]i$ transient. In GH3 cells, but not nonexcitable cells, the initial Ca^{2+} spike was followed by a slower and more prolonged increase in $[Ca^{2+}]i$ that depended on the activity of L-type Ca^{2+} channels and was often associated with an increase in the frequency of $[Ca^{2+}]i$ oscillations. This second phase displayed a bell-shaped dependence on TRH dose. These Ca^{2+} response patterns are partially responsible for the biphasic TRH secretory response.

S14.3

STRUCTURE-FUNCTION RELATIONSHIPS OF THE THYROTROPIN-RELEASING HORMONE (TRH) RECEPTOR. M.C. Gershengorn, J.H. Perlman, D.R. Nussenzveig. Div. of Molecular Medicine, Dept. of Medicine, Cornell Univ. Medical College, New York, NY, USA, 10021

The TRH receptor (TRH-R) is a member of the seven transmembrane-spanning, guanine nucleotide-binding protein-coupled receptor (GPCR) family. Like other GPCRs, TRH-R contains distinct domains that are involved in binding, G protein coupling and internalization. We have begun to identify these domains within TRH-R. By creating site-specific mutants of TRH-R and using a series of TRH analogs, we find that binding of the pyroGlu residue of TRH is localized to amino acids within the putative third transmembrane alpha helix. In experiments with other TRH-R mutants, we have identified residues within several transmembrane helices and in the third intracellular loop which are necessary for productive coupling to G protein. And, in studies using a series of other TRH-R mutants we have shown that signalling for receptor internalization are present in the carboxyl terminal tail of TRH-R. Thus, we have begun to determine the structure-function relationships of different regions/residues of TRH-R that will permit the construction of a molecular model of TRH-R activation and regulation.

S14.SC1

PULSATILE TSH SECRETION IN ADDISON'S DISEASE (AD); EFFECT OF GLUCOCORTICOID SUBSTITUTION.

J. Hangaard*, M. Andersen, E. Grodum, O. Koldkjaer, P.B Poulsen, C. Hagen
Dept. of Endocrinology, Odense University Hospital and Dept. of Clinical Chemistry Sønderborg Hospital, Denmark.

Glucocorticoids are known to inhibit TSH secretion, but the mechanism is uncertain. Opioid peptides probably play no role in basal TSH secretion, but are involved in the stress induced fall in TSH. The purpose of this study was to examine the changes in serum TSH level and pulsatility pattern during normal, low and high plasma cortisol levels in well treated patients with AD. These results were compared also to the TSH secretion pattern of normal controls. Eight normal controls (age 22-32 year) and twelve euthyroid patients with AD were studied; seven women (age 30-69 yrs) and five men (age 43-53 yrs). None received any medication beside their usual substitution therapy. Blood samples were obtained every 10 min. from 8.00 am until 6.00 pm. on three occasions. **A**: 24 h. infusion of a normal physiological dose of cortisol (mean p-cortisol 357 nmol/l); **B**: 24 h. placebo infusion (mean p-cortisol 32 nmol/l) and **C**: 24 h. infusion of a high dose of cortisol (mean p-cortisol 850 nmol/l). TSH pulsatility were analyzed by the PDS computer program. During normal plasma cortisol level, the AD patients had similar basal TSH levels and TSH pulsatility compared to normal controls. During test B compared to test A, the mean basal TSH levels increased significantly ($p<0.01$) in all AD patients (**2.0** mlE/l ± 1.6 and **1.0** mlE/l ± 0.5 respectively), and the TSH pulse frequency increased nonsignificantly ($0.05<p<0.10$), (**3.4** ± 2.5 and **5.2** ± 2.7 respectively) but the peak amplitude did not change (**0.240** mlE/l ± 0.059 and **0.267** mlE/l ± 0.151 respectively). During test C compared to test A, the mean basal TSH levels decreased significantly ($p<0.01$) (**0.4** mlE/l ± 0.2 and **2.0** mlE/l ± 1.6 respectively), and the pulse frequency decreased significantly ($p<0.01$) (**0.3** ± 0.9 and **3.4** ± 2.5 respectively). Stimulation test with 10 μg TRH showed a TSH response of 684%, 503% and 863% in test A, B and C respectively. These results suggest that cortisol has a direct inhibitory effect on thyrotropic neurons at pituitary level which superimpose the inhibitory opioid tonus during acute stress.

S14.SC2

EFFECTS OF TRH AND TRH-LIKE PEPTIDES ON THE ANTERIOR PITUITARY CELL PROLIFERATION IN RATS.*

M. Pawlikowski, D. Słowińska-Klencka
Institute of Endocrinology, Medical University of Łódź,
Poland, PL 91-425

Although the effect of TRH on the anterior pituitary mitotic activity has been reported in the seventies (Pawlikowski and Kunert-Radek, End. Exper. 1975, 9, 135) its involvement in the control of pituitary cell growth is still considered as controversial. The present paper deals with the effects of a single dose (100 μg/kg b.w.) of TRH or of TRH-like tripeptides pGlu-His-Gly-OH (colon mitosis inhibitor, CMI) and pGlu-His-Gly-NH_2 (CMI-NH_2) on the anterior pituitary cell proliferation in adult male rats. The incorporation of bromodeoxyuridine (BrDU) into cell nuclei was used as the index of cell proliferation. It was found that TRH and CMI-NH_2 but not CMI increased the BrDU labelling of the anterior pituitary cell nuclei 12 hours after the peptide administration. These findings support the hypothesis of the positive control of the anterior pituitary cell proliferation by TRH, and, possibly, by some other TRH-like peptides.

*Supported by the Committee of Scientific Research of Poland, Grant No 403379101

S15.1

NITRIC OXIDE, NEUROPEPTIDES AND PITUITARY HORMONE SECRETION. **Satya P. Kalra and Juan J. Bonavera, Department of Neuroscience and Physiology, University of Florida College of Medicine, Gainesville, FL 32610**

Nitric oxide (NO) is a novel, gaseous biological messenger molecule which is enzymatically formed from L-arginine by nitric acid synthase (NOS), a constitutive Ca^{2+}-calmodulin-dependent enzyme in the central nervous system. Since NOS exists in several hypothalamic sites, we investigated the role of NO in regulation of pituitary LH and prolactin secretions. The results of a series of *in vivo* and *in vitro* studies with either NOS inhibitors or NO generator compounds, revealed that NO efflux in the hypothalamus is critical for the intermittent ultradian bursts and for extended surges of these pituitary hormones. Additionally, stimulation of NO efflux by intermittent administration of NO generating L-arginine methyl ester, reinstated the proestrous pattern of pituitary LH activation in estrogen-primed ovariectomized rats. Further investigations revealed that NOS inhibitors blocked the excitatory effects of N-methyl-D-aspartate (NMDA) on hypothalamic GnRH secretion, thus reinforcing the tenet that the NMDA receptor-NO link plays a facilitatory role in the two modalities of pituitary LH secretion. These findings, taken together with the knowledge that NO is an unorthodox, diffusible neurotransmitter, imply that the excitatory effects of NO, both at presynaptic and postsynaptic elements, may also underlie the synchrony in pituitary LH and prolactin secretions.

S15.2

REGULATION OF PARTICULATE GUANYLATE CYCLASE ACTIVITY BY ANGIOTENSIN II. **S.P. Bottari, INSERM U. 244, DBMS/BRCE, C.E.N.G. 38054 Grenoble France**

Angiotensin II (AII) binds to two pharmacologically distinct receptor subtypes, AT1 and AT2. Whereas AT1 receptors mediate most of AII' s known biological effects through G-protein coupled pathways, the functional role and signalling mechanism of AT2 receptors, which do not appear to be functionally coupled to G-proteins, is still unclear. Both receptors mediate a decrease of cellular cGMP levels. However, whereas the AT1 receptor does so by stimulating phosphodiesterase activity through a Ca++/calmodulin dependent pathway, the AT2 receptor mediates the inhibition of ANP responsive particulate guanylate cyclase (pGC) activity. While investigating the signalling mechanisms of AT2 receptors, we found that this receptor induces a rapid dephosphorylation of phosphotyrosine residues of specific proteins in the 70 to 150 KDa range in PC12W cells. This proteintyrosinephosphatase (PTPase) activity was further characterized using the synthetic substrate para-nitrophenyl phosphate (pNPP). Dephosphorylation of pNPP in response to Ang II is not affected by GDP ßS or GTPγS, neither by depletion of solubilized membrane preparations from G-proteins by lectin affinity chromatography. Interestingly, we found the Ang II induced inhibition of pGC to be blocked by the PTPase inhibitors Na3VO4 and phenylarsine oxide. These observations suggest that the AT2 receptors decreases cellular cGMP by inhibiting pGC through a G-protein independent pathway which involves the activation of a PTPase.

S15.3

NEUROENDOCRINE MECHANISMS IN CARDIOVASCULAR REGULATION. Thomas Unger* and Juraj Culman. Department of Pharmacology, University of Kiel, 24105 Kiel, Germany.

The existence of the brain renin-angiotensin system (RAS) has been firmly established. Evidence has accumulated that the brain RAS acts and is regulated independently of the hormonal RAS. The brain RAS has been implicated in central osmoregulatory and cardiovascular control mechanisms. Biological actions of angiotensin II (ANG II) are mediated by two subtypes of angiotensin receptors, referred to as AT1 and AT2, respectively. ANG II-containing pathways in the circumventricular organs (CVO) and in the paraventricular (PVN) and supraoptic (SON) hypothalamic nuclei, brain areas involved in central cardiovascular regulation and control of body fluid and electrolyte homeostasis, have been described. Stimulation of circumventricular ANG II receptors engenders a distinct pattern of cardiovascular, endocrine and behavioural responses, including blood pressure increase, attenuation of baroreceptor reflex, drinking, natriuresis and release of pituitary hormones such as vasopressin (AVP), oxytocin, and ACTH. We have shown that catecholaminergic and angiotensinergic pathways in the PVN and SON mediate the ANG II-induced release of AVP. Activation of AT1 receptors in the CVO leads to the release of ANG II in the PVN and SON. ANG II then stimulates vasopressinergic neurons via release of noradrenaline (NA) from catecholaminergic terminals. NA in turn acts on postsynaptic $\alpha 1$ and $\alpha 2$ adrenoceptors in the PVN and on $\alpha 1$ adrenoceptors in the SON located on vasopressinergic neurons to promote the vasopressin release. As the VP release is controlled by the PVN and SON, the ANG II-NA interaction in these two areas contributes to central blood pressure regulation and volume control.

S15.SC1

DIRECT REGULATION OF HYPOTHALAMIC CORTICOTROPIN RELEASING HORMONE NEURONS BY ANGIOTENSIN II (AII). G. Aguilera, W.S. Young, A. Kiss, A Bathia, B. Akbasak. DEB, NICHD and LCB, NIMH, NIH, Bethesda, Maryland, USA

The role of AII in the control of the hypothalamic pituitary adrenal (HPA) axis was studied in the rat by examining the regulation and cellular localization of AII receptors in the PVN and the effect of AII on CRH mRNA levels. While autoradiographic analysis of ^{125}ISar^{1},Ile^{8}]AII binding showed equal density of type-1 AII receptors (AT_1-R) in the parvicellular and magnocellular divisions of the PVN, in situ hybridization showed that AT_1-R mRNA levels in the PVN were high in the parvicellular and low in the magnocellular pars. Double-labeling hybridization using digoxin-labeled CRH, VP and oxytocin probes and ^{35}S-labeled AT_1-R cRNA probes showed AT_1-R mRNA in cells stained for CRH mRNA, but not in VP or oxytocin cells. AT_1-R mRNA in the PVN markedly increased 4 hr after a single i.p. hypertonic saline (HS) injection or 1 hr immobilization, and remained elevated at lower levels after 14 days repeated stress. In addition, CRH mRNA levels in the PVN were increased to similar levels following a single i.c.v. injection of 50 ng AII or i.p HS injection stress. The differential distribution of AT_1-R and AT_1-R mRNA in the PVN indicates that while AII directly modulate CRH neurons through receptors in PVN perikarya, regulation of magnocellular function is partly indirect via receptors associated with afferent innervation to the PVN. The data support a role of AII in the regulation of the HPA axis during adaptation to stress.

S15.SC2

CLINICAL IMPLICATION OF THE LOCAL ADRENAL RENIN-ANGIOTENSIN SYSTEM. K. Rácz*, F. Pinet, J-M. Gasc, E. Gláz+, P. Corvol. INSERM U36, College de France, Paris, France, 75005; *+2nd Dept. of Semmelweis University, Budapest, Hungary, H1088.

The presence of the two components of the renin-angiotensin system (RAS) was investigated in human normal (n=5) and pathologic adrenal tissues (n=33) to study possible differences in the coexpression of renin and angiotensinogen in tissues of cortical and medullary origin. Renin, prorenin and angiotensinogen levels were measured and the relative levels of renin and angiotensinogen mRNAs were determined by Northern blot analysis. Renin concentrations in normal and pathologic adrenals were 30-fold higher than those in the plasma of normal subjects, except for a Cushing's adenoma, which had an extremely high renin content. All adrenal tissues contained high proportions of active renin (between 56 and 87%), suggesting a likely conversion of prorenin to renin within these tissues. Renin mRNA was detected in each group of adrenal tissues, even in aldosterone-producing adenoma and hyperplastic tissue from idiopathic hyperaldosteronism. The relative level of renin mRNA was significantly correlated with the renin content. Angiotensinogen and its mRNA were detected in all normal and pathologic adrenals and, among all adrenal tissues, pheochromocytomas showed the highest angiotensinogen mRNA levels. However, the increased mRNA level in these tissues was not accompanied by a parallel increase in tissue angiotensinogen concentration. Since the translability of angiotensinogen mRNA was verified by in vitro cell-free translation, the low level of angiotensinogen compared to the relatively high amount of angiotensinogen mRNA suggested a lack of storage of this protein in adrenal cells. These studies demonstrate that human normal and pathologic adrenal tissues coexpress renin and angiotensinogen and that the local adrenal RAS may play a yet undefined role in the pathophysiology of the adrenal gland.

S16.1

X CHROMOSOME-LINKED KALLMANN'S SYNDROME (*KAL*): EXPRESSION OF THE *KAL* GENE IN THE CHICKEN EMBRYO

R. Legouis[1], J.-P. Hardelin[1], C. Ayer-Le Lièvre[2], C. Petit[1]*

[1]Unité de Génétique Moléculaire Humaine, Institut Pasteur, 25 rue du Docteur Roux, 75724 Paris Cedex 15, France.

[2]Institut d'EmbryologieCellulaire et Moléculaire, 49 bis avenue de la Belle Gabrielle, 94736 Nogent-sur-Marne Cedex, France.

The human *KAL* gene is responsible for the X chromosome-linked Kallmann's syndrome, which consists of an association between hypogonadotropic hypogonadism and anosmia. The disease may be due to a defect in the embryonic migratory pathway of GnRH-synthesizing neurons and olfactory axons from the olfactory pits up to the brain. The human and chicken *KAL* genes have been isolated. From the deduced amino acid sequences, we have postulated that the KAL protein is an extracellular matrix component with putative antiprotease and adhesion functions. Using *in situ* hybridization, we studied the *KAL* gene expression during embryonic development in the chicken. From embryonic day 2 (ED2) to ED8, the *KAL* gene is expressed in various endodermal, mesodermal, and neurectodermal derivatives, whereas the expression from ED8 is almost entirely restricted to definite neuronal populations in the central nervous system, most of which still express the gene after hatching. According to such a spatio-temporal pattern of expression, we suggest that the *KAL* gene is involved both in morphogenetic events and in neuronal late differentiation. With respect to the olfactory system, the *KAL* gene is expressed in the mitral cells of the olfactory bulbs from ED8 on. In contrast, no expression of the *KAL* gene is detected either in the embryonic olfactory epithelium or in the surrounding nasal mesenchyme. Therefore, we suggest that Kallmann's syndrome results from a central olfactory target cell defect.

S16.2

QUALITATIVE AND QUANTITATIVE STUDIES OF EXTRACRANIAL GnRH-IMMUNOREACTIVE NEURONS DURING ONTOGENETIC DEVELOPMENT. G.Sétáló. Dept. of Anatomy, University Medical School, Pécs, Hungary, H-7643.

Ontogenetic development of the GnRHir neuron system was studied with ICC in the rat and in the amphibian Clawed toad (Xenopus laevis) employing polyclonal mGnRH antibodies in both studies, and polyclonal as well as monoclonal cGnRHII antibodies in the amphibian study. In the Clawed toad, the study was repeated following uni-, or bilateral ablation of the olfactory placode during developmental stages 29-35. In the rat, quantitative data about the distribution of GnRHir neurons on subsequent days of the intrauterine life period indicated their shifting from the olfactory placode to forebrain areas. Unilaterally placodectomized toads studied with the use of both mGnRH and cGnRHII antibodies following their metamorphosis did not exhibit side differences in the number and distribution of the GnRHir cells and nerve fibers. These findings indicate that GnRHir neuroblasts differentiating on one side in the olfactory placode are able to inhabit both sides of the forebrain in the course of their migration. (Supported by Grant OTKA T6260)

S16.3

REMOVAL OF OLFACTORY PLACODE FAILS TO DEVELOP GnRH NEURONS IN THE FOREBRAIN IN THE CHICK EMBRYO. [1]Y. Arai, [1]S. Murakami, [2]S. Akutsu, [1]M. Kamiya, [1]Miyakawa, [1]T. Seki, [2]Y. Kuwabara. Depts of [1]Anatomy and [2]Ob-Gyn, Juntendo University School of Medicine, Hongo, Tokyo 113, Japan

We have found that both olfactory nerve fibers and GnRH neurons are strongly immunopositive to an embryonic form of NCAM(NCAM-H) during the time of neuronal migration in vivo and in vitro. However, this strong NCAM-H immunoreactivity in the GnRH neurons disappear after the GnRH neurons move into almost the same position as in the adult brain. Olfactory placodectomy fails to develop GnRH- and NCAM-H-expressing neurons as well as NCAM-H-expressing olfactory nerve fibers. Since NCAM-H is highly polysialylated and less adhesive, this diminished adhesiveness of NCAM-H may be responsible for creating space between the cells and the fibers to facilitate neuronal migration.

When the epithelial cells of the placode are labeled with DiI, the labeled cells sequentially appear in the olfacytory nerve, the rostral forebrain, and the septo-preoptic area. Furthermore, double staining for DiI and GnRH demonstrates that DiI-labeled neurons co-express GnRH. These results provide evidence for the actual migration of GnRH neurons from the olfactory placode to the septo-preoptic area during the development.

S16.4

ONTOGENY AND MIGRATION OF LHRH NEURONS IN HUMAN EMBRYOS. M. Schwanzel-Fukuda (Rockefeller University, New York); P.M.G. Bouloux (Royal Free Hospital, London); J.-P. Hardelin and C. Petit (Pasteur Institute, Paris).

LHRH neurons originate in the epithelium of the medial olfactory pit and migrate into the brain along a migration route formed by the central processes of the vomeronasal and terminal nerves. Originally demonstrated in mice, the migration of LHRH cells has been shown to take place in a variety of vertebrates, including humans. This migration route is rich in neural cell adhesion molecule (NCAM) immunoreactivity, and is formed before LHRH neurons are detected. In 29-31 day old embryos, NCAM-immunoreactive cells are seen in the epithelium of the medial olfactory pit and emerge to form a cellular aggregate in the mesenchyme between the nasal epithelium and the rostral forebrain. Antibodies to a polysialylated form of NCAM (PSA-NCAM) showed no immunoreactivity in the nasal mesenchyme at these ages. In 41-42 (but not 38-39) day old human embryos, LHRH-immunoreactivity was detected in cords of cells in the nasal mesenchyme, just outside of the epithelium of the medial olfactory pit, in the "ganglion terminale" and caudal margin of the cellular aggregate and at the basal lamina of the medial forebrain, caudal to the developing olfactory bulb. In these embryos, NCAM was present in all parts of the migration route. In contrast, PSA-NCAM was seen in specific parts of the migration route: in fascicles in the nasal mesenchyme, in fine fibers along the caudal margin of the cellular aggregate and extending into the forebrain, but not in the cellular aggregate below the rostral forebrain.

S16.SC1

SPATIAL EXPRESSION OF KAL GENE mRNA IN THE DEVELOPING HUMAN FOETUS.

*V M Duke[1] P J D Winyard[2] H Dewchand[2] A S Woolf P V Thorogood[2] P-M G Bouloux[1]
[1]Academic Department of Medicine, Royal Free Hospital School of Medicine, London, England NW3 2PF and [2]Developmental Biology Unit, Institute of Child Health, London.

The X-linked form of Kallmann's Syndrome (KS-hypogonadotrophic hypogonadism and anosmia) results from a migratory defect with failure of a common developmental pathway, namely the development of olfactory bulbs and migration of Gonadotrophin Releasing Hormone (GnRH) neurones from the olfactory placode to the forebrain. This is based on post mortem examination of a 19 week old male foetus with KS and two age and sex matched controls; the foetus with KS had no olfactory bulbs and GnRH neurone migration had arrested at the cribriform plate. The KAL gene has been localised to Xp22.3 and expression in humans has been demonstrated by Reverse Transcriptase PCR in liver, brain, muscle and kidney; Southern blotting alone being unsuccessful due to low copy number. We have demonstrated expression of the KAL mRNA in foetal material using in situ hybridisation. The 2.3Kb cDNA was used to generate S^{35} labelled sense and antisense riboprobes which were allowed to hybridise overnight to paraffin fixed sections of human foetal tissue ranging from 7 to 10 weeks gestation.. The slides were washed stringently then dipped in photographic emulsion and exposed for five days.

Expression was seen in the olfactory bulbs, the retinal neuroepithelium, extrinsic ocular muscles and in the developing mesonephros and ureteric bud. In contrast the whole embryo showed expression of a ubiquitous house-keeping gene. These findings correlate with previous in situ hybridisation studies performed on chick embryos where KAL expression was found in the retina, cerebellar Purkinje cells and mitral cells of the olfactory bulb.

Our findings to date are consistent with established theories concerning the defect in the olfactory and GnRH system as well as the unilateral renal agenesis seen in 50% of patients with X-linked KS. The KAL gene clearly has an important role in the development of the human urogenital and central nervous systems.

SI 1

GROWTH HORMONE AND IGF-1: THERAPEUTIC IMPLICATIONS.

Mary Lee Vance, University of Virginia, Charlottesville, VA 22908 USA

Potential therapeutic uses of growth hormone (GH) and insulin like growth factor-1 (IGF-1) are numerous, several of which are undergoing clinical trials. Some potential clinical uses of GH include replacement therapy in adults with GH deficiency, severe catabolic illness (e.g., burns, trauma, surgical recovery), aging, obesity, infertility and osteoporosis. Potential clinical uses of IGF-1 are less well defined but include severe catabolic illness, growth retardation secondary to GH resistance, obesity and diabetes. The combination of GH and IGF-1 treatment has also been proposed for with the rationale of preventing GH-induced hyperglycemia and amplifying the anabolic effect of both agents. With any new therapy, the questions of efficacy, outcomes and safety must be addressed by appropriate clinical studies. It now appears that GH replacement in adults has beneficial effects on body composition (increased muscle mass, decreased fat mass), and perhaps improving muscle strength in some, but the long-term effects and ultimate outcomes regarding morbidity and mortality are not known. This will require years of study before a definitive answer is possible. Information on potential therapeutic uses of IGF-1 is more limited, but it may be of greatest use when combined with GH therapy. Since IGF-1 suppresses endogenous GH secretion, it likely lessens GH's anabolic effects.

SI 2

THE SYNDROME OF GROWTH HORMONE DEFICIENCY (GHD) IN ADULTS AND THE EFFECTS OF GH REPLACEMENT.

P.H. Sönksen*, A. Weissberger, F. Salomon, R.C. Cuneo, G.A. McGauley, K. Verikiou and C. Lowy. Department of Endocrinology, Division of Medicine UMDS, St Thomas' Hospital, London SE1 7EH.

Although GH has long been known to possess potent anabolic, lipolytic and diabetogenic properties, its importance in maintaining health in adults had not been appreciated until recently when the results of several placebo-controlled trials of GH replacement became available. Adults with GHD receiving optimum replacement therapy with other hormones are disadvantaged but rarely complain of their problems. When carefully compared with matched controls, adults with GHD have significantly impaired quality of life (particularly loss of energy and vitality but also social isolation and low mood), altered body composition (reduced lean body mass, increased fat mass, particularly central fat), reduced muscle strength and exercise performance, increased plasma cholesterol and (unlike children with GHD) insulin resistance. There is epidemiological evidence to suggest that the unfavourable lipid profile is reflected in a reduced quantity of life with a twofold increase in cardiovascular mortality rates in both sexes. There are now four published placebo-controlled studies of GH replacement in adults with GHD and the results are remarkably consistent. The quality of life problems are completely relieved, body composition changes dramatically and rapidly. Strength and exercise performance are normalised, as is the lipid profile. Longer term studies indicate that continuous GH replacement is required to maintain these beneficial effects. Side effects are mild, reversible and dose-related. Conclusions: GH replacement in adults with GHD leads to marked improvement in quality of life in the majority of cases. It seems that life-long replacement therapy is required but further research on optimum doses and monitoring of efficacy is needed.

SI 3

Abstract not received

P1.1

LOCALIZATION AND FUNCTIONAL IMPLICATIONS OF AXONAL mRNA IN THE HYPOTHALAMO NEUROHYPOPHYSEAL SYSTEM OF RAT. G.F. Jirikowski*, T. Skutella, J.C. Probst. Dept. of Neuroendocrinology, Max Planck Institute of Psychiatry, Clinical Inst. Munich, Germany D 80804.

Transcripts encoding the hypothalamic peptides vasopressin, and oxytocin as well as the katecholamine synthesizing enzyme tyrosine hydroxylase were localized in the magnocellular hypothalamic nuclei, the median eminence and the posterior pituitary lobe of rats. With nonradioactive in situ hybridization, it could be demonstrated that these mRNA sequences are located in axonal varicosities. Electron microscopy indicated that these mRNAs are associated with a fraction of the large secretory vesicles. Osmotic stimulation increased within 15 min cytoplasmic hybridization signal in the magnocellular perikarya, which was not observed, when animals had been pretreated with colchizine, to block axonal transport. Pretreatment with a potent polymerase II Inhibitor however failed to block increase of transcriptional message upon short term osmotic challenge.
It is likely that hypothalamic transcripts are under certain conditions stored in axons, perhaps compartimentalized in secretory vesicles. Our findings indicate that specific stimulation facilitates immediate retrograde transport of mRNA and consecutive translation, perhaps to replenish depleted peptide pools, prior to de novo transcription of the respective message.

P1.2

VASOPRESSIN GENE EXPRESSION IN THE PARAVENTRICULAR NUCLEUS OF SPONTANEOUSLY HYPERTENSIVE RATS (SHR) IN RESPONSE TO DEHYDRATION AND REHYDRATION

M.J.A. Rocha, M.F.Callahan, P.Rucker, K.Vrana and M. Morris. Bowman Gray School of Medicine Winston -Salem, NC 27103, USA

Although there is no known cause of primary (essential) hypertension, disturbances in the control of fluid/electrolyte homeostasis have often been associated with this and other forms of hypertension. Vasopressin (VP) is believed to play a role in hypertension because it affects fluid and electrolyte balance, has potent vasoconstrictor effects, and modulates cardiovascular reflexes. In this study, we evaluated the effect of dehydration and rehydration on VP secretion and VP gene expression in male spontaneously hypertensive (SHR) rats and their normotensive controls, Wistar Kyoto (WKY). The animals were submitted to dehydration for 48 hr followed by 0, 1 hr or 6 hr rehydration period before being sacrificed. Plasma, pituitary and paraventricular (PVN) VP was determined by RIA. VP mRNA levels in the PVN were evaluated by slot blot. Plasma and PVN VP content showed similar changes upon dehydration and rehydration in both SHR and WKY animals. Dehydration produced a depletion of neurohypophyseal VP in the controls with no change observed in the SHR. For peptide mRNA the SHRs showed a more than 2 fold increase in PVN VP mRNA. This was followed by a rapid rebound in mRNA levels after 1 hr of rehydration. In contrast there were no changes in VP mRNA in the controls. The SHRs appear to be more sensitive to changes in volume and osmolality, responding with rapid changes in VP mRNA levels. This data shows that there are differences between the hypertensive and normotensive strains in the way that they regulate peptide secretion..

P1.3

TRANSGENIC EXPRESSION OF DOMINANT INHIBITORS OF THE CAMP AND PROTEIN KINASE C PATHWAYS IN RAT MAGNOCELLULAR NEURONS. S.J. Waller*, Q. Zeng, D. Murphy. Institute of Molecular and Cell Biology, National University of Singapore, 10 Kent Ridge Crescent, Singapore 0511.

In magnocellular neurons, the response of the rat vasopressin gene to osmotic stimuli is two fold: an upregulation of transcription of the VP gene results in increased levels of the VP mRNA, and an increase in the extent of polyadenylation of the VP transcript is exhibited. Temporal, pharmacological and anatomical experiments have shown these responses to be independently regulated, and although the precise mechanisms mediating these effects are unknown, several lines of evidence suggest roles for the cAMP-dependent protein kinase (PKA) and/or protein kinase C (PKC) signal transduction pathways. In order to examine further the contribution of these second messenger systems to the physiological regulation of the VP gene, we have cloned two proteins proposed to be inhibitory to these protein kinases. PKAI, a previously characterised protein inhibitor of PKA, was cloned from a rat brain cDNA library. A novel cDNA sequence encoding pPKCI, a putative inhibitor of PKC, was cloned from a bovine brain cDNA library. Sequence analysis of pPKCI revealed considerable (60%) homology at the nucleotide and amino acid levels with a protein of unknown function from the cyanobacteria Synechococcus. We have subsequently cloned related sequences from rat, mouse and chinese cabbage, and experiments are underway to define the roles of these highly conserved relatives of pPKCI.
Transgenic rats expressing PKAI and pPKCI in the vasopressinergic magnocellular neurons of the hypothalamus have been generated, by inserting the cDNAs encoding PKAI and pPKCI into a genomic rat VP fragment, previously shown by us to direct cell specific and highly inducible expression of reporter genes to these cells in transgenic rats. The effects of these inhibitors on the regulation of magnocellular neuron function following osmotic stimulation are being examined.

P1.4

GENE-EXPRESSION OF ARGININE VASOTOCIN IN OVARIAN AND UTERINE TISSUES OF CHICKEN: N. Saito[1]*, R. Grossmann[2]. [1]Dept. Animal Physiology, Nagoya University, Nagoya Japan, 464-01 [2]Institute for Small Animal Research (FAL), Celle, Germany.

The hypothalamus is the classical site of synthesis for arginine vasotocin (AVT) as neurohypophyseal hormone in the chicken. However, high concentrations of AVT were measured in ovarian tissues by RIA. Surprisingly, northern blot analysis failed to detect measurable amounts of AVT mRNA even after mRNA enrichment. In this study we have applied the highly sensitive polymerase chain reaction (PCR) to measure AVT specific mRNA. Hypothalamic tissue as well as the four largest ovarian follicles (F_1-F_4) and the shell gland (uterus) of adult chickens were collected 4 hr before and 4 hr after oviposition. Follicular tissues were separated into granulosa, theca interna and theca externa cell layers. The uterine tissues were separated into myometrium and endometrium. AVT specific 5' and 3' primers (kindly provided by Dr. Richard Ivell, IHF, Hamburg) and Vent DNA polymerase were used to amplify the cDNA reversly transcripted from mRNA (30 cycles at successively 95°C, 55°C and 72°C, each for 1 min). Semiquantitative comparison of mRNA levels between different tissue were made. The PCR products were detected in all tissues used, however, the amounts in ovarian and uterine tissues were about 50 to 1000 times lower than that found in the hypothalamus. These data suggest that AVT in the ovary and the uterus may have autocrine or paracrine function, although the low level of AVT gene expression does not point to a specific function of ovarian/uterine AVT during oviposition and/or ovulation.

P1.5

MUTATION OF ACIDIC AMINO ACIDS IN THE MOUSE GnRH RECEPTOR REVEALS THAT GLU^{301} DETERMINES BINDING SPECIFICITY FOR ARG^{8} IN MAMMALIAN GnRH. R.P. Millar[1*], C.A. Flanagan[1], I.I. Becker[1], J.S. Davidson[1], I.K. Wakefield[1], W. Zhou[2], and S.C. Sealfon[2], [1]M.R.C. Regulatory Peptides Research Unit, University of Cape Town Medical School, Observatory, 7925, South Africa; [2]Fishberg Center in Neurobiology and Department of Neurology, Mount Sinai School of Medicine, New York.

Arg^{8} of mammalian GnRH is necessary for high affinity binding to mammalian GnRH receptors. Substitution of Arg^{8} with neutral amino acids results in decreased affinity. This suggested that the positively-charged Arg may interact with a negatively-charged acidic residue in the receptor. We therefore mutated acidic residues, Glu^{8}, Glu^{90}, Asp^{98}, Glu^{111}, Asp^{185}, Asp^{292}, Glu^{294} and Glu^{301} in the extracellular and transmembrane domains of the mouse GnRH receptor (GnRHR) to corresponding Asn or Gln residues and found that the [Gln^{301}]-GnRHR, expressed in COS-1 cells, exhibited low affinity for mammalian GnRH (K_d, $1.2 \times 10^{-6} \pm 7.4 \times 10^{-8}$ M) and did not distinguish it from analogues with substitutions for Arg^{8}. The mutant receptor affinity for GnRH was similar to the affinities of the wildtype GnRHR for analogues in which Arg^{8} is substituted. Even when the binding affinities of the analogues were increased by introduction of a conformational constraint in position 6, the mutant receptor did not exhibit preference for Arg in position 8. However, the [Gln^{301}]-GnRHR, like the wildtype GnRHR, did distinguish between GnRH and analogues which contain substitutions in positions 5, 6, 7 and 10. Thus the mutant receptor retains the specificity of the wildtype GnRHR for substitutions of GnRH residues other than Arg^{8}.

These data show that the Glu^{301} residue of the mouse GnRHR determines binding specificity for Arg in position 8 in GnRH, and may constitute part of the GnRH binding site in which there is an interaction between these residues.

P1.6

MUTAGENESIS OF N-GLYCOSYLATION SITES IMPAIRS EXPRESSION BUT NOT AFFINITY OF THE GnRH RECEPTOR. J Davidson[*a], C Flanagan[a], W Zhou[b], I Becker[a], R Elario[a], W Emeran[a], S Sealfon[b] and R Millar[a]. MRC Regulatory Peptides Research Unit[a], University of Cape Town Medical School, Observatory 7925, South Africa; Fishberg Center in Neurobiology and Dept. of Neurology[b], Mount Sinai School of Medicine, New York, NY10029.

The GnRH receptor (GnRHR) belongs to the 7-transmembrane receptor superfamily and is coupled via the G-protein G_q to phospholipase C. It was previously proposed that glycosylation of the GnRHR played an essential role in ligand binding. GnRHRs cloned from four species contain two conserved consensus sequences (N-X-S/T) for N-glycosylation (N18 and N102), in the extracellular domains. In addition the rodent receptors have a non-conserved site (N4). We mutated these asparagines in the mouse GnRHR to glutamines and determined the effects on ligand binding and phospholipase C activation in transfected COS-1 cells.

After photoaffinity labelling of the expressed receptors with ^{125}I-azidobenzoyl-D-lys^{6}-GnRH, the N18Q and N4Q mutants showed lower apparent MW on SDS-PAGE, while the N102Q receptor showed normal mobility. This indicates that the GnRHR is glycosylated at N4 and N18 but that N102 is not utilized as a glycosylation site.

Binding studies showed that the N4Q, N18Q and N102Q receptors were expressed to 54%, 39%, and 77% respectively of the wild type level. Binding affinities of all 3 mutant receptors were indistinguishable from wild type, indicating that carbohydrate moieties are not involved in the ligand binding site.

Inositol phosphate production assays showed that all the glycosylation site mutants were capable of normal signal transduction. The N18Q and N4Q mutants showed decreased maximal responses, consistent with decreased receptor expression on the cell surface.

These results show that mutation of N-linked glycosylation sites does not affect ligand binding affinity or signal transduction of the GnRHR. The results suggest, however, that glycosylation at N4 and N18 sites is necessary for normal GnRHR expression. The role of glycosylation in this peptide receptor resembles the ß-adrenergic receptor, and differs from the TSH receptor where glycosylation is essential for high affinity ligand binding.

P1.7

RETINOIC ACID REGULATES GnRH RELEASE AND GENE EXPRESSION IN THE RAT HYPOTHALAMIC FRAGMENTS AND GT1-7 CELLS IN VITRO. S. Cho, H. Cho and K. Kim*. Department of Molecular Biology and Center for Cell Differentiation, Seoul National University, Seoul 151-742 KOREA

Gonadotropin-releasing hormone (GnRH) plays a pivotal role in the regulation of mammalian reproduction and development. One of the recent finding that a putative retinoic acid responsive element (RARE) is present in the 5' flanking region of the rat GnRH gene (Kepa et al., Nucleic Acid Res. 20:1393-1399, 1992) led us to examine a possible role of retinoic acid (RA) in the regulation of GnRH neurons. Using hypothalamic fragments derived from long-term ovariectomized rats and GT1-7 cells, the effect of RA on GnRH release and gene expression was assessed. Increasing concentration of RA significantly increased GnRH release in a dose-dependent manner. RA-evoked GnRH release rapidly ensued within 30 min and then returned basal levels. During a 2 hr incubation, RA significantly decreased GnRH mRNA levels in a dose-dependent manner. Gel shift analysis showed that the cell extracts from the POA-MBH fragments as well as GT1-7 cells contained putative transcription factors which specifically bind to RARE of the rat GnRH gene promoter. These findings suggest that RA may play an important role in the regulation of GnRH gene expression and secretion.

P1.8

LEVELS OF GnRH, GnRH mRNA AND GnRH RECEPTOR mRNA FOLLOWING CASTRATION AND TESTOSTERONE REPLACEMENT IN THE MALE RAT I.I. Becker[1*], M. Jakubowski[2], M. Tsutsumi[3], C.A. Flanagan[1], P.D.W. Davies[1], S. Sealfon[3], R.P. Millar[1] and C.M. Dutlow[1], [1]M.R.C. Regulatory Peptides Unit, University of Cape Town Medical School; [2]Beth Israel Hospital, Boston and [3]Mount Sinai School of Medicine, New York

We examined the effect of surgical castration and testosterone (T) replacement on levels of hypothalamic GnRH and GnRH mRNA and pituitary GnRH receptor (GnRHR) mRNA in relation to serum LH levels. In addition, we examined the effect of chemical castration, using GnRH antagonist treatment on GnRHR gene expression. Adult male rats were sacrificed on days 1, 3, 9, 15 and 21 postcastration; intact rats were used as controls. Other rats received either T replacement (0.5mg/day/100g weight) or vehicle beginning on day 21 postcastration and sacrificed 1, 4 or 7 days later. As expected, serum LH increased rapidly after castration and was suppressed by T replacement. GnRH content decreased from 3.8 $\pm$0.4 ng/H in intact animals to 1.4 $\pm$0.2 ng/H by day 9 postcastration. T increased GnRH content to 2.4 $\pm$0.3 ng/H after 7 days of treatment. GnRH mRNA increased from 306 $\pm$38 fg/H in intact males to 727 $\pm$61 fg/H by day 9 postcastration, then decreased to 422 $\pm$45 fg/H by day 21. T had no significant effect on GnRH mRNA. GnRHR mRNA increased from 12.12 $\pm$3.19 pg/P in intact animals to 35.79 $\pm$4.79 pg/P by day 9 postcastration. T significantly decreased GnRHR mRNA levels. Treatment for 8h with GnRH Antagonist resulted in a decline in serum T level and a 67% decrease in GnRHR mRNA compared to control rats.

The decrease in GnRH content after castration reflects depletion of the decapeptide stores due to increased secretion, and the initial postcastrational rise in GnRH mRNA levels may reflect an increase in GnRH biosynthesis to replenish the decapeptide stores. The subsequent decline in GnRH mRNA levels between days 9 and 21 may represent a transition to a new steady state of lower GnRH biosynthesis and secretion rates. Lower GnRH release at this stage would be compatible with increased pituitary sensitivety, i.e., receptor upregulation. GnRH plays a major role in the postcastrational rise of GnRHR mRNA, as was determined by the effect of GnRH antagonist. We suggest that the postcastrational rise in LH secretion is caused primarily by pretranslational upregulation of GnRHR due to increased GnRH secretion.

P1.9

ADMINISTRATION OF TESTOSTERONE INDUCES C-FOS IN THE NEONATAL FEMALE RAT HYPOTHALAMUS.

F.Stylianopoulou*, M.Giannakopoulou, University of Athens, P.O.Box 14224, Athens 11510, Greece.

Administration of testosterone to female rats during the first days of life results in defeminization and masculinization of their brain. The effect of testosterone is mainly exerted at the hypothalamus,and in particular at the sexual dimorphic nucleus (SDN). In an effort to elucidate the molecular mechanisms underlying these effects, we examined the expression of the protooncogene c-fos in the hypothalamus of 2 day old female rats exposed to testosterone. C-fos is an early-induced gene, whose induction is considered an index of neuronal activity. Using Northern analysis, we showed that administration of testosterone propionate to 2 day female rats increased c-fos mRNA levels in the hypothalamus. In situ hybridization and immunocytochemistry revealed that the increase in c-fos mRNA and protein levels were localised in the SDN. Administration of the antiandrogen cyproterone acetate together with testosterone prevented the induction of c-fos. Our results show that testosterone acting through the androgen receptor induces c-fos transcription. The fos protein in turn would affect the transcription of other genes, by binding to AP1 sites in their promoters. The aromatase gene could be such a gene since we show that testosterone increases aromatase enzyme activity in the neonatal rat hypothalamus.

P1.10

INHIBITORY EFFECTS OF STEROIDS ON GONADOTROPHIN-RELEASING HORMONE -I mRNA AND NEURONE NUMBERS.

Sharp, P.J., Dunn, I.C., Sang, H.M., [1]Mess, A., [1]Gladwell, R.T., AFRC Roslin Institute, Roslin, Midlothian, EH25 9PS and [1]University of Reading, Reading, RG6 2AJ, U.K.

The mechanism of action of inhibitory steroids on GnRH neurone function is not fully understood, partly because measurements of GnRH mRNA in steroid-manipulated mammalian models have produced conflicting results. The objective of the study was to further understanding of the steroid regulation of the GnRH neurone using the domestic cockerel. Chicken GnRH-I mRNA was measured using competitive RT-PCR and GnRH-I cells were counted after localisation by immunocytochemistry using antibodies which recognise the GnRH-I pro-peptide.

Cockerels were castrated/sham operated at 3 weeks of age and killed at 9 weeks of age. Oestradiol benzoate (0.5mg/kg) or oil was administered intra-muscularly on four alternate days before death. Total RNA was extracted from each hypothalamus and reverse transcribed before PCR analysis using GnRH-I specific primers. Immunohistochemistry was performed on 70µm Vibratome sections.

Treatment	**GnRH-I mRNA (moles/hypothalamus x10^{-18} ± S.E., n=8)**	**GnRH-I neurones (Nos./hypothalamus ± S.E., n=5)**
Castrate control	8.3±1.4	1324± 57
Intact	3.7±0.5 **	700±142 **
Castrate + oil control	5.0±0.7	1985±101
Castrate + oestradiol	2.3±0.3 **	1128± 87 ***

** *P<0.01*; *** *P<0.001 compared with control.*

Castration significantly increased GnRH mRNA and the visible numbers of GnRH cell bodies (See Table). These effects of castration were reversed by oestrogen. This steroid is thought to inhibit GnRH release in the cockerel, being derived from testosterone by aromatisation within the hypothalamus. It is concluded that oestrogen may regulate the function of GnRH neurones by altering mRNA content and GnRH synthesis. The effect of oestrogen may be mediated by a change in the number of active GnRH neurones.

P1.11

NEONATAL ESTROGENIZATION: WHAT ELSE DOES IT IMPAIR IN THE FEMALE BRAIN?

V.K. Patchev*, S. Hayashi, *Dept. Neuroendocrinology, Max Planck Institute of Psychiatry, 80804 Munich, Germany and Dept. Anatomy & Embryology, Tokyo Metropolitan Institute for Neuroscience, Tokyo 183, Japan.

Neonatal administration of supraphysiological doses of estrogen to female rats results in irreversible alterations in gonadal axis function and sexual behaviour. These effects of estrogen have been ascribed to its "organizing" action on neuroendocrine mechanisms involved in gonadal regulation. Since gonadal steroids reportedly affect the function of the hypothalamo-pituitary-adrenal (HPA) axis, we examined the possibility that neonatal estrogenization (NE) produces long-term effects on the expression of hypothalamic neuropeptides and hippocampal glucocorticoid receptors involved in HPA regulation. NE was associated with increased levels of mRNAs coding for CRH and AVP in the PVN, POMC in the ARC, and proenkephalin in several brain regions. The expression of type II glucocorticoid receptors (GR) was decreased in the hippocampus of NE rats. In an attempt to prove that the described effects resulted from the neonatal exposure to estrogen, we compared the response of these parameters to estrogen treatment in ovariectomized adult normal and NE rats. The initially observed differences persisted after removal of the gonads, and subsequent supplementation of normal rats with estrogen resulted in changes in CRH and AVP mRNAs which resembled those in NE animals. POMC gene expression was uniformly suppressed by estrogen in both groups. Striking differences between normal and NE rats were observed in the responsiveness of GR mRNA to estrogen treatment. The results suggest that i) increased production of opioids and their secretagogues, such as CRH and AVP, might contribute to the suppression of gonadal function in NE rats; ii) NE might be associated with altered HPA regulation, and iii) neonatal exposure to supraphysiological estrogen levels may have a "mal-organizing" effect on several neuroendocrine regulatory mechanisms, which may account for a myriad of dysfunctions outside of the reproductive system.

P1.12

EXOGENOUS ESTROGEN ACTS DIFFERENTLY ON PRODUCTION OF ESTROGEN RECEPTOR IN THE PREOPTIC AREA AND THE MEDIOBASAL HYPOTHALAMIC NUCLEI.

C.Orikasa*, S.Hayashi Dept. of Anatomy and Embryology, Tokyo Metropolitan Inst. for Neuroscience, 2-6 Musashidai, Fuchu, Tokyo 183, Japan.

Estrogen receptor (ER) mediates action of estrogen as a transcription factor, which initiates *de novo* protein synthesis and eventually regulates neuronal function. Being related to the control of reproductive function, the arcuate (ARH) and the ventromedial (VMH) hypothalamic nuclei, as well as the preoptic nucleus (PON), contain numerous ER. We investigated influence of exogenous estrogen on ER-mRNA and ER protein molecules in these nuclei in the newborn female rats. Pups have received daily injections of 10 ug estradiol benzoate (EB) for 5 or 10 consecutive days from the day of birth and killed on days 6 or 11. ER was examined by *in situ* hybridization- and by immuno-histochemistry for gene and protein levels. Both ER-mRNA and ER protein were suppressed by EB in ARH and VMH. In PON, on the contrary, EB suppressed ER protein, but not ER-mRNA. These observations suggest that the ER-mRNA signals detected in PON do not represent normal ER-mRNA. This mRNA, however, might still maintain base sequences detectable by the cRNA probes we used. In VMH and ARH, in contrast, ER-mRNA seemed to be suppressed directly, and then ER protein synthesis eventually decreased. Thus, EB seemed to act on the different steps of gene expression between PON and VMH/ARH. All these mechanisms may contribute to irreversible changes in the specific sets of genes involved in neuronal function.

P1.13

COMPARISON OF REGIONAL AND DEVELOPMENTAL CHANGES OF mRNA LEVELS ENCODING AROMATASE CYTOCHROME P450 AND 5α-REDUCTASE IN THE RAT BRAIN. M.E. Lauber* and W. Lichtensteiger, Inst. of Pharmacology, Univ. of Zürich, 8057 Zürich, Switzerland.

Sex hormones play a crucial role in many aspects of development and sexual differentiation of the rat brain. 17β-estradiol (E2), for example, determines a number of sexually dimorphic functions, whereas 5α-dihydrotestosterone (DHT) appears to be involved only in some aspects of sexual differentiation but might be more important for myelinization. Peripheral-derived testosterone is converted to E2 and DHT by the enzymatic actions of aromatase cytochrome P450 (*CYP19*) and 5α-reductase, respectively. In order to better understand the role of E2 and DHT, we have investigated regional and developmental changes of mRNA levels encoding *CYP19* and 5α-reductase employing the *in situ* hybridization technique to male fetuses and offspring of time-pregnant Long Evans rats. At gestational day (GD) 16 (GD 1 = 24 hours after mating), moderate aromatase mRNA levels were only detected in the preoptic/hypothalamic area. At GD18 and GD20, high levels of aromatase mRNA were observed in preoptic and hypothalamic regions as well as in limbic structures (bed nucleus of the stria terminalis and medial amygdala). At postnatal day (PN) 2 and during further development (PN6, PN15 and adult), aromatase mRNA in the preoptic/hypothalamic area decreased to much lower levels, but remained high in the limbic structures. mRNA encoding for 5α-reductase could already be detected at GD 16 and was maintained at comparable levels throughout further development. 5α-reductase mRNA expression appeared uniformly distributed throughout the whole brain, except for the neuroepithel where higher mRNA levels could be detected. These results demonstrate that aromatase cytochrome P450 mRNA is expressed in regions where local estrogen synthesis is required for the establishment of sexually dimorphic functions. In addition, the time course and regional distribution of 5α-reductase mRNA expression might not only link 5α-reductase activity with myelinization, but also provide evidence for additional developmental functions, e.g. cell proliferation.

P1.14

SEXUAL DIMORPHISM AND SEX STEROID MODULATION OF GLIAL FIBRILLARY ACIDIC PROTEIN (GFAP) mRNA AND IMMUNOREACTIVITY LEVELS IN THE RAT HYPOTHALAMUS. J.A. Chowen*, S. Busiguina and L.M. García-Segura. Instituto Cajal, 28002 Madrid, Spain.

Sex steroids influence the morphology and physiology of the hypothalamus, both during development and in adulthood, resulting in endocrine functions that are sexually dimorphic and modulated by the steroid environment. Although sex steroids are known to modulate neurons, it is now clear that glia are also influenced by these hormones. Since glia appear to be involved in the proliferation, survival, migration and maturation of neurons, as well as changes in synaptic connectivity, it follows that hormonal modulation of glia may mediate some of the steroid effects on neurons. To better understand this phenomenon, we have studied the effects of testosterone (T), both neonatally and during adulthood, on the mRNA levels and immunoreactivity surface density (ISD) for the glia specific protein, GFAP. As shown below, males had significantly higher GFAP mRNA levels and ISD than females in the hypothalamic arcuate nucleus (ANOVA: $p<0.0001$). Both adult and neonatal castration of males significantly reduced GFAP mRNA levels and ISD. Neonatal and adult T treatment increased both of these parameters in both sexes.

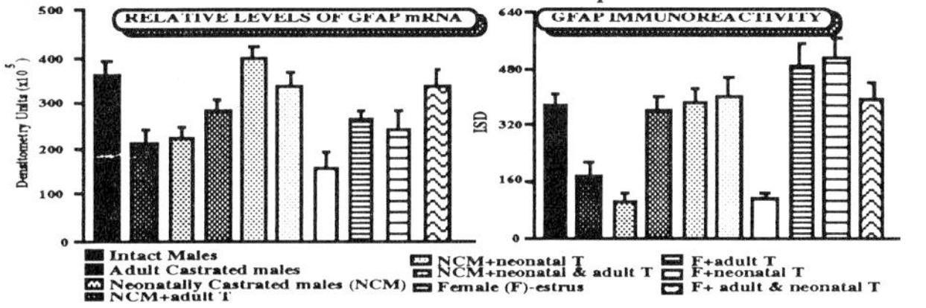

These data suggest that glia are significantly influenced by both the neonatal and adult sex steroid environment and that some of the steroid effects on neurons may be mediated, at least in part, through modulation of glia.

P1.15

EXPRESSION OF Gα SUBUNITS mRNAs IN HUMAN PROLACTINOMAS. L. Caccavelli, D. Dewailly, C. Kordon, P. Jaquet, A. Enjalbert. ICNE-UMR 9941 CNRS, Université Aix-Marseille II, Service Endocrinologie et Diabétologie, CHR Lille, U 159 INSERM Paris, France.

Somatic mutations in Gsα and Gαi2 subunits have been described in various adenomas but none of there mutations was found in prolactinomas. Nevertheless in bromocriptine resistant prolactinomas dysfunctions occur at the level of the dopamine D2 receptor. Resistance was associated with a decrease of D2 dopaminergic binding sites as well as level of mRNA, but also with alteration of dopamine inhibition of adenylate cyclase.

We have investigated whether instead of mutations, the G protein expression could be modified in these prolactinomas. Quantitative RT-PCR was used to measure Gαo, Gαi2 and Gαs mRNA levels. Resistant prolactinomas expressed less mRNAs encoding for Gαi2 than bromocriptine sensitive adenomas whereas Gαo and Gαs mRNA levels were not affected. Moreover in bromocriptine sensitive prolactinomas Gαi2 mRNA levels were correlated with D2 dopamine receptors mRNA levels. Such correlation was not observed in resistant prolactinomas.

It is concluded that resistance to bromocriptine therapy could be accounted by reduced expression of D2 dopamine receptors as well as Gi2 proteines, known to mediate the coupling with adenylate cyclase.

P1.16

PITUITARY ADENYLATE CYCLASE-ACTIVATING POLYPEPTIDE (PACAP)/ VASOACTIVE INTESTINAL PEPTIDE (VIP)RECEPTOR SUBTYPES IN RAT TISSUES :INVESTIGATION OF RECEPTOR BINDING AND MOLECULAR IDENTIFICATION BY CHEMICAL CROSS LINKING.
M. SONE,*D. M. SMITH,**I. GOZES,& *S. R. BLOOM. Tohoku University School of medicine,Sendai 980,Japan.*RPMS,London W12 ONN,UK. **Tel Aviv University,Israel.

Receptors for PACAP have been subdivided into type I receptors (PACAP specific) and typeII receptors (bind PACAP and VIP with approximately equal affinity).Using rat brain stem as a tissues containing type I receptors and rat lung as a tissue containing type II receptors we investigated the binding of ^{125}I labelled PACAP,VIP and helodermin to these tissues and by chemical cross-linking the relative molecular weight of the receptors. Type I receptors showed an Mr of 58,000 with typeII having an Mr of 54,000. The difference in molecular weight was still apparent after deglycosylation of the receptors indicating that type I and II receptors are different proteins.We also studied a hybrid (VIP- neurotensin) VIP receptorantagonist which was unable to displace type I receptors (K_i >10 μM)but was effective at type II receptors and propose that this peptide could be used to differentiate between PACAP effects via the two receptor subtypes. ^{125}I-helodermin has been used as a specific ligand for high affinity VIP site.We found in stomach fundus a higher number of helodermin binding sites (767 fmol/mg protein) than VIP binding sites (346 fmol/mg protein)indicating the possibility of a novel as yet uncharacterized receptor.The Mr of this site was 55,000.

P1.17

GHRH AND SRIH IMMUNOREACTIVITY IN THE BRAIN OF DWARF TH-hGH TRANSGENIC MICE. B. J. Collins*, S. B. Cichy, M. Szabo, and L. A. Frohman. Department of Medicine, Michael Reese Hospital and University of Illinois at Chicago, Chicago IL USA 60616.

The TH-hGH transgenic (tg) mouse expresses the human growth hormone (hGH) gene in the central nervous system at sites of tyrosine hydroxylase (TH) synthesis, suppressing endogenous mGH and producing a dwarf phenotype. Previous studies demonstrating hGH expression in hypothalamic arcuate and periventricular (PeVN) nuclei, areas containing growth hormone releasing hormone (GHRH) and somatostatin (SRIH) neurons involved in the control of pituitary GH secretion, suggested that the neuronally expressed hGH exerts negative feedback at these loci. Recent studies in our laboratory have demonstrated a 65% reduction in hypothalamic GHRH mRNA of TH-hGH mice, as revealed by Northern blotting. The present study reports immunocytochemical evidence of altered GHRH and SRIH expression in the brain of the TH-hGH tg mouse. Female mice injected with 20 µg colchicine 24 h prior to sacrifice were perfused with heparinized saline followed by Zamboni's fixative (2% paraformaldehyde and picric acid in PB). Twenty µm coronal sections were thaw mounted, incubated with rabbit polyclonal antibodies to GHRH and SRIH, and immunostained by the ABC method (Vectastain) with DAB/peroxide visualization. Wild-type (wt) controls exhibited abundant GHRH staining of cell bodies in the arcuate nucleus, while tg mice had only a few stained cells. The pattern of fiber staining was similar in both, and corresponded to published data. Somatostatin cell staining was increased in the PeVN of tg mice, but the difference from wt mice was less pronounced than that for GHRH in the arcuate nucleus. We conclude that hypothalamic hGH expression in the tg mouse reduces pituitary mGH secretion primarily by suppressing GHRH production.

P1.18

DIFFERENTIAL EXPRESSION OF TYPE-1 ANGIOTENSIN II (AngII) RECEPTOR SUBTYPES IN THE RAT HYPOTHALAMUS AND ANTERIOR PITUITARY. **Z. Lenkei, C. Morea, A. Enjalbert, P. Corvol, C. Kordon, C. Llorens-Cortes*. INSERM U36, College de France and INSERM U159, Paris, France.**

AngII is involved in the regulation of the secretion of several anterior pituitary hormones, acting both directly at the anterior pituitary and indirectly on the hypothalamus. Most of these actions are mediated by the type-1 AngII receptor (AT1). Recently cDNAs for two AT1 receptor subtypes (AT1a and AT1b) have been cloned. Close similarities in their pharmacological properties make it difficult to differentiate them by binding studies. In order to study their distribution and regulation, we have developed two approaches for estimating the expression of their respective mRNAs: 1) specific quantification by reverse transcriptase polymerase chain reaction amplification in the presence of a 63 bp deleted AT1 receptor mutatnt cRNA as an internal standard; 2) visualization by in situ hybridization using specific cRNA probes. Predominant expression of AT1 receptor mRNA (85%) has been found in brain sites which control prolactin, ACTH or LH secretions, such as the subfornical organ, the vascular organ of the lamina terminalis, the preoptic area, the paraventricular and arcuate nuclei. In contrast, strong AT1b receptor mRNA expression (80%) was detected in the anterior lobe of the pituitary. Analysis of normal pituitary cells separated on unit gravity gradients or of pituitary cell lines (AtT-20, GH4C1, GC, aT3) shows that the AT1b receptor subtypes mRNA is predominantly expressed in lactotropes and corticotropes. These results indicate that neuroendocrine effects of AngII are mediated by different receptor subtypes at the hypothalamic and pituitary level. This may have functional consequences since gene expression of both receptor subtypes appears differentially regulated. (Llorens-Cortes et al., Submitted to J. Biol. Chem.)

P1.19

EFFECT OF MATERNAL ADRENALECTOMY ON HYPOTHALAMIC CRF AND GLUCOCORTICOID RECEPTOR mRNA AND ANTERIOR PITUITARY POMC mRNA SYNTHESIS IN MALE AND FEMALE NEONATES. I. Halasz*, F. Aird and E. Redei. Departments of Psychiatry and Pharmacology, University of Pennsylvania, Philadelphia, PA, USA 19104-6141.

We studied the effect of maternal glucocorticoids on steady state levels of hypothalamic CRF and glucocorticoid receptor (GR) mRNA and anterior pituitary POMC mRNA by adrenalectomizing dams prior to the functioning of the fetal pituitary-adrenal axis. Time pregnant Sprague-Dawley rats were adrenalectomized (ADX) or sham-adrenalectomized (SHAM) on day 8 of gestation. Messenger RNA levels were measured by northern blotting in male and female offspring on days 1, 7, 14 and 21 of age. CRF and GR mRNA levels increased with age in both male and female offspring equally, peaking at day 14 and decreasing by day 21. Maternal ADX had no effect in male offspring, but CRF and GR mRNA levels were increased on days 7 and 14 in female offspring of ADX dams. Both CRF and GR mRNA synthesis returned to SHAM levels by day 21. Anterior pituitary POMC mRNA levels show a significant but transient increase on day 7 in both males and females. Maternal ADX increased POMC mRNA levels of male offspring on day 7 and of female offspring on day 21. Overall, male offspring had higher levels of POMC mRNA than females. These data suggest that a potentially important developmental event occurs in the neonatal hypothalamic-pituitary axis between days 7 and 14 of age. Furthermore, the lack of maternal glucocorticoids influences hypothalamic CRF and GR expression only transiently, but seems to have prolonged effect on POMC expression in the female offspring. (Supported by AA07389)

P1.20

GLUCOCORTICOIDRECEPTORS IN THE BRAIN ARE NOT DOWN-REGULATED BY GLUCOCORTICOIDS IN RABBITS. R.B.Xu, J.Wang, J.X.Tan. Dept. of Pathophysiology, Second Military Med. Univ. Shanghai, P.R.China, 200433.

In our previous work, it has been reported that the glucocorticoid receptor(GR) and GRmRNAof brain was not altered when the plasma level of glucocorticoids(GC) was maintained at stress concentration, whereas the GR and GRmRNAin peripheral organs, such as liver, spleen etc. was decreased markedly in rats (J Steroid Biochem 1989; 32:99-104; Academic J Second Military Univ1990; 11:393-397). In the present work, 5mg/kg b.w. of dexamethasone phosphate was pulse injected intravenously in the rabbits, and decapitataed 4 hours latter, GR was determined by Scatchard analysis in lung and one point analysis in brain cytosol, using [3H]dexamethasone(Dex) as the ligand. The specific bindings in the control and Dex injected group (n=6 for each group) were 46.4+10.5 and 25.5+5.2fmol/mgprotein for lung cytosol(p<0.001), 51.3+7.8 and 50.6+6.9 fmol/mgprotein for brain cytosol. These results further indicated that GC down-regulate GR in various peripheral organs but not the GR in the brain in both rabbits and rats.

P1.21

CLINICAL SURVEY AND KALIG-1 MUTATION SCREENING IN PATIENTS WITH KALLMANN SYNDROM.

B. Heye, K. Kellner, J. Schopohl[1*], M. Laska[2], J. Stemmler[1], B. Incerti[3] A. Ballabio[3], T. Meitinger Abteilung Pädiatrische Genetik, Kinderpoliklinik, [1]Medizinische Klinik, [2]Institut f. Med. Psychologie, Klinikum Innenstadt, LMU-München, [3]Baylor College of Medicine, Houston

Hypogonadotropic hypogonadism with anosmia (Kallmann Syndrome) is clinically and genetically heterogenous. Clinical investigation in 20 KS patients and 15 patients with idiopathic hypogonadotropic hypogonadism (IHH) included standard endocrinological methods, ultrasound of the abdomen, the modified Munich smell test (MOD), magnetic resonance imaging (MRI) and neurological examination. Complete anosmia was found in all patients with KS, while MRI findings demonstrated either aplasia or hypoplasia of the olfactory bulbs. In 8 of 15 IHH patients, the smell test was within the lower range of normal distribution, the MRI showed normal olfactory bulbs with two exceptions. Renal agenesis and mirror movements were found to be restricted to X-linked KS.

To obtain information about the mutation pattern of the KALIG-1 gene which is known to be mutated in X-linked forms of KS, a mutation screening was performed in 51 unrelated KS patients. Within 5 familial (X-linked) cases, a 2bp deletion in exon 9 and two stop mutations were detected. No mutations were found among sporadic cases by SSCP (single strand conformation polymorphism) analysis of all 14 exons. These results indicate that mutations in KALIG-1 are rare among sporadic cases and that the majority of sporadic cases with these conditions are probably autosomal.

P1.22

GLUCOSE INHIBITS THE GH RESPONSE TO GHRH OR ARGININE IN NORMAL SUBJECTS BUT NOT IN OBESE PATIENTS.

M. Procopio, S. Grottoli, M. Maccario, S.E. Oleandri, G.M. Boffano, F. Camanni, E. Ghigo. Department of Clinical Pathophysiology, Div. of Endocrinology,University of Turin, C.so Dogliotti 14, 10126, Torino, Italy.*

Glucose has an inhibitory effect on GH secretion in normal man, reducing the somatotrope responsiveness to many stimuli. Many data suggest that this inhibitory effect of glucose is likely mediated by increase of hypothalamic somatostatin release. It is well known that GH secretion is reduced in obesity, though its pathogenesis is still unclear. Interestingly, it has been recently reported that the low GH secretion in obese subjects is resistant to the inhibitory effect of somatostatin. To study the sensitivity of somatotrope cells to inhibitory influences in obesity, in 14 obese patients (OB, 24-41aa, BMI, mean ± SEM, 37.2 ± 1.8 kg/m^2) and in 14 normal subjects (NS, 26-33 aa, BMI 21.2 ± 1.5 kg/m^2), we studied the effect of oral glucose load (100 g) on the GH response to GHRH (1 mcg/kg iv) or arginine (ARG, 0.5 g/kg iv), which likely acts via inhibition of hypothalamic somatostatin release. Basal GH levels were lower in OB than in NS (0.3 ± 0.1 vs 2.5 ± 0.7 µg/L, $p<0.001$) while IGF-I levels were similar in both groups (155.8 ± 19.6 vs 145.3 ± 8.2 µg/L).The somatotrope responsiveness to GHRH or ARG was clearly lower in OB than in NS (172.4 ± 33.6 vs 479.5 ± 83.9 µg/L/h, $p<0.005$ and 155.1 ± 39.7 vs 625.1 ± 139.1 µg/L/h, $p< 0.02$, respectively). Noteworthy, the GH response to GHRH was clearly reduced by glucose in NS (260.8 ± 38.3 vs 479.5 ± 83.9 µg/L/h, $p<0.03$) but not in OB (193.7 ± 39.4 vs 172.4 ± 33.6 µg/L/h). Similarly, glucose blunted the GH response to ARG in NS (294.8 ± 46.3 vs 625.1 ± 139.1 µg/L/h,$p<0.05$) but not in OB (121.1 ± 43.4 vs 155.1 ± 39.7 µg/L/h). In conclusion, our results show that in obesity, not only somatotrope cells are less responsive to GHRH as well as to stimuli acting through the CNS, but even less sensitive to the inhibitory influence of glucose. The results agree with animal data suggesting that the inhibitory influences on GH secretion are operative only when the somatotrope secretory function is normal.

This study was partially supported by a grant of MURST.

P1.23

INHIBITION OF LIPOLYSIS BY ACIPIMOX IMPROVES THE SOMATOTROPE RESPONSIVENESS IN OBESITY.

S. Grottoli, M. Maccario, M. Procopio, GM Boffano, S.E. Oleandri, F. Camanni, E. Ghigo.

Department of Clinical Pathophysiology, Div. of Endocrinology, C.so Dogliotti 14, University of Turin, 10126, Turin, Italy.

Increased free fatty acid (FFA) levels could play a role in the pathogenesis of GH hyposecretory state of obesity. To address this point we studied the effect of acute (500 mg po) and prolonged (750 mg/day for 4 days) administration of an anti-lipolytic drug, acipimox (ACX), on the GH response to GHRH (1µg/kg iv), alone or combined with arginine (ARG, 0.5 g/Kg iv), in 13 obese females (18-57 yr, BMI: 37.5 ± 1.7 kg/m^2). GH responses to GHRH alone or combined with ARG were lower than in22 age-macthed controls (AUC: 207.0 ± 96.3 vs 1242.5 ± 194.5 and 605.9 ± 217.5 vs 3362.6 ± 386.0 µg/L/h, $p<0.01$). ACX deeply reduced baseline FFA levels. Acute ACX enhanced the GH response to GHRH (531.8 ± 184.9 vs 235.8 ± 91.1, $p<0.01$) without affecting that to GHRH+ARG (673.7 ± 168.7 vs 547.4 ± 147.6). Prolonged ACX furtherly enhanced GH response to GHRH (1156.0 ± 483.6) and increased the response to GHRH+ARG (1581.3 ± 380.8 vs 680.0 ± 228.8, $p<0.05$). These results show that the reduction of FFA levels clearly increases the reduced somatotrope response to GHRH in obesity. After prolonged treatment the effect of ACX is more marked and additive with that of arginine. Thus, elevated FFA levels play an important role in causing GH hyposecretion in obesity.

This study was partially supported by a grant of M.U.R.S.T.

P1.24

POSTOPERATIVE EVALUATION OF GROWTH HORMONE RESERVE IN PATIENTS WITH CRANIOPHARYNGIOMAS

L. De Marinis*, C.Fiumara, A.Mancini, C.Anile° and G. Maira^
Institutes of Endocrinology and °Neurosurgery, Catholic University, Rome, and ^Neurosurgery,University of Perugia

The functional evaluation of pituitary-thyroid and pituitary-adrenal axis and of post-pituitary reserve are usually considered in pre- and post-operative management of craniopharyngioma patients, in the view of a replacement therapy after surgery. Recent reports,however, have underlined the meaning of GH in adult subjects and its role in processes other than growth.

We have therefore tested the GH response to GHRH in 10 subjects, 3 males and 7 females, aged 14-43 ys, who underwent neurosurgical intervention for craniopharyngioma (8 transcranial and 2 transphenoidal surgery). The tests (GHRH 1-29, 50 µg i.v.) were performed 10-96 months after the intervention.

In 9 of 10 patients the GH response was abolished or blunted (basal 0.58±0.22 ng/ml, peak 2.66±0.87 ng/ml); only one patient had a peak response greater than 10 ng/ml (28 ng/ml). Mean IGF-I levels were 173±56.9 ng/ml. This suggests that a relevant number of these patients can develop a GH deficiency after surgery. These results underline the importance of a pre- and post-operative evaluation of GH secretion and reserve even in adult patients undergoing neurosurgical intervention on the hypothalamus-pituitary system.

P1.25

THE GHRH-PYRIDOSTIGMINE TEST (GHRH-PYT) IN NORMAL SUBJECTS AND PATIENTS WITH PITUITARY LESIONS: CORRELATION WITH THE INSULIN TOLERANCE TEST (ITT). M. Andersen, J. Hangaard, T.B. Hansen, J. Bertelsen, C. Hagen. Departments of Endocrinology and Clinical Chemistry, Odense University Hospital, Denmark.

The importance of GH in adults, emphasizing the need for a safe, reliable and simple test for GH-deficiency. We have established the normal range for max GH concentration after the administration of pyridostigmine 120 mg orally followed at 60 min by the injection of GHRH 1 μg/kg i.v.. Bloodsamples at 0, 20, 30, 60 and 90 min. GH was measured by a RIA assay (Pharmacia). 40 normal subjects, 8 men ≤ 40 yrs, 8 men > 40 yrs, 8 premenopausal women (PW), 8 PW using oral contraceptives and 8 post-menopausal women were included. Men ≤ 40 yrs had higher ($p < 0,05$) GH response than PW. In 7 normal subjects the optimum dose of pyridostigmine was determined using 0, 10, 60 and 120 mg doses. The optimum dose was found to be 120 mg. The mean GH response for normal subjects was 139 mU/l (± 63 mU/l SD, range 46-318).
In 39 adult patients, 17 women and 22 men with a mean age of 44 yrs (range 19-61) with pituitary lesions 2 tests (GHRH-PYT and a standard ITT) were performed at least 48 hours apart. 36/39 of the patients had an abnormal GH response during the GHRH-PYT and 3 patients had a normal response. There was a significant correlation between the GH responses during GHRH-PYT and ITT ($r = 0.82$, $p < 0,01$). 36/39 patients had similar responses during GHRH-PYT and ITT. 3 patients had normal GH responses during ITT, but an abnormal response during GHRH-PYT. During more than 150 GHRH-PYT no severe side effects have been observed.
These data demonstrate that the GHRH-PYT is safe with only few side effects and correlate to a high degree with results obtained during ITT.

P1.26

GROWTH HORMONE (GH) RESPONSE AFTER DEXAMETHASONE STIMULATION IN HYPERTHYROID PATIENTS: EFFECT OF LONG TERM ANTITHYROID DRUGS. A.Kendereški*, D.Micić, M.Šumarac, S.Zorić, Dj.Macut, D.Manojlović, C.Dieguez#, F.Casanueva#. Institute for Endocrinology, 11000 Belgrade, Yugoslavia and # Endocrine Section, Department of Medicine, Faculty of Medicine, Santiago de Compostela, Spain

Thyroid hormones may alter neuroregulation of GH secretion. Acute administration of corticosteroids increases GH secretion. The aim of our study was to investigate GH response to Dexamethasone (DEX) in hyperthyroidism before and after thiamazole therapy. Thirteen hyperthyroid patients (43.53+/-3.72 yrs; BMI: 22.88+/-0.62 kg/m2) were studied before (T4: 287.0+/-20.8 nmol/l) and after (T4: 124.93+/-11.66) long term therapy (thiamazole 20-40 mg/d for 12+/-0.9 months) and compared with age and sex matched control group. GH (RIA Delphia, mU/l) was measured after DEX (4 mg i.v.) and GHRH (1 mcg/kg i.v.), in a separate study, before and after antithyroid therapy. There was no significant difference in GH response between controls and hyperthyroid patients after DEX (basal: 1.48+/-0.45 vs. 2.15+/-0.66; peak: 11.16+/-2.72 vs.7.84+/1.78; AUC: 1604.74+/-284.55 vs. 1384.79+/-211.89 mU/l/min) as well as after GHRH (basal: 2.01+/-0.72 vs 3.70+/-0.98; peak: 22.54+/-7.67 vs 13.35+/-2.19; AUC: 1695.53+/-537.95 vs 1555.31+/-214.48). Before and after therapy GH response to DEX (basal: 0.91+/-0.29; peak: 6.36+/-1.79; AUC: 1008.2+/-175.94) and to GHRH (basal: 3.78+/-2.42; peak: 20.21+/-11.46; AUC: 1021.8+/-349.57) were not significantly different. In conclusion, neither hyperthyroidism nor long term thiamazole therapy did not impair GH response to DEX stimulation in middle aged subjects.

P1.27

EFFECT OF GROWTH HORMONE REPLACEMENT THERAPY ON MAXIMAL OXYGEN UPTAKE AND CARDIAC STRUCTURE
R. Nass*, R.M. Huber, V. Klauss, O.A. Müller and C.J. Strasburger.
Medizinische Klinik, Klinikum Innenstadt (LMU), München, Germany
Only limited data exist concerning the effect of human growth hormone (hGH) replacement on physical work capacity and cardiac structure and function in patients with hGH deficiency of adult onset. A 6 months double blind placebo controlled trial was started with twenty patients aged 28 to 60 years, all showing a peak hGH response of less than 2 ng/ ml to insulin induced hypoglycaemia or to an arginine stimulation test and IGF 1 levels below the normal range. The growth hormone dose of 12.5 µg per kilogram body weight was self administered daily subcutaneously. In the verum group the V02 max data expressed per kg body weight (ml/ min/ kg bw) showed an increase from 23.2±2.4 to 30.0±2.3 ($p<0.01$) in the verum group, whereas the V02 max data expressed per lean body mass (ml/ min/ kg lean body mass) did not change significantly in either group. The maximal ventilation (l/min ± SE) increased in the rhGH group from 53.4 ± 6.3 to 59.4 ± 6.0 ($p < 0.05$) whereas in the placebo group no significant changes could be observed. The maximal power output (Watts ± SE) increased significantly ($p<0.01$) from 192.5 ± 13.5 to 227.5 ± 11.5 in the verum group but remained constant in the placebo group. Maximal systolic blood pressure, diastolic blood pressure as well as heartfrequency did not change significantly after six months growth hormone treatment. Cardiac structure (left ventricular posterior wall, interventricular septum thickness, left ventricular mass, left ventricular end systolic dimension, left ventricular end-diastolic dimension) as well as cardiac function did not change significantly after six months treatment in either group; only left ventricular mass showed a slight but not significant increase after six months treatment. We conclude that hGH replacement in hGH-deficient adults improves oxygen uptake and exercise capacity. These improvements in pulmonary parameters might be due to an increase in respiratory muscle strength and partly due to the changes in muscle volume per se observed under hGH replacement therapy. Furthermore hGH treatment shows no significant effects on cardiac function and structure.

P1.28

REDUCED GROWTH HORMONE RELEASE IN PARKINSON'S DISEASE
Strollo F., Fabbrini G.*, Cella S.°, Di Piero V.*, Bollanti L., Strollo G., Morè M., Ciarmatori A. and Riondino G. INRCA., Endocrine Unit, Rome; * 5th Neurology Clinic, Rome University; ° Dpt of Medical Pharmacology , Milan University, Italy.

Dopamine (DA) stimulates GH secretion in humans; pituitary GH content at least partly results from DA-dependent endogenous GHRH release (other mechanisms involving ACh-modulated SRIF release coming also into play). TRH is known to increase DA turnover within the CNS in the animal; a slight GH-stimulating effect of TRH was described in normal subjects, possibly due to TRH-induced hypothalamic DA turnover increase occurring n the human too. The aim of our study was to verify the hypothesis of a DA-enhancing role of TRH in the elderly by comparing GH response to GHRH and to TRH in normal aged subjects and in Parkinson's disease patients (PDP), that may be viewed as spontaneous experimental models of impaired central DA tonic release.
8 newly diagnosed PDP 57 to 78 yrs of age and 16 age-matched healthy subjects (HS) underwent GHRH test for GH (1 μg/Kg i.v.) and TRH test for TSH and GH (200 μg i.v.) in the morning after overnight fast. 6 age-matched healthy subjects were used as controls (CS) for spontaneously occurring GH fluctuations, by injecting saline instead. GH and TSH were measured by highly sensitive IRMA methods at 30', 0', 30', 60' 90' and 120' during the tests.
Saline: no significant TSH or GH changes were found in CS. TRH: TSH response to TRH was normal and baseline GH was comparable in both HS and PDP, but GH peak and cumulated concentrations were higher in HS than in PDP or CS ($p<0.02$).GHRH: GH response was blunted in PDP as compared to HS, both in terms of peak and cumulated concentrations ($p<0.05$).Our results seem to indicate that (1) the chronically occurring impairment of DA tonic relase within the CNS in PDP is associated with a lower GH responsivity to both GHRH and TRH as compared to normal subjects and that (2) TRH-induced GH secretion might depend on functional integrity of DA containing nerve endings. Our results are therefore in agreement with findings concerning the pro-dopaminergic properties of TRH in animals.

P1.29

GH AND CATECHOLAMINE RESPONSES TO CLONIDINE IN PATIENTS WITH HYPOGONADISM BEFORE AND DURING THERAPY G. Del Rio, *A. Velardo, G. Zizzo, M. Procopio, F. Coletta, C. Carani., E. Ghigo. Cattedra di Endocrinologia, Università di Modena, 41100 Modena, Cattedra di Endocrinologia, Università di Torino, 10126 Torino, Italia.

Clonidine did not induce cardiovascular and GH responses in castrated rats and a normal pattern of response is restored after testosterone therapy. We studied the cardiovascular, catecholamine and GH responses to clonidine administration (300 µg per os) in 8 males with hypogonadism (HS) (age 32±5 years) before and after 3 months of testosterone treatment (250 mg im every 21 days) and in 8 control subjects (CS). Plasma Norepinephrine (NE), Epinephrine (E) and GH were determined toghether with systolic (SBP), diastolic blood pressure (DBP) and pulse rate (PR) for three hours. Basal plasma NE levels were lower in HS patients before therapy than in CS (125±31 vs 196±44 pg/ml, respectively; $P<0.05$). We observed an incresease in plasma NE levels of HS after testosterone treatment (185±33 pg/ml; $P<0.05$ vs before). The basal levels of GH, E, SBP, DBP and PR were not different between HS before and after therapy and CS. The peak of GH after clonidine was similar in HS both before and after therapy (8.1±2.6 vs 7.8±2.8 ng/ml respectively; P=NS). The decrease in plasma NE during clonidine was significant (ANOVA F=13; $P<0.005$) and similar both before and after therapy (46 ±9% vs 50±10% respectively; P=NS) and comparable to that of CS (42±8%). Clonidine administration induced a decrease in SBP values (F=12, $P<0.001$) that was similar in HS both before and after therapy and in CS (F=0.2, P=NS). Clonidine affected DBP values (F=10, $P<0.001$) both before and after therapy but did not affect PR both before and after therapy (F=1, P=NS). These data show for the first time in humans that in conditions of low testosterone secretion a decreased sympathoadrenergic tone is present but this phenomenon is not linked to modifications in the α2-mediated GH, cardiovascular and catecholamine responses.

P1.30

CYCLOSPORIN A AND FK506 ARE POTENT ACTIVATORS OF ANTERIOR PITUITARY POMC

K.E.Sheppard
Baker Medical Research Institute, Prahran, Vic. Australia

Recent studies have shown that the immunosuppressant drug cyclosporin A (CsA) can inhibit in vivo ACTH release, and have suggested that the drugs action is mediated via inhibition of cytokine activation of the HPA axis. To determine if CsA has a direct effect on POMC expression and peptide secretion we have compared the corticotrope tumour cell line (AtT20) with rat anterior pituitary (AP) cultures. In addition we also assessed the role of the immunosuppressant FK506. Both CsA and FK506 induced a dose-dependent increase in ß-endorphin (ß-EP) secretion from AtT20 cells and primary AP cultures. Acute (60min) treatment with 10µM FK506 or 1µM CsA induced a maximal 5 fold increase in ß-EP secretion and a 2 fold increase in POMC heteronuclear RNA (hnRNA). In addition to stimulating basal ß-EP secretion, FK506 enhanced CRF, PMA and Bay K induced secretion. Although both immunosuppressant drugs bind proteins that can associate with the glucocorticoid receptor (GR), neither CsA or FK506 had an effect on GR binding, nuclear translocation, or function (as measured by the ability of dexamethasone (DEX) to suppress CRF-stimulated ß-EP release). In preliminary experiments DEX pre-treatment was able to diminish the FK506 induced increase in both POMC hnRNA levels and peptide secretion suggesting that the mechanism of action is partly inhibited by glucocorticoids. These studies suggest that both CsA and FK506 can act directly on the corticotrope cell to stimulate both POMC gene expression and ACTH secretion, but have no effect on the ability of glucocorticoids to bind GR and repress this stimulation invitro.

We would like to thank Fujisawa for kindly supplying FK506.

P1.31

TRH STIMULATES GONADOTROPIN RELEASE IN PATIENTS WITH ACROMEGALY S.Damjanović*, V.Popović, M.Petakov, M.Đurović, Institute of Endocrinology, Belgrade University Medical School, 11000 Belgrade, Serbia

TRH is known to induce paradoxical responses of pituitary hormones in some patients with pituitary tumours. We studied TRH induced response of gonadotropin and free α-subunit(SU) in 29 patients with acromegaly(**A**), mean age 44.7 yr. Hypopituitarism(**HP**) was present in 5 patients and 10 had hypergonadotropism(**HG**). Levels of FSH, LH and α-SU were analyzed in randomized study after placebo (0.9% saline s.c.) and TRH (200 µg iv) administration on separate days. During the placebo samples were taken hourly for 24 h. In TRH test samples were taken 20 and 60 min after TRH administration. FSH and LH concentrations were determined by IRMA (MAIA clone, Serono S.p.A.) and free α-SU level by commercial RIA (Biomerica, Inc., N. Beach, USA). Cross-reaction with intact hFSH, hLH, hTSH and hCG is less than 0.2%. MANOVA with repeated measures was used for data evaluation. During 24 h there was no significant changes in LH (F=0.6; p=0.9) and α-SU (F=0.5; p=0.9) concentrations. Changes in FSH concentration (F=2.5; $p<0.001$) were detected between 14 00 h and 19 00 h. TRH induced significant FSH and LH rise, basal vs 20 min. (9.0 ± 0.2 vs 11.0 ± 0.2 mIU/ml; F=4.5, p= 0.044) and (3.3 ± 0.2 vs 5.0 ± 0.3 mIU/ml; F=10.9, p=0.003) respectively. The same pattern of response is found in patients with **HG** and **HP**. In comparison with others, they had significantly higher/lower gonadotropin levels. α-SU rose from basal (0.3 ± 0.2 mIU/ml) to (0.6 ± 0.2 mIU/ml; F=9.7, p=0.004) at 20 and to (0.5 ± 0.2 mIU/ml; F=8.1, p=0.008) at 60 min of TRH test. The pattern of response and the le-vel of α-SU is unaffected by **HP**. The higher levels of α-SU are in patients with HG (F=8.8; p=0.006) but the same type of response as well as in other patients is found. Paradoxical gonadotropin response to TRH in **A** could be associated with plurihormonal pituitary tumours and tumorous origin of TRH induced gonadotropin release. Does the elevated level of α-SU *per se* marks plurihormonal tumour should be elucidated.

P1.32

SERUM CONCENTRATIONS OF PRL, TSH AND LH IN IDDM PATIENTS: EFFECT OF DOPAMINE (DA) INFUSION.

E. Grodum, J. Hangaard, L. Christensen, E. Haug, C. Hagen, Department of Endocrinology, Odense University Hospital, Odense, Denmark, and The Hormone Laboratory, Aker Hospital, Oslo, Norway.

Earlier studies point toward increased dopaminergic activity/sensitivity in women with IDDM which to some extent may explain the raised incidense of menstrual irregularities among these patients. The purpose of this study was to examine whether the influence on pituitary hormone secretion in female IDDM patients of a small dose of DA (0.4 µg/kg/min) differs from controls. And if so, whether this abnormal effect is exerted at the hypothalamic and/or the pituitary level. Eight women with IDDM (age 22 - 45 yrs) and 8 normal women (age 22 - 32 yrs) were studied in the early follicular fase. The duration of diabetes was 18.5 yrs (5 - 37). None of the subjects had other diseases or recieved medication influencing the hormones measured. Blood samples were obtained every 10 min. from 7.30 am. until 5.30 pm. on two occations during 9½ hrs infusions of either DA or placebo. In this study we have evaluated the serum levels of PRL, TSH and LH during the last 2½ hrs. In the control group DA infusion did not change the LH level, but TSH and PRL decreased significantly. In diabetics LH levels decreased with 31 % compared to controls 11 %; $p < 0.05$. The decrease in TSH level was in the diabetics 44 % and in the controls 29 %; $p < 0.05$. The PRL level in diabetics decreased with 68 % compared to 59 % in controls; $p > 0.05$. Dopamine exerts its effect on LH on the hypothalamic level, on TSH on both the hypothalamic and the pituitary level and on PRL only on the pituitary level. These results suggest that diabetics are more sensitive to a small increase in DA concentration at the hypothalamic level and probably not at the pituitary level. Patients with IDDM may have a defect blood-brain barrier.

P1.33

EFFECTS OF HEXARELIN (EP 23905-MF 6003) ON CIRCULATING PRL LEVELS IN NORMAL SUBJECTS AND IN ACROMEGALIC PATIENTS.
E. Palmieri, G. Casati, L. Guglielmino, O. Biella, G. Gambino, M. Arosio G.Faglia.
Institute of Endocrine Sciences, University of Milano, Ospedale Maggiore IRCCS, Milano, Italy.

His-D-2-Methyl-Trp-Ala-Trp-D-Phe-Lys-NH2 (Hexarelin) is a new synthetic GH-releasing peptide (GHRP) analogue able to stimulate GH secretion in man. While GHRP has been demonstrated to significantly increase serum PRL levels in normal subjects, but to reduce TRH-stimulated PRL increase, there are no data on the effects of hexarelin on PRL secretion. Therefore, we studied the effects of the administration of 1 µg/Kg hexarelin by iv bolus on PRL release in 6 normal subjects (5 women and 1 man aged 26-29 yr) and in 7 normoprolactinemic acromegalic patients (5 women and 2 men aged 30-65 yr, 4 untreated and 3 previously unsuccessfully operated on), characterized by high IGF-I, (129.8±45.3 nmol/L mean ± SD) and GH 11.1±10.7 µg/L) levels. In addition, the effect of the administration of hexarelin on TRH-stimulated PRL secretion was evaluated in 5 normal subjects. In healthy individuals hexarelin did not significantly modify serum PRL levels (from 6.7±2 to 9.5±3.0 µg/L, *p*:NS). On the contrary a significant PRL increase was seen in all acromegalic patients (from 8.7± 6 to 13.5±6 µg/L, *p*<0.01). The peak of serum PRL was observed 15 min after the drug injection, and was contemporary to GH peak. In normal subjects the associated administration of hexarelin and TRH elicited a PRL percent increase significantly greater than that observed after TRH alone (709±432% vs 436±290%, p< 0,05). In conclusion, these preliminary data suggest that the effects of hexarelin on PRL secretion are different from those previously described for GHRP. The present data show that in normal subjects hexarelin does not cause a significant serum PRL increase but it is able to potentiate the TRH-induced PRL secretion. Moreover, hexarelin is able to provoke PRL release in acromegalic patients. The mechanism of action of this drug on PRL release remains to be clarified.

P1.34

GROWTH HORMONE SECRETORY RESPONSE TO HEXARELIN (His-2-Me-D-Trp-Ala-Trp-D-Phe-Lys-NH2) IN THALASSEMIC PATIENTS AND CONTROLS. V.Markussis[1], A.Botsis[2], S.Alexopoulos[2], G.Mortzos[2], *H.Moschoyannis[1], V.Lenaerts[3], R.Deghenghi[3], G.Tolis[1].
[1]Hippokration Hospital, [2]401 General Army Hospital, Athens, Greece and [3]Europeptides, Argenteuil, France.

Growth hormone (GH) secretion in Thalassemia Major (TM) has been described as an example of "neuroregulatory dysfunction". This study compared the GH secretory response to the novel secretagogue Hexarelin in patients with TM and normal controls. Nine (5 males) patients were studied, aged 22 (14-29) yrs. Five were below the 3rd centile for height and two had delayed bone age and Tanner stage. Ten normal controls, aged 21.6 (20-26), were also studied. All subjects received 1 mcg/kg (IV) Hexarelin (Europeptides) and GH was measured at time 0, 30, 60, 120 min. Fasting GH values were lower in the thalassemic group (x±SEM)(1.2±0.39 vs 7.7±2.2 ng/ml, p<0.01), as were IGF-1 (165.0±44.2 vs 272.7±20.2 ng/ml, p<0.05) and IGFBP-3 (2.30±0.27 vs 4.71±0.24 mcg/ml, p0.001) levels. In response to Hexarelin, significant increases in GH levels were observed in both groups. Peak levels were observed 30 min after the administration of the peptide. There was no difference between patients and controls in GHmax (35.7±5.8 vs 38.8±4.3 ng/ml), D-GH (34.5±5.6 vs 31.0±3.2 ng/ml) or GH-area under the curve (67.2±11.7 vs 73.0±11.2 ng/ml.h) after Hexarelin. The GH releasing potential was independent of sex and IGF-1/IGFBP-3, ferritin levels. Patients with TM exhibit lower GH/IGF-1 and IGFBP-3 levels compared to healthy subjects, which is suggestive of a downstream defective somatotropic function. The prompt response of GH producing cells to Hexarelin, with maximum levels indistinguishable from that of controls, suggests a potential therapeutic indication for this potent secretagogue.

P1.35

NEUROENDOCRINOLOGICAL AND METABOLIC MODULATION OF THE GROWTH HORMONE-RELEASING ACTIVITY OF HEXARELIN IN MAN. L. Gianotti, E. Arvat, M. Maccario, M. Procopio, S. Grottoli, B.P. Imbimbo, V. Lenaerts, R. Deghenghi, F. Camanni, E. Ghigo, Div. of Endocrinology, Dept. of Clin. Pathophysiol., Univ. of Turin, Italy; Med. Dept., Mediolanum Farmaceutici, Milan, Italy; Europeptides, Argenteuil, France.

Hexarelin (HEX) is a synthetic GH-releasing hexapeptide (His-D-2-methyl-Trp-Ala-Trp-D-Phe-Lys-NH2) whose mechanism of action has never been studied in man. We investigated the neuromodulation of the GH-releasing activity of HEX in 18 normal males (24-31 yrs). In these subjects we studied the interaction of HEX (2 µg/kg i.v.) with GHRH (2 µg/kg i.v.), somatostatin (2 µg/kg/h i.v.), pirenzepine (0.6 mg/kg i.v.), pyridostigmine (120 mg p.o.) arginine (0.5 g/kg i.v.), glucose (100g p.o.) or lipid-heparin infusion (250 mL of a 10% lipid solution + 2,500 U heparin), factors known to influence GH secretion. In study I, the GH response to HEX was higher than that to GHRH (AUC: 4693±691 vs 1494±102 µg/min/L, P<0.01) and their coadministration potentiated GH release (7395±450 µg/min/L, P<0.05). Somatostatin abolished the GH response to GHRH (363±89 µg/min/L, P<0.01), while it only blunted that to HEX (1314±297 µg/min/L, P<0.05). In study II, pyrenzepine only blunted the GH response to HEX (1931±446 vs 4586±674 µg/min/L, P<0.05) while pyridostigmine and arginine did not modify it (5169±771 and 4743±774 µg/min/L). In study III, both glucose and lipid-heparin infusion only blunted the HEX-induced GH release (2237±564 and 2141±253 vs 4586±674 µg/min/L, p<0.05) while they strongly inhibited the GHRH-induced GH rise (391±61 and 237±31 vs 1305±65 µg/min/L, p<0.01). In conclusion, the GH-releasing activity of HEX is greater than that of GHRH and they act synergistically. Differently from GHRH, the effect of HEX is only blunted by somatostatin, pirenzepine, glucose and free fatty acids and is not potentiated by pyridostigmine or arginine. In man, HEX and GHRH have a different mechanism of action and the potent GH-releasing activity of HEX is partially refractory to inhibitory modulation by somatostatin and metabolic inputs.
This study was supported by a grant from Europeptides, France, and Mediolanum Farmaceutici, Italy.

P1.36

EFFECTS OF HEXARELIN, A SYNTHETIC HEXAPEPTIDE, ALONE AND COMBINED WITH GHRH OR ARGININE ON GH SECRETION IN NORMAL ELDERLY SUBJECTS. E. Arvat, L. Gianotti, S. Grottoli, B.P. Imbimbo, V. Lenaerts, R. Deghenghi, F. Camanni, E. Ghigo. Div. of Endocrinology, Dept. of Clin. Pathophysiol., Univ. of Turin, Italy; Medical Dept., Mediolanum Farmaceutici, Milan, Italy; Europeptides, Argenteuil, France.

Growth hormone (GH) secretion undergoes an age-related decrease though the secretory pool of somatotrope cells is preserved in human ageing. We verified the age-related effect of the maximally effective dose of hexarelin (HEX, 2 µg/kg i.v.), a synthetic hexapeptide, alone or with GHRH (2 µg/kg i.v.) or arginine (ARG,0.5 g/kg i.v.), which likely inhibits hypothalamic somatostatin. We studied 13 young males (Y, 24-30 yrs) and 16 normal elderly males (E, 65-84 yrs). Basal IGF-I levels in E were lower than those in Y (114.5±18.7 vs 211.5±19.1 µg/L, p<0.001). In study I (Y=7, E=8), HEX induced GH rise higher in Y than in E (AUC: 2424.3±300.7 vs 1046.6±337.4 µg/L/h, p<0.001). GHRH elicited a GH response lower than that induced by HEX both in Y (759.7±46.6 µg/L/h, p<0.02) and in E (281.3±43.3 µg/L/h, p<0.02). GHRH potentiated the somatotrope responsiveness to HEX both in Y (4009.4± 331.6µg/L/h, p<0.02) and in E (1872.7±294.8 µg/L/h, p<0.04). The GH response to HEX+GHRH was lower in E than in Y (p< 0.001). In study II (Y=6, E=8), HEX induced a GH response higher in Y than in E (2409.6±334.0 vs 824.6±229.7 µg/L/h, p<0.001). ARG did not increase the GH response to HEX in Y (2371.7±387.2 µg/L/h) while potentiated it in E (2069.3±528.5 µg/L/h, p<0.001). The GH response to HEX+ARG was lower than that to HEX+GHRH in Y (p<0.03) but not in E. Our data show that: a) the effect of HEX on GH secretion is age-dependent but even in elderly subjects it releases more GH than GHRH; b) the activity of HEX is potentiated by GHRH to a lesser extent in elderly while it is enhanced by arginine only in ageing. Thus, HEX unlikely acts modulating GHRH and/or somatostatin release. A somatostatinergic hyperactivity, absolute or relative to GHRH hypoactivity, is likely present in ageing.
This study was supported by CNR, Europeptides and Mediolanum Farmaceutici.

P1.37

DESMOPRESSIN (DDAVP) DOES NOT MODULATE ACTH AND CORTISOL RESPONSE TO OVINE CORTICOTROPHIN RELEASING HORMONE (CRH) IN ANOREXIA NERVOSA (AN) PATIENTS.

L.Foppiani, M.Giusti, P.Sessarego, S.Valenti and G.Giordano. DISEM Cattedra di Endocrinologia, University of Genova, I 16132 Genoa, Italy.

Recently, Malerbi et al.(1993) have demonstrated that iv DDAVP administration can stimulate ACTH and cortisol release in patients with Cushing's disease but not in normal subjects. In this study we evaluated the effect of DDAVP (10 μg iv), CRF(1μg/kg/bw iv) and DDAVP+CRH in AN. Seven AN women (age range: 18-37 years; BMI: 13-21 kg/m^2) and 7 normal cycling women age matched were studied. ACTH (34±6 pg/ml) and cortisol (197±14 ng/ml) peaks after CRH were significantly lower in AN than those found in controls (96±22 pg/ml; 329±60 ng/ml). Neither in AN patients nor in controls DDAVP was able to modify ACTH-cortisol circadian decline. DDAVP priming did not change ACTH response to CRH (the peak was 37±5 pg/ml in AN and 92±17 pg/ml in controls). After DDAVP+CRH cortisol pattern was unchanged (peak: 194±14 ng/ml) in AN and slightly reduced (270±32 ng/ml) in controls.

Our data are in agreement with literature's ones (Brambilla et al 1993), showing that the ACTH-cortisol response to CRF is blunted in AN. Moreover, we confirm that V2-receptors are slightly involved in the ACTH-cortisol regulation in normal subjects and indicate that AVP receptors are probably normal at the pituitary level in AN and without any influence on the alterations in the hypothalamic-pituitary-adrenal function known to be present in AN.

P1.38

PULSATILITY OF FSH AND LH IN CUSHING'S DISEASE

M.Drezgić*, Z.Penezić, S.Vujović, M.Stojanović, J.Bjekić, V. Rajković. Institute of Endocrinology, KCS, Belgrade, Yugoslavia

The basal levels of LH and FSH as well as their responses to GnRH stimulation in Cushing's disease are normal. Reduced LH pulse frequency and amplitude may result from inhibiting action of CRH on GnRH pulse generator. A combined event of central CRH and serotonergic overactivity and peripheral acyclic estrogen feedbeck may be operative, accounting for the development of chronic anovulation. In order to assess the influence of chronic glucocorticoid excess on FSH and LH pulsatile secretion we have evaluated 6 females with clinical and biochemically proven pituitary dependent Cushing's disease, subsequently confirmed by histology. The average age (aa) of patients was 41+/-11.1y, BMI 36.0+/-1.9kg/m^2, with irregular menstrual cycles. In the control group there were 10 females, aa of 28.3+/-4.4y, BMI 21.8+/-1.2kg/m^2, with regular menstrual cycles. Blood sampling was performed every 10 min from 2pm to 8pm during the luteal phase. Serum concentrations of FSH and LH were determined by RIA (INEP). Statistic analysis were done by Pulsar peak identification algorithm. Comperison of resoults by Student T test have shown statistically significant diference ($p<0.05$) in number and amplitude of LH pulses. All other diferences are statistically insignificant ($p>0.05$).

	pulse No	frequency	amplitude	inter-p.
FSH	1.0+/-0	0.0028	0.66+/-0.33	0+/-0
contr.	1.2+/-0.4	0.0033	9.0+/-18.0	52+/-116
LH	1.6+/-1.1	0.0055	2.8+/-1.5	93+/-100
contr.	2.9+/-0.3	0.008	0.9+/-0.12	152+/-12

P1.39

HYPERACTIVITY OF THE HYPOTHALAMIC-PITUITARY-ADRENAL (HPA) AXIS IN WOMEN WITH ABDOMINAL OBESITY: DISSOCIATION BETWEEN CRF-AVP AND PSYCHOMETRIC STIMULATORY TESTS.

R. Pasquali*, B. Anconetani, M. Biscotti, F. Casimirri, V. Vicennati, AM Morselli-Labate. Inst. Clin. Medicine 1, S. Orsola Hosp., Alma Mater Univ. of Bologna, Italy.

We have previously demonstrated that women with abdominal obesity may have hyperactivity of the HPA axis. In this study we examined whether they may also have peculiar hormonal and psychological response to psychometric tests, comparable, in some way, to that elicited by pharmacological stimulation. Two groups of seven age-matched obese women with peripheral (P-BFD) and abdominal (A-BFD) body fat distribution (classified by using abdominal CT scan) and a group of five control normal weight women, randomly underwent different tests: a) CRF (h-CRF, Clinalfa, Switzerland), (100 μg) plus AVP (Pitressin, Parke-Davis, Germany) (0.3 I.E.) iv bolus; b) CRF 1 μg/kg b.w.) + AVP (0.005 I.E./kg b.w.) iv bolus; c) standardized psychometric test (performed by completing puzzles and mental calculation, both divided into easy and difficult tasks); and, d) a control saline test. Cortisol, ACTH, pulse rate (PR), blood pressure (BP) were measured at regular intervals throughout each test; the Kellner Symptom Questionnaire (SQ) was also administerd both before and at the end of each test. In both the CRF+AVP tests, A-BFD women showed significantly higher ACTH and cortisol levels than P-BFD and controls. On the contrary, neither cortisol nor ACTH changed significantly during the psychometric test nor were significant differences found during this test between the three groups. Moreover, PR, BP and SQ changes during each test showed no significant difference between the groups. We conclude that the hyperactivity of the HPA axis we further demonstrated in women with abdominal obesity cannot be reproduced during a standardized psychometric stimulation thus suggesting that different neurondocrine mechanisms are involved.

P1.40

CORTICOTROPIN RELEASING HORMONE, INTERLEUKIN-6 AND SERUM AMYLOID A CONCENTRATIONS IN SYNOVIAL FLUIDS OF PATIENTS WITH RHEUMATOID ARTHRITIS.

T. Nishioka*, H. Kurokawa, T. Takao, Y. Kumon, K. Nishiya, K. Nakatani, K. Hashimoto. Second Dept. of Internal medicine, Kochi Medical School, Nankoku, Kochi 783, and Misato Marin Hospital, Kochi 780, Japan

It is well known that such cytokines as IL-1, IL-6 and TNF-α are related to various inflammatory response like fever and the production of acute phase protein and also related to the regulation of HPA axis. To define the relationship between HPA axis and the cytokines in patients with rheumatoid arthritis (RA), we measured the concentrations of corticotropin releasing hormone (CRH) and interleukin-6 (IL-6) or serum amyloid A protein (SAA) which is one of acute phase proteins in plasma and synovial fluids of 26 patients with RA (14; treated with low dose prednisolone, 12; treated with NSAIDs or DMARDs) and 18 patients with osteoarthritis (OA). CRH and IL-6 levels in synovial fluid of patients with RA were significantly higher than those of patients with OA. CRH and ACTH levels in plasma in RA were significantly lower than those in OA. SAA levels in both plasma and synovial fluid were significantly higher in RA than in OA. SAA levels were weakly correlated with the levels of CRH and IL-6 in synovial fluid, whereas there was no correlation between CRH and IL-6 levels in synovial fluid. It is possible that CRH and IL-6 have a role in producing SAA in synovial fluid. It was also shown that the regulatory mechanism of synovial CRH secretion was different from those of plasma CRH and ACTH as there were no significant correlations between them.

P1.41

CORTICOTROPIN-RELEASING FACTOR (CRF) INCREASES HUMAN SERUM GALANIN (GAL) LEVELS IN PREPUBERTAL SUBJECTS.

G. Ceresini[*], G. Valenti[*], E.H. Meade[†], S. Bernasconi[¶], L. Ghizzoni[¶], I. Merchenthaler[†], A. Negro-Vilar[†] & F.J. López[†]. Chair of Ger.[*] and Ped.[¶], Univ. Parma, Italy and FMS-RNS[†], LMIN, NIEHS, RTP, NC 27709, USA.

Human GAL (hGAL) is a 30-amino acid molecule with an acid-free C-terminal residue. Galanin has received attention as a neuroendocrine regulator, since it has been shown to modulate hypothalamic-pituitary axis functions. In humans, GAL has been localized to corticotrophs, suggesting that it could be secreted into blood stream concomitantly with ACTH. We have evaluated pituitary responsiveness to human CRF (hCRF) in normal prepubertal children (age 6.0 ± 1.8 y). After an overnight fast, subjects were injected intravenously with either saline, hCRF (1 µg/Kg b.w., bolus injection) or ACTH (1 µg/Kg b.w. infused over 15 min). The saline-treated group was divided into two subgroups which were subjected to either a bolus injection or a 15 min infusion of saline. Blood samples were collected at -30, -15, 0, 5, 15, 30, 60, 90, 120 min and at -30, -15, 0, 60, 120 min for the hCRF and ACTH test, respectively. Plasma or serum samples were assayed for cortisol or ACTH using commercially available RIA kits. Human GAL levels were measured in a direct RIA using a specific sheep anti-hGAL serum (FMS-FJL #21-3). Administration of hCRF in prepubertal children increased ACTH secretion and, more importantly, significantly elevated serum hGAL levels. The effect of hCRF on hGAL was specific, since ACTH administration did not alter hGAL concentrations, even though significantly increased plasma cortisol levels were observed. The data clearly indicate that hCRF enhances hGAL secretion in prepubertal children. Therefore, our results provide evidence to support the notion that hCRF-induced activation of corticotrophs leads to concomitant secretion of hGAL and ACTH.

P1.42

CHANGES IN CEREBRAL BLOOD FLOW AND PLASMA CATECHOLAMINES DURING ORTHOSTATIC HYPOTENSION.

*Y. Nishioeda[1], K. Hayashida[2], Y. Ishida[2], M. Tsushima[1], Y. Harano[1], M. Takamiya[2] and I. Ninomiya[3]. Dept. of Internal Medicine[1] and dept. of Radiology[2], National Cardiovascular Center, Osaka, Japan, 565. Dept.of Physiology[3], Institute of Health Sciences, Hiroshima University, Hiroshima, Japan, 730.

The role of central command as the regulator of plasma catecholamines during orthostatic hypotension (OH) was examined in the "active standing test" of 21 patients with normal brain MRI who complained faintness. In this test, cerebral blood flow (CBF) using Technetium-99m-HMPAO Brain SPECT were evaluated together with plasma norepinephrine(NE), epinephrine, dopamine, blood pressure and heart rate. Brain SPECT showed a decrease in activity of the frontal area immediately after standing in 6 out of 7 OH patients (OH group). The result indicated that CBF in the frontal area decreased at the onset of upright posture. On the other hand, in 14 patients without OH (non-OH group), decrease in CBF were not detected. Basal NE levels were 485 pg/ml and 441 pg/ml in the OH and non-OH groups, respectively. At the onset of upright posture, NE did not increase in the OH group but increase significantly by 20% of the basal NE level in the non-OH group and difference in % change of NE between two groups was significant (p>0.01). Our results suggest that the decrease in CBF in the frontal area is a key factor leading OH due to a lack or delay of sympathetic activation by central command at the onset of upright posture.

P1.43

THE PITUITARY-THYROID AXIS IN INSULIN DEPENDENT DIABETES MELLITUS (IDDM).

P.C.Eskildsen,* I.Jensen, Medical Dept., Köge County Hospital, DK 4600 Köge, Denmark.

Abnormalities of the TSH secretion and of thyroid function in patients with IDDM typically reflect glycemic dysregulation. We wanted to evaluate the pit.-thyr.axis in IDDM pat. in good glycemic control. 48 clinically euthyroid IDDM PAT. (DIAB),11F + 37M,age 20-63yr (mean 44), weight 76.8±2.0(SE) kg, diabetes duration 19.3±1.6yr, with a HbA1c level of 7.9 ±0.2% were compared with 28 age, sex and weight matched controls (CON). Serum TSH (detect.lim.0.05 mU/l),total+free T4 and T3, thyroid peroxidase-ab (TPO-ab), prolaktin (PRL) and cortisol (C) were measured in blood sampled at morning in non-fasting state. The DIAB showed compared to CON increased TSH(1.18±0.1 vs 0.88±0.08mU/l,p=0.04), decreased total T4(85.5±2.1 vs 90.7±3.8nmol/l,p=0.03)and increased free T3(7.3±0.2 vs 6.6±0.2pmol/l,p=0.03), but all within normal limits. Serum levels of free T4, total T3 and PRL were normal and identical in DIAB and CON, while serum C was significantly elevated in DIAB (424±19 vs 323±21 nmol/l,p= 0.001). Among DIAB no correlation occurred between serum TSH and C, and serum TSH, T4 and T3 were uninfluenced by the presence of TPO-ab(in 7 DIAB vs 1 CON), duration of diabetes, occurrence of microalbuminuria and autonomic/sensoric neuropathy. Conclusively the study showed a normal functioning pit.-thyr.axis in DIAB in good glycemic control but indicated an increased deiodination of T4 to T3 with an increased TSH feed back. The increased C level may have some influence on the pit.-thyr.axis in IDDM.

P1.44

INVOLVEMENT OF THYREOLIBERIN (TRH) IN THE REGULATION OF ANTERIOR AND POSTERIOR PITUITARY HORMONES IN MAN.

F. Laczi*, M. Vecsernyés, J. Gardi, I. Pávó, J. Julesz, Endocrine Unit, A. Szent-Györgyi Medical University, Szeged, Hungary, 6720.

The role of TRH demonstrated in the neurohypophysis (NH) has not been clarified. Increased plasma AVP levels have been observed in peripheral hypothyroidism of animals and man. Exaggerated hypothalamic TRH secretion has also been reported in this disease. These data suggest some role of the TRH in the regulation of NH function. In the present study, the effects of TRH (200 µg iv bolus injection) on plasma arg-8-vasopressin (AVP), oxytocin (OT), thyrotropin (TSH), prolactin (PRL) and corticotropin (ACTH) were investigated in 6 healthy individuals, 4 patients with peripheral hypothyroidism and 1 suffering from partial central diabetes insipidus (DI). Before and 30, 60, 90 and 120 min after TRH administration, antecubital venous blood samples were collected for hormone RIAs. TRH increased the plasma AVP, OT, TSH, PRL and ACTH levels of healthy subjects. The basal levels of AVP but not those of OT were increased in hypothyroidic patients, which phenomenon seems to be dependent of the severity of the thyroidal hypofunction. Hypothyroidics displayed blunted AVP and OT reactions to TRH. Both basal and stimulated TSH levels were found to be elevated in hypothyroidism; and the stimulability of PRL of these patients was enhanced. Basal plasma ACTH proved to be lower than normal in 3 of 4 hypothyroidism patients and was increased by TRH load. In our case with central DI due to osmoreceptor failure, TRH provoked an AVP response similar to those of healthy controls. The present data suggest that TRH may participate in the ACTH and neurohypophysial hormone regulation possibly involving the baroreceptor system. Supported by OTKA, grant No.s. 1350 and T-6223, and ETT, grant No. T-92/1990.

P1.45

ASYMMETRIC TEMPORAL LOBE MODULATION OF LUTEINIZING HORMONE SECRETION. A.G. Herzog, A.E. Coleman, F.W. Drislane, D.S. Schomer. Harvard Neuroendocrine Unit, Beth Israel Hospital, Boston, MA 02215, USA

Reproductive endocrine disorders are unusually common among men and women with epilepsy. We investigated the possibility that altered temporolimbic modulation of hypothalamopituitary function may promote the development of these disorders and that lateralized cerebral and hypothalamic asymmetries may be responsible for the association of different reproductive disorders with left and right temporal lobe epilepsy (TLE). The pulsatile secretion of luteinizing hormone (LH) over 8 hours during concommitant EEG recording was evaluated in 12 men and 11 women with unilateral TLE and 11 male and 10 female normal controls. LH pulse frequency was significantly more variable ($p < 0.05$) in men and women with TLE than in controls. In men, right temporal epileptiform activity was associated with significantly greater LHPF than left (R/L: 6/3; $p < 0.05$). In women, left temporal epileptiform activity was associated with significantly greater LHPF than right (L/R: 6/3; $p < 0.05$). Paroxysmal unilateral slowing had opposite effects. The findings suggest that the laterality and nature of temporal lobe paroxysmal discharges may be important determinants of LHPF and the development of particluar reproductive endocrine disorders.

P1.46

BRAIN MRI AND OLFACTORY THRESHOLD IN THE DIFFERENTIAL DIAGNOSIS OF HYPOTHALAMIC HYPOGONADISM. P. Travaglini, T. Re, M. Farabola*, G. Broich**, C. De-Min, S. Borgato, S. Mantovani, P. Beck-Peccoz and G. Faglia. *Institute of Endocrine Sciences, and Departments of *Neuroradiology and **ENT, Ospedale Maggiore IRCCS, University of Milan, 20122-Milan, Italy.*

Anatomical, functional and genetic abnormalities may lead to dysfunction of GnRH-secreting neurons and hypothalamic hypogonadism (HH). The above neurons originate from the olfactory placode and migrate into the brain with olfactory nerves. In X-linked Kallmann syndrome (KS), mutations of a specific gene encoding for neuronal cell adhesion molecule(s) prevent cells and nerves of the olfactory placode to migrate in the brain. This results in alterations of olfactory bulbs, tracts and sulci, anosmia and hypogonadism which are characteristic of KS, but are absent in other forms of HH. In the present study, we evaluated the effectiveness of high resolution brain MRI (thin, T1-weighted and coronal sections) and olfactory threshold (standard sniff-test and diluition test) in the differential diagnosis of HH. One 44-yr-old woman with primary amenorrhea and 3 men aged 16, 42 and 47 years were studied. Basal LH [0.3 ± 0.1 (SD) U/L] and FSH (0.7 ± 0.2 U/L) levels were low in all patients and increased to 3-11 U/L and 2-7 U/L, respectively, in response to 3 consecutive GnRH boli (100 μg every 2 hour). Two patients (16- and 47-yr-old) complained of subjective hypoosmia and were therefore diagnosed as having KS. All had normal hypothalamic-pituitary structures and lack of obstructive disease of nasal cavities. MRI showed a normal olfactory system in all but the 16-yr-old man who had absence of olfactory bulbs, tracts and right-side sulcus. In this patient however the olfactory threshold was normal, while true hypoosmia was documented only in the 42-yr-old man with subjectively reported normal sense of smell.

In conclusion, our data highlight the current difficulties in the differential diagnosis of the various forms of HH. The discrepancies among the clinical picture, the brain MRI and the olfactory threshold recorded in the present study, point to the necessity of including in the differential diagnosis of HH also appropriate genetic studies in order to clarify the variable phenotypic appearance of hypothalamic hypogonadism.

P1.47

BETA ENDORPHIN LEVELS DURING THE MENSTRUAL CYCLE IN WOMEN WITH PREMENSTRUAL SYNDROME (PMS)
S.Vujović,Z.Penezić,M.Drezgić,V.Rajković,J.Bjekić, D.Slijepčević. Institite of Endocrinology,KCS, Belgrade,Yugoslavia.

The aim of this study was to determinate ß endorphin (BE) levels in PMS and control group.According to modified Moos questionarre we formed group of 60 women with severe PMS, mean age of 29 +/-5y.,BMI=21,9 +/-1,2 kg/m^2,with regular cycles.There were 60 women in control group,25 +/-6 years old,BMI=23,6 +/-4,with regular cycle.Blood samples for FSH,LH,PRL,BE,estradiol and progesteron were obtained on 7th,14th,and daily from 21st-28th day and detectid by RIA. Statistic analysis were done by Wilcoxon Mann-Whitney test. We found significantly lower concentrations of BE in PMS group,compared to controls on 21st day (42,2 +/-10,3 pg/ml v.s. 190,0 +/-24,8 pg/ml,z=2,02,p<0,05),while there were no difference on 28th day (78,0 +/-7,6 v.s. 64,2 +/-12,4; p>0,05).While in the PMS group BE rised from 21st-28th day in controls it felt down progressivly.

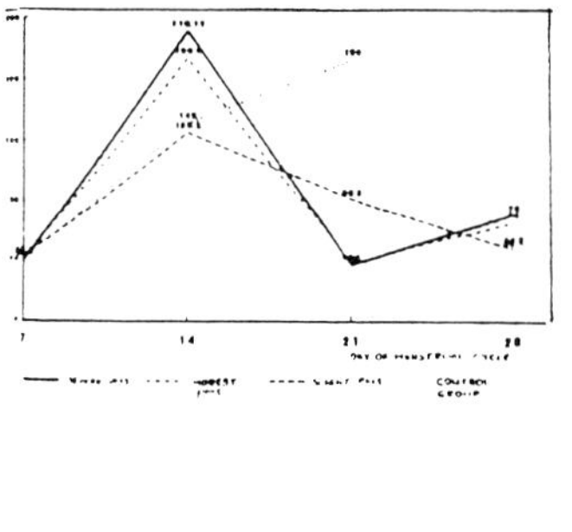

Our data indicated direct influence of relative hyperestrogenia,high E2/P ratio,relative hyperprolactinaemia, without significant changes in gonadotropin levels on ß endorphin levels prior to menstruation in PMS group.

P1.48

THE EFFECT OF CORTICOLIBERIN (CRH) ON GONADOTROPIN HORMONE RELEASING HORMONE (GnRH) HYPOTHALAMIC NEURONAL SYSTEM DURING PREOVULATORY PERIOD IN THE EWE. J. Polkowska*, F. Przekop. The Kielanowsky Institute of Animal Physiology and Nutrition, Jablonna. Poland.

The effect of continuous infusions of the synthetic CRH into the 3rd ventricle of the brain of ewes during proestrus (15th and 16th days) on the immunoreactive (ir)GnRH neuronal system and pituitary LH-cells were studied. The control animals (saline infusions) were decapitated together with experimental ones (CRH infusions) on the day of estrus (18th day), but before the ovulation. None of the experimental sheep displayed estrous acitivity and have ovulated on that day. Hypothalamic GnRH and pituitary LH were analysed by immunocytochemistry, plasma LH by radioimmunoassay. The GnRH center in CRH-treated ewes situated in the preoptico-septal area was well organized. Numerous irGnRH perikarya filled with dense ir material and rich network of irGnRH axons were observed. However, irGnRH stores in the nerve terminals of the median eminence were poorly seen as compared to the controls. In the pituitary gland, the hyperplasia of LH-cells was observed, but the plasma concentration of LH was low and did not exceed the basal level. These results show that CRH blocks the preovulatory LH surge in the ewe, but does not impair the synthesis of GnRH and LH. It is suggested that CRH can affect GnRH neuronal system possibly via suppression of axonal transport of this neurohormone.

P1.49

EFFECTS OF CONTINUOUS AND PULSATILE ADMINISTRATION OF A POTENT ANALOG OF GHRH(1-30)-NH_2 ON GROWTH RESPONSES IN RATS TREATED WITH MONOSODIUM GLUTAMATE. M. Kovács*, A. Fáncsik, E. Hrabovsky, I. Mező, I. Teplán, B. Flerkó. Dept. of Anatomy, University Medical School, Pécs, Hungary, 7643 and Inst. of Biochemistry, Semmelweis University Medical School, Budapest, Hungary, 1444.

To assess the efficacy of a potent GHRH analog (D-Ala^2,Nle^{27},Gaba^{30}-GHRH(1-30)-NH_2) in the treatment of GH deficiency, we investigated the effects of chronic administration of A-495 on growth responses in MSG-lesioned rats. Basal serum GH concentrations, GH responses to bolus injections of GHRH, as well as acceleration of body gain and linear growth were compared after long-term continuous and pulsatile administration of A-495. Treatment with MSG reduced the body weight and linear growth of the animals (-22% and -11%, respectively), the basal serum GH concentration (-66%), and the GHRH-induced GH responses (-61%). Repetitive administration of 10μg daily doses of A-495 for two weeks restored the normal GH responsiveness to GHRH and induced acceleration of body gain and linear growth, by which MSG-treated animals achieved the growth of normal controls. However, basal serum GH concentrations were only modestly enhanced. Continuous infusion of A-495 at the same daily dose resulted in slight increases in the GHRH-induced GH rises, moderate acceleration of body gain, but no changes in linear growth and basal serum GH concentrations. In conclusion, our results demonstrate that chronic treatment with GHRH is able to fully restore the blunted sensitivity of the GHRH-induced GH secretory response of MSG-lesioned rats. Although, both continuous and pulsatile administrations of GHRH are useful in the treatment of the hypothalamic GHRH deficiency syndrome, pulsatile administration is more effective at the same daily dose. The growth response appears to be related to the magnitude of the GHRH-stimulated rise in GH levels rather than basal GH concentrations. Present results demonstrate the therapeutic usefulness of our new GHRH analog. (Supported by grants OTKA-2994 and ETT-T-569/90).

P1.50

EVALUATION OF THE THERAPEUTIC EFFICACY OF SUPERACTIVE ANALOGUES OF LHRH ON BREAST AND PROSTATE CANCER ANIMAL MODELS. R.M.G. Nair*, G.K. Nambiar, Fairwell Thomas¶, School of Sciences & Technology, Savannah State College, Savannah, GA 31404 and NHLBI¶, NIH, Bethesda, MD, USA.

Potent agonists and antagonists of LHRH were specially designed by computer modelling and synthesized. The therapeutic efficacies of the most potent agonist(s) and antagonist(s) were studied on WF female rats bearing MT-W9a (KIM) mammary tumor, Copenhagen males or Nobel males bearing Dunning R3327H or 2PR-121 D prostate adenocarcinoma. His^2-Me-D-Ala^6-Des-Gly^{10}-LHRH-ethylamide (agonist), N-acetyl-D-β-Nal-p-Cl-D-Phe-3-pyridyl-D-Ala-Ser-N-ε-nicotinoyl-Lys-N-ε-nicotinoyl-D-Lys-Leu-N-ε-isopropyl-Lys-Pro-D-Ala-NH_2 (antagonist) were administered i.m., b.i.d. (0.025mg dose) to the experimental groups. Control animals received only saline. Reduction of the tumor size and cell doubling time, disappearance of the serum estrogen or testosterone levels, decrease in the proportion of aneuploid cells from tumor aspirates by flowcytometry, and percentage inhibition of specific oncogenes if any, in comparison with control groups were performed weekly. Statistical analysis of the data indicated that the antagonist(s) was the most efficient in tumor reduction (98%, p-value <.001) after 45 days' treatment. The agonist-treated groups showed an initial increase in the tumor volume and cell aneuploidy, but later the proliferation mitigated (95% reduction). Although the chronic administration of the agonist down-regulates the LH and FSH receptor sites on the gonads, the effect of the transient elevation of the gonadotropins may have a decisive role on the reduction of the therapeutic value of this group of superactive analogues, as evidenced by our experimental findings.

P1.51

RAT PAROTID GLAND TISSUE IS ABLE TO ASSUME PITUITARY FUNCTIONS UNDER HYPOTHALAMIC EXTRACTS IN CULTURE.

P. Fernández, B. Granados, C. Ariznavarreta, A. Rodriguez-Ramos, P. Gil-Loyzaga, A., J.A.F. Tresguerres.
Depts of Physiology and Morphology. Medical School. Univ. Complutense. Madrid. Spain.

Parotid tissue transplanted to the sella turcica after hypofisectomy has been shown to partially assume the pituitary functions in vivo. To asses this morphofunctional change in vitro parotid glands were carefully removed from 2 days old female Wistar rats and submitted to mechanical dissection, followed by collagenase, trypsin and hyaluronidase digestion in a test tube. Cells were cultured in RPMI medium, in 24 well dishes for one week allowing to stabilize. Culture wells were divided into 4 different groups of 12 wells each. 1.Controls were cultured in the presence of medium suplemented with 10% fetal calf serum. 2.Were submitted twice a day to the influence of rat hypothalamic extracts (0.5 /hypothalamus/well dissolved in 50 µl of medium). 3.Were submitted to lamb hypothalamic extracts (1:100 hypothalamus, well/dissolved in 50 µl of medium) and 4.treated similarly to 3 but with a 1:100 dilution of an LHRH antibody. The cultures were followed for 3 weeks with samples of the culture medium being obtained every 3 1/2 days. Group 2 showed a dramatic increase in LH values starting 3 1/2 days after the treatment with rat hypothalamic extract as compared to controls. This increase was mantained over the 3 studied weeks. Group 3 showed also an increase in LH production but the amount reached was significally lower than in group 2, thus indicating the existence of species specific inductors of morphofunctional changes. Group 4 showed significantly lower levels than in group 3 indicating that LHRH plays also an important role in the differenciation process. This work has been possible through FIS 92/475

P1.52

SYSTEMIC GROWTH HORMONE-RELEASING HORMONE (GHRH) ENHANCES SLEEP IN INTACT AND HYPOPHYSECTOMIZED RATS. F. Obál Jr. (1)*, R. Floyd (2), J.M. Krueger (2), Dept. Physiology, A. Szent-Györgyi Medical University, Szeged, Hungary 6720 (1), and Dept. Physiol., University of Tennessee, Memphis, TN, USA, 38163 (2)

Intracerebral GHRH promotes non-rapid eye movement sleep (NREMS) and REMS (Obál et al., 1986, 1988, Ehlers et al., 1986, Nistico et al., 1987) whereas an antagonist (Obál et al., 1990) or antibodies to GHRH (Obál et al., 1992) decrease sleep. Iv GHRH reportedly enhances sleep in human subjects under certain conditions (Steiger et al., 1992, Kerkhofs et al., 1993). In the present experiments, GHRH was iv injected to intact and hypophysectomized rats chronically implanted with EEG electrodes and brain thermistors for sleep recording and an intracardial catheter for blood sampling. The rats received GHRH at light onset (AM group, 0.05 μg/kg) or 6 h after light onset (PM group, 0.05, 0.5, 5.0 μg/kg; n=6-10 for rats for each dose). Sleep-wake activity was recorded for 24 h whereas GH was determined (RIA) from the blood sampled at 15 min intervals for 1.5 h postinjection. Physiological saline was injected on the baseline day. GHRH promoted NREMS in the PM group; the effect decreased when the dose was increased. Each dose enhanced REMS. GH was dose-dependently stimulated. In hypophysectomized rats, GHRH continued to stimulate NREMS and failed to enhance REMS. GHRH did not promote sleep in the AM group, and the GH response was also attenuated in these rats indicating a "time of the day" effect. It is concluded that the NREMS promoting activity of GHRH is not mediated via GH. In contrast, GH is involved in the enhanced REMS after GHRH.

P1.53

ON THE ROLES OF SRIF AND GRF IN GH SECRETORY DYNAMICS OF THE MUTANT DWARF RAT. G.S. Tannenbaum*, J. Turner, M. Lapointe, W. Gurd. Departments of Pediatrics, Neurology and Neurosurgery, McGill University, Montreal, Quebec, Canada H3H 1P3.

To elucidate the mechanism(s) underlying the impaired GH secretion of the mutant dwarf rat (Dw), we 1) characterized spontaneous and GRF-stimulated GH secretory profiles, 2) assessed the possible involvement of endogenous SRIF, and 3) examined the SRIF/GRF interaction in adult male Dw (a gift from Dr. R. Clark, Genentech, Inc.) and age-matched Lewis control rats. Spontaneous 6-hour plasma GH profiles of free-moving Dw rats revealed a 7-fold reduction in both GH pulse amplitude (14.9±3.0 vs. 108.5±14.0 ng/ml; $P<0.001$) and mean 6-h plasma GH level (2.6±0.2 vs. 18.7±2.0 ng/ml; $P<0.001$), although the 3.2 h period between GH secretory episodes was unchanged. While Dw rats exhibited a 6- to 10-fold lower GH response to GRF stimulation, they continued to show a cyclical pattern of responsiveness when challenged at GH peak versus trough times. Passive immunization of Dw rats with SRIF antiserum failed to alter either GH peak amplitude, GH trough values or mean 6-h plasma GH levels when compared to Dw control rats administered normal sheep serum. Pretreatment of Dw rats with the long-acting SRIF analog, octreotide, failed to potentiate GH responsiveness to GRF; moreover, the SRIF-14-induced post-inhibitory rebound release of GH was 26-fold less in Dw rats than that observed in controls ($P<0.001$). These results demonstrate that: 1) the ultradian GH rhythm is preserved in the Dw rat suggesting that SRIF/GRF secretion continues to be cyclical in this model; 2) while the Dw rat is GRF and SRIF responsive, endogenous SRIF/GRF release is low; and 3) the impairment in GH secretion of the Dw rat is not due to increased SRIF tone but primarily a reflection of reduced pituitary GH production.

P1.54

TRANSIENT CEREBRAL OEDEMA FOLLOWING PITUITARY STALK LESION IN RATS. Cs. Varga, I. Rojik, *S. Csáti, **M. Vecsernyés, ***G. Makara, F.A. László. Dept. of Comparative Physiology, Attila József University of Sciences, *First Dept. of Medicine, **Endocrine Unit and Research Laboratory, Albert Szent-Györgyi Medical University, Szeged; ***Institute of Experimental Medicine, Hungarian Academy of Sciences, Budapest, Hungary.

The acute stage of head injury or transsphenoidal pituitary surgery are frequently associated with the development of the syndrome of inappropriate antidiuretic hormone secretion (SIADH), aggravating the clinical signs of cerebral lesion (1). In these cases, damage of the hypothalamoneurohypophyseal tract (HNHT) must be taken into consideration (2).

For study of the role of HNHT impairment in the development of SIADH, pituitary stalk lesion was electrolytically performed in rats (3). Daily water consumption, urinary output, sodium excretion, plasma osmolality and sodium concentration, arginine vasopressin (AVP) (4) and corticosterone levels (5), brain water and electrolyte contents were examined in rats with pituitary stalk lesion. At the end of the experiments, the brain was studied histologically to establish the location of the lesions. Pituitary stalk lesion produced a classic triphasic water metabolism disturbance: transitory polyuria and polydipsia (1st phase), an oliguric interphase (2nd phase), and permanent polyuria (3rd phase). During the oliguric interphase, increased sodium excretion, decreased plasma osmolality and corticosterone level, transient hyponatriaemia, and increases in brain water and sodium contents were detected. Cerebral oedema was accompanied by elevated vasopressin levels inappropriate for the plasma sodium level, inappropriately concentrated urine, water retention, and natriuresis. The transient hyponatriaemia occurred 2-3 days after lesioning and returned to normal by days 5-7, which corresponds to the second phase of the triphasic response in rats.

The results permit the conclusion that AVP released from the damaged HNHT, including the posterior pituitary, plays an important pathogenetic role in the development of transitory cerebral oedema following pituitary stalk lesion.

1. Zerbe, R.L., Stropes, L., Robertson, G.L.: Annu. Rev. Med. 31, 315-327, 1980.
2. Ultmann, M.C., Hoffman, G.E., Nelson, P.B., Robinson, A.G.: Neuroendocrinology, 56, 803-811, 1992.
3. László, F.A., de Wied, D.: J. Endocrinol. 36, 125-137, 1966.
4. Laczi, F., Iványi, T., Julesz, J., Janáky, T., László, F.A.: Acta Endocrinol. 113, 168-174, 1986.
5. Mihály, K., Makara, G.B., Stark, E.: Proc. Symp. Anal. Steroids, (ed: Görög, S.) Budapest: Acad. Press, 217-221, 1981.

P1.55

EFFECTS OF V_1 AND V_2 VASOPRESSIN ANTAGONISTS ON THE DEVELOPMENT OF CEREBRAL OEDEMA IN RATS WITH EXPERIMENTAL SUBARACHNOID HAEMORRHAGE. F.A. László, Cs. Varga, *L. Baláspiri, **T. Dóczi. Dept. of Comparative Physiology, Attila József University of Sciences, *Dept. of Medical Chemistry, Albert Szent-Györgyi Medical School, Szeged; **Dept. of Neurosurgery, Medical School, Pécs, Hungary.

The acute phase of subarachnoid haemorrhage (SAH) is frequently associated with an impaired water metabolism and a disposition to cerebral oedema (1,2). For study of the pathogenesis of brain oedema, an experimental model of SAH was created in the rat (3). The diuretic curves after water loading, the brain water and electrolyte contents and the plasma and cerebrospinal fluid arginine vasopressin (AVP) levels (4) were examined in rats with SAH. Furthermore, it was investigated whether the highly specific V_2 antagonist $d(CH_2)_5D$-$Ile^2Ile^4Ala^9AVP$ or the pressor (V_1) antagonist $d(CH_2)_5Tyr(Me)AVP$ (5) can prevent the development of cerebral oedema in experimentally induced SAH.

Following a water load, a significant water retention and increases in brain water and sodium contents were observed after cerebral bleeding. Plasma and cerebral fluid AVP levels were also elevated following SAH. When the V_2 antagonist was administered immediately after water loading, water retention could not be detected in rats with SAH. The higher brain water accumulation with an accompanying increase in the sodium content was totally prevented by simultaneous administration of the V_2 antagonist. On the other hand, the water retention and cerebral oedema were not influenced by administration of the V_1 antagonist.

There results demonstrate that AVP plays important roles in the development of an impaired water metabolism and cerebral oedema following experimental SAH, and the cerebral oedema is significantly reduced by the administration of a highly specific V_2 antagonist, suggesting a new approach to the treatment of cerebral oedema.

1. Zerbe, R.L., Stropes, L., Robertson, G.L.: Annu. Rev. Med. 31, 315-327, 1980.
2. László, F.A., László, F.Jr., de Wied, D.: Pharmacol. Rev. 43, 73-108, 1991.
3. Dóczi, T., László, F.A. Szerdahelyi, P., Joó, F.: Neurosurgery 14, 436-444, 1984.
4. Laczi, F., Iványi, T., Julesz, J., Janáky, T., László, F.A.: Acta Endocrinol. 113, 168-174, 1986.
5. Manning, M., Sawyer, W.H.: J.Lab.Clin.Med. 114, 617-632, 1989.

P1.56

DUAL RECEPTOR REGULATION OF RAT PINEAL MELATONIN SECRETION. Z. Rekasi*, V. Csernus, B. Mess. Dept. of Anatomy, University Medical School, Pecs, Hungary, 7643.

Pineal function is known to be regulated by ß-adrenergic receptors coupled to adenylate cyclase activity associated with serotonin N-acetyltransferase (NAT) induction. Recent studies have demonstrated that vasoactive intestinal peptide (VIP) also stimulates cAMP accumulation and NAT activity in the rat pineal gland. We examined the effects of norepinephrine (NE, 10^{-7}-10^{-5} M) and VIP (10^{-7}-10^{-5} M) on melatonin (MT) release from perifused rat pineal glands. Both NE and VIP stimulated MT synthesis and release in a dose-dependent manner above 10^{-7} M concentration. The kinetics of MT responses after NE or VIP exposures were similar. The MT production reached the maximum value after a relatively long lag (2 to 3 h) when NE or VIP applications had been stopped and it returned to basal values after 5 to 6 h. The effects of NE and VIP in doses tested were not additive. The VIP- stimulated MT secretion was not influenced by propranolol (10^{-5} M), while the NE-evoked MT response was reduced significantly by this ß-adrenergic receptor antagonist. In contrast, an effective VIP receptor antagonist (10^{-5} M) could markedly decrease the VIP-induced MT production but the magnitude of MT response after combined application of NE with VIP receptor antagonist remained unchanged. These data provide further evidence that in addition to sympathetic nervous system, peptidergic nerve fibers might influence pineal indole metabolism via specific receptors. (Supported by grant from the Hungarian National Science Foundation OTKA 1168).

P1.57

MODIFICATION OF CHICKEN SERUM MELATONIN LEVEL BY CORTICOSTERONE AND EXOGENOUS MELATONIN. K. Skwarlo-Sonta★+, A. Gladysz +, Z. Koter▪. +Dept. of Animal Physiology, University of Warsaw, and ▪Institute of Aviation Medicine, Warsaw, Poland.

The aim of study was to evaluate the magnitude of changes evoked in chicken pineal gland activity by the treatment with exogenous corticosterone (CS), and/or melatonin (MEL), both agents having well established influence on immune system function. Pineal gland activity was measured by serum MEL level determined by RIA twice over a 24 hr period (at mid-day and mid-night) in 5-week-old cockerels kept from hatching in L:D=12:12 light conditions. Chickens were treated with CS in drinking water or as sc injections for 7 consecutive days. Two days after beginning of CS treatment chickens were immunized ip with sheep red blood cells (SRBC) and then some of them received sc injections of different MEL doses for 5 days or/and naloxone (NX, an opioid antagonist), 2 hr before the end of light or at the beginning of light period. Control birds were injected with saline (PBS). The day after last injection, chickens were sacrificed and serum was prepared and stored in -20°C until assay. Morning injections of both PBS or CS slightly diminished and those of MEL increased serum MEL without effect on the nocturnal/diurnal (N/D) ratio, an index of the circadian rhythm of pineal gland function. CS alone administerd in drinking water exerted similar effect, whereas additional treatment with MEL, administered 2 hr before the end of light strongly modified both the serum MEL level and its circadian rhythm (diminished N/D ratio) in a dose-dependent manner. Influence of NX was less-well pronounced and did not antagonize the effect of MEL, whereas the effect of PBS injections was ambiguous. The effect of highest MEL dose without previous CS administration was smaller and did not disturbe N/D ratio. It is concluded that in chicken CS (stress?) modifies the feedback regulatory mechanism between peripheral MEL level and pineal gland function.

P1.58

DEVELOPMENT AND LIGHT SENSITIVITY OF THE *IN VITRO* MELATONIN SECRETION PATTERN FROM AVIAN PINEAL GLAND. *V. Csernus, M. Ghosh and B. Mess**. Dept. Anatomy Univ. Med School Pécs, Hungary, and (M.G.) Dept. of Zoology, Banaras Hindu Univ., Varanasi, India.

Melatonin secretion from the pineal glands, *in vivo*, shows a characteristic circadian pattern, controlled by the environmental lighting conditions. The peak of the melatonin level is in the middle of the dark phase. Unlike the mammalian glands, avian pineals exhibit circadian alteration in N-acetyl-transferase (NAT) activity and of melatonin release even *in vitro*. To study the factors of the formation and maintenance of this rhythmicity, melatonin production of the chicken pineal gland was monitored in a long-term perifusion system. The eight to 10 week old pineal donor chickens were kept under normal lighting condition or exposed to continuous light or darkness before sacrifice. The tissue fragments in the superfusion column were also subjected to various lighting regimes *in vitro*. Spontaneous, circadian melatonin rhythm could not be influenced by keeping the pineal donor birds in constant light or constant dark environment for two weeks before sacrifice. Circadian melatonin rhythm developed even if the chickens were kept under continuous illumination from hatching to sacrifice. Constant illumination or continuous darkness, *in vitro*, do not extinguish only modify the circadian melatonin rhythm (reduced amplitude). It was concluded that the avian pineal gland has a genetically coded circadian rhythm which develops and is maintained without cyclic illumination and can only be slightly modulated by long-term changes in environmental lighting conditions.

(Supported by grant from the Hungarian National Science Foundation, **OTKA 1168.**)

P1.59

MELATONIN(Mel)-INDUCED INHIBITION OF LUTEINIZING HORMONE (LH)RELEASE FROM PARS TUBERALIS(pt)MEDIATE LH-RELEASING HORMONE(LH-RH) RELEASE BY SHORT-LOOP NEGATIVE FEED-BACK OF LH. K,Nakazawa.* K,Suzuki, T, Makino. S.M.McCann.** *Dept. of Obstetrics and Gynecology, Keio University School of Medicine Tokyo 160 JAPAN. **Dept. of Physiology, UT South-Western Medical Center, Dallas, TX 75235.

The highest concentration of Mel receptor is in the pt. We hypothesized that Mel action on the hypothalamus may be mediated via the pt by altered release of LH. To test this hypotesis we incubated median eminence (ME)-pt complex from male rats in vitro. LH-RH or LH released into the medium was measured by radioimmunoassay. Mel induced a dose - related, significant stimulation of LH-RH release.This concentration of Mel also significantly lowered the release of LH. The increased release of LH-RH induced by 10^{-5}M Mel was completely blocked by the addition of LH(50ng/ml),which had no significant effect on LH-RH release. Rat LH anti serum (1/1800) significantly elevated LH-RH output, whereas normal rabbit serum at similar dilution was without effect. The results support the hypothesis that LH released from the pt diffuses to the LH-RH terminals in the ME and suppresses LH-RH release. Mel acts on its receptors in the pt to inhibit LH release, thereby stimulating the release of LH-RH from the terminals in the ME.

P1.60

REPRODUCTIVE ACTIVITY IN THE MALE SYRIAN HAMSTER IS SENSITIVE TO THE PHASE OF THE MELATONIN SIGNAL. B. Pitrosky, R. Kirsch, B. Vivien-Roels, I. Georg-Bentz*, B. Canguilhem* and P. Pévet, CNRS-URA 1332 "Neurobiologie des fonctions rythmiques et saisonnières", and *Institut de Physiologie, Faculté de Médecine, Université Louis Pasteur, 67000 STRASBOURG, FRANCE.

The pineal gland is directly involved in conduction of photoperiodic information to the brain, via the daily pattern of melatonin (MEL) secretion. The duration of MEL secretion is proportional to the duration of dark period. Whatever the photoperiod is, MEL synthesis occurs always 3 or 4 hrs after the onset of dark period. It is well known that 1) pinealectomy abolishes the daily rhythm of plasma MEL and prevents gonadal regression observed in Syrian hamsters maintained under short photoperiod (SP), and 2) daily MEL infusions, that reproduce the pattern of MEL secretion in SP, induce gonadal atrophy in pinealectomized hamsters. To determine the relative importance of the duration or of the phase of the MEL signal in the control of reproductive activity, a daily infusion protocol (for 8 weeks) was used in pinealectomized hamsters, where all infusions started 3.5 hrs after the onset of darkness. Long duration of MEL infusion (10 hrs) induced a complete gonadal atrophy whereas short duration infusion (5 hrs) was completely ineffective (testis weight: 0.81±0.23 and 2.97±0.24 g, respectively). When the animals were infused with two times 2.5 hrs separated by 3 hrs, they presented a gonadal atrophy (testis weight: 0.70±0.31g) similar to that observed with a 10 hrs infusion. On the contrary, gonadal regression did not occur when the two periods of infusion were separated by 5.5 hrs (testis weight: 2.43±0.51g). Measurement of plasma MEL during the infusion and separation periods revealed that MEL reached physiological values during the infusion period (70±14 pg/ml plasma) and falled to daytime values (10±1 pg/ml plasma) 1 hr after the end of an infusion period. This confirms that, in our experimental conditions, there were two separate MEL peaks in the plasma. We report here that 1) reproductive activity of the male Syrian hamster can be inhibited with cumulative short duration of MEL infusion (two times 2.5 hrs separated by 3 hrs), and 2) these effects can not be due to a time additive action of the two MEL pulses since MEL falls to daytime levels between the infusion periods. These results demonstrate that periods of sensitivity to MEL exist, which are important for the action of MEL in transducing photoperiodic information.

P1.61

DIRECT ACTION OF MELATONIN, INFUSED INTO THE THIRD BRAIN VENTRICLE, ON PROLACTIN SECRETION IN ANESTROUS SHEEP. T. Misztal, K. Romanowicz, B. Barcikowski. The Kielanowski Institute of Animal Physiology and Nutrition, 05-110 Jabłonna near Warsaw, Poland.

Ringer-Locke (RLS), or melatonin (MS) solution, 100 ug/100 ul/1h, were infused into the third brain ventricle in 8 one-year-old Polish Lowland ewes during the period of seasonal anestrus (April-May). The infusions were performed via the ss cannulae between 14.00-18.00h. Peripheral blood samples were collected during the period of 10 hrs. (from 12.00 to 22.00) at 30 min. intervals. The concentrations of melatonin (MLT) and prolactin (PRL) were measured by RIA. At days when RLS was infused, the mean daily concentration of MLT was 94.3 ±14.5 pg/ml, and the natural raise of the hormone secretion (up to 200 pg/ml) was noted after the sun set. The average peak concentration of PRL at evening was 177.9±8.6 pg/ml. After 30 min. of MLT treatment, the mean concentration of MLT increased, reaching plateau 1264.4±155.4 pg/ml that remained during the next hours of the infusion. After 30 min. from the begining of MLT treatment, the mean concentration of PRL increased by about 50% as compared to the concentration found during the infusion of RLS (138.2±11.3 pg/ml) or to the concentration noted before the infusion of MLT (149.2±29.7 pg/ml). This enhanced concentration of PRL remained at the level 215.8±16.1 pg/ml during 3 hrs. The results show that MLT stimulates the PRL secretion in ewes during anestrus.

P1.62

EFFECT OF MELATONIN OF THE CIRCADIAN BODY TEMPERATURE RHYTHM AND UTERINE METABOLISM DURING ALTERED PHOTOPERIODS. F. Spencer*, E. Dunbar. Biology Dept. and Health Research Center, Southern University, Baton Rouge, LA 70813, U.S.A.
The pineal hormone, melatonin, was investigated to determine its effect on the circadian rhythm of body temperature and on uterine function following the induction of the deciduoma. Female Sprague-Dawley rats (220-260g) were kept under photoperiodic conditions: 12L:12D (control); 8L:16D and 16L:8D (experimentals) under light intensity of 30.5 ft. candles and ambient temperature of 21±2 C. Decidualized pseudopregnancy (PG) was induced by cervical stimulation (cs), followed by surgical uterine traumatization on day 4 of post-cs leucocytes. Concomitantly, bio-telemeters were surgically implanted in the upper abdominal cavity. Injections of melatonin (1mg/kg/day) were given subcutaneously on days 5-9 PG at 2 hours before and 2 hours after the dark phase. The body temperature was monitored (days 9-10 PG) and analyzed by Dataquest computation. Uterine protein and progesterone were assayed on day 10PG. Results indicated that melatonin promoted significant modifications ($p<0.05$) in the body temperature profiles and parameters (mesor, amplitude and acrophase) and significantly affected uterine protein and progesterone ($p<0.05$) on the altered photoperiods, especially in 8L:16D.

P1.63

TRANSCRIPTION OF *ICER*, AN EARLY RESPONSE REPRESSOR OF THE NEUROENDOCRINE AXIS, IS MARKEDLY ENHANCED BY CYCLOHEXIMIDE *IN VITRO* AND *IN VIVO*. S.L. Coon, P.H. Roseboom and D.C. Klein. Section on Neuroendocrinology, Laboratory of Developmental Neurobiology, NICHD, National Institutes of Health, Bethesda, Maryland, 20892, USA .

The newest member of the CREM family of transcription factors to be identified is ICER, a strong and inducible repressor of cAMP regulated promoters, which is highly expressed in neuroendocrine tissues. In the rat, ICER expression is highest in the pineal gland, where it is induced at night by NE acting through cAMP. Thus ICER negatively autoregulates its own transcription. Accordingly, we report here that the protein synthesis inhibitor (PSI), cycloheximide, augments the induction of ICER transcription by NE in cultured pineal glands. Interestingly, cycloheximide (CHX) by itself induces accumulation of ICER transcripts in less than one hour and levels continue to rise for at least 6 hours. In contrast, other PSI's, such as anisomysin, puromycin, emetine, and exotoxin A, have no apparent effect on the level of ICER transcripts, indicating that induction by CHX is not due to inhibition of protein synthesis. In addition, *in vivo* administration of CHX increases ICER transcript levels in pineal, pituitary and adrenal glands, but not in other tissues. Thus, CHX regulates ICER expression through a novel pathway that is selectively functional in neuroendocrine tissues.

P1.64

NOCTURNAL SERUM MELATONIN LEVELS IN WOMEN WITH PCOD. C.T. Erel, H. Seyisoglu, T. Irez, U. Colgar, E. Ertüngealp. Dept of Obstet. & Gynecol, Cerrahpasa Faculty of Medicine Istanbul/Turkey

We have investigated if there is a nocturnal change of melatonin mainly secreted by pineal gland in women with polycystic ovarian disease (PCOD). Woman with PCOD (n=5) and normal subjects (n=3) were included. The blood was sampled between 20.00 and 08.00 by two hours intervals. The serum melatonin levels were determined by RIA in both groups. In PCOD group, the nocturnal mean melatonin peak value was 172/74 pg/ml and the secretion pattern was irregular. Whereas in the control group, the mean peak value was 217, 30 pg/ml and reached its peak value at 24.00. The mean serum melatonin levels at 02.00 and 06.00 a.m. were 34,5 pg/ml, 16,84 pg/ml for women with PCOD and 2,46 pg/ml, 0,69 pg/ml for normal subjects, respectively. When we compared the two groups in terms of serum melatonin levels, we found a significant increase in women with PCOD at 02.00 and 06.00 (p<0.05). We could not find any significant change at the other hours. We assume that melatonin can have an important impact on aetiology of PCOD by both dopaminergic and opioidergic mechanisms.

P1.65

INVOLVEMENT OF DIFFERENT CYTOKINES ON THE ENDOTOXIN-STIMULATED HYPOTHALAMO-PITUITARY-ADRENAL (HPA) AXIS FUNCTION.

R. Hadid* (1), E. Spinedi (1), J-M Dayer (2), G. Grau (3), R-C Gaillard (1). (1) Division of Endocrinology and Metabolism, Department of Medicine, CHUV, CH-1011 Lausanne, (2) Division of Immunology, Department of Medicine, HCUG, CH-1211 Geneva, and (3) Department of Pathology, Geneva University Medical Center, CH-1211 Geneva, Switzerland.

Controversy exists within the literature regarding the role of different cytokines on the endotoxin (LPS)-stimulated hypothalamo-pituitary-adrenal (HPA) axis activity. The discrepancies may be related to the fact that the effects of cytokines vary during the time after LPS administration. This study was performed in order to determine the role of 3 differents cytokines, tumor necrosis factor alpha (TNF), interleukin-1 (IL-1) and IL-6, on the HPA axis response at 2 and 6 h after LPS injection. Adult male BALB/c mice were injected i.p. with 25 µg of LPS or saline. Among them, groups of 6-8 mice were injected (i.p.),12 h before endotoxin treatment, with antibodies against either TNF, IL-1 or IL-6. Mice were then killed after 2 or 6 hours after LPS administration. Plasma ACTH and corticosterone (B) concentrations were measured by specific assays. Our results showed that none of the antibodies used modified the LPS-induced ACTH and B levels 2 hours after administration. In contrast 6 hours after endotoxin injection, TNF and IL-1 antibodies significantly inhibited B secretion in blood , and in addition TNF antibody significantly decreased plasma ACTH levels. In preliminary experiments, IL-6 antibody had no effect on LPS-elicited stress hormone rise in plasma at any time-period studied. In summary, we observed that TNF and IL-1, but not IL-6, could be involved in the early response of the HPA axis under the endotoxic shock; however, the effect of the quenching of these cytokines was only observed 6 h after endotoxin administration.

P1.66

PURIFICATION AND IN VITRO TRANSLATION OF RAT CORTICOTROPHIN-RELEASING FACTOR FROM THYMIC CELLS.

E. W. Hillhouse* & N.G.N. Milton, Department of Molecular Pathology, University College London and *Department of Medicine, University of Bristol.

We have recently demonstrated a role for a thymic derived corticotrophin-releasing factor (CRF) in the immune responses to pyrogenic interferon inducers. In the present study we sought to purify and characterize the biological nature of this peripheral CRF. Rat thymic cells were activated in vitro with polyinosinic: polycytidylic acid [poly (I) poly (C)]. Poly-A+ mRNA was isolated from activated cells and subjected to in vitro translation using a rabbit reticulocyte lysate system. Thymic CRF was affinity purified from either culture medium or in vitro translation extracts on a monoclonal anti-CRF column and subjected to size exclusion HPLC, SDS-PAGE analysis and immunoassay using an enzyme amplified immunometric assay (EAIA) for rat CRF. In vitro translation showed that poly-A+mRNA from poly (I) poly (C) activated thymic cells produced ir-CRF. Chromatography of the form released into culture medium showed the presence of a 31kDa protein which could be reduced with 2-mercaptoethanol, to a 15kDa protein. This material displayed CRF immunoreactivity and bioactivity and was able to stimulate the release of ACTH and PGE_2 from the rat anterior pituitary gland.

P1.67

NEUROENDOCRINE AND NEUROPHARMACOLOGICAL STUDIES ON BRAIN-IMMUNO-ENDOCRINE INTERACTIONS IN RATS.

J.M.H.M. Reul*, A.C.E. Linthorst. Max Planck Institute of Psychiatry, Clinical Institute, Department of Neuroendocrinology, 80804 Munich, FRG.

During disease a balanced interaction between the brain, immune system and the HPA system is critical to maintain homeostasis. I.p. lipopolysaccharide (LPS) injection stimulates macrophages and other immune cells to produce cytokines such as IL-1ß, IL-6 and TNF-*α*, which are thought to affect brain function. The combined use of *in vivo* microdialysis and biotelemetrics permits a detailed study of neuropharmacological and autonomic changes in freely moving animals. In addition, we established to continuously monitor HPA system activity by measurement of free corticosterone levels in the dialysate. We observed that i.p. LPS produced a marked dose-dependent increase in the activity of the raphe-hippocampal serotonergic system, as evidenced by elevated extracellular hippocampal levels of serotonin (5-HT) and its metabolite 5-hydroxyindoleacetic acid (5-HIAA). These changes were accompanied by rises in free corticosterone levels and body temperature, and signs of sickness behavior, such as reduced locomotor activity, curled body posture and piloerection. These effects could be largely mimicked by i.c.v. IL-1ß injection, whereas i.c.v. pretreatment with the IL-1 receptor antagonist (IL-1ra) blocked all effects of IL-1ß, except the pyrogenic response. These data may point to an important role of the hippocampus in the processing of immune stress. To study further the role of this limbic brain structure, we applied IL-1ß directly into the hippocampus (or neocortex as a control) via the microdialysis probe. It was found that IL-1ß in the hippocampus, but not in the neocortex, increased local 5-HT levels, and most interestingly, produced fever and a marked activation of the HPA system. We postulate that the hippocampus plays a principal role in the coordination of neuroendocrine, autonomic and behavioral responses after an immune challenge. (Supported by VW I/68 430).

P1.68

INTERLEUKIN-1-INDUCED RELEASE OF PROSTAGLANDIN E2 IN THE RAT HYPOTHALAMUS IS MEDIATED BY INTERLEUKIN-1 TYPE-II RECEPTORS.

A. Mirtella, G. Pozzoli, L. Parente*, P. Preziosi and P. Navarra. Institute of Pharmacology, Catholic University Medical School, Rome and *IRIS Research Center, Siena, Italy.

In the present study, we have investigated whether the increase of prostaglandin E2 (PGE2) release induced by interleukin-1 (IL-1) from acute rat hypothalamic explants (Navarra <u>et al</u>., Neuroendocrinol. 56: 61, 1992) is mediated by the activation of IL-1 type-II receptors. IL-1β (50 ng/ml) was given alone or in the presence of 10 µg/ml of a monoclonal antiserum raised against human type-II receptor (ALVA 42).

Data are expressed as the mean (± SEM, n=9) ratios of PGE2 released in the presence of test substances in 20-min incubations to that released in the previous 20 min. ** P<0.01 vs Control. Control: 1.55 ± 0.10; IL-1β, 50 ng/ml: 2.05 ± 0.10**; ALVA-42, 10 µg/ml: 1.55 ± 0.09; IL-1β + ALVA-42 as above: 1.75 ± 0.08.

This finding suggests that some effects of IL-1 in the hypothalamus, such as increased PGE2 release, might be mediated by type-II receptors.

Supported by CNR, grant 93.00357.CT04

P1.69

PERIPHERAL AND CENTRAL EXPRESSION OF INTERLEUKIN 6 IN LPS-TREATED RATS. B. Schöbitz*, G. Pezeshki, E.R. de Kloet[1], F. Holsboer and J.M.H.M. Reul, Max Planck Institute of Psychiatry, Clinical Institute, 80804 Munich, Germany and [1]Leiden-Amsterdam Center for Drug Research, Division of Medical Pharmacology, University Leiden, The Netherlands.

Nonspecific activation of the immune system by bacterial constituents, such as lipopolysaccharide (LPS), is associated with rapid induction of the pleiotropic cytokine interleukin 6 (IL6). It has been observed that the magnitude of the inflammatory response to LPS in a given tissue is reflected by the IL6 or IL6 mRNA level. The cytokine activates lymphocytes and induces the hepatic acute-phase reaction and contributes to neuroendocrine, behavioural and metabolic changes during infections. We studied the distribution of IL6- and IL6 receptor mRNAs in the brain of healthy rats by *in situ* hybridization. Both messages were found in neurons in hippocampus, hypothalamus, cerebellum and other brain areas. Northern blot analyses were performed with RNA isolated from spleen, adrenals, pituitary gland, hypothalamus, hippocampus and cerebellum of rats injected intraperitoneally with LPS. A rapid induction of IL6 mRNA was observed in peripheral organs, whereas no increase could be measured in the brain. However, when IL6 was injected directly into the lateral ventricle of the rat brain, IL6 mRNA was induced in cortex, hippocampus and hypothalamus, but also in spleen. We conclude that peripherally administered LPS does not cause a significant inflammatory response in the brain. The central effects of IL6 during systemic infection seem to be caused by mechanisms that do not involve transcription of the IL6 gene. However, under conditions when LPS appears in the CNS, e.g. during bacterial meningitis, the brain is probably capable to synthesize large amounts of the cytokine.

P1.70

INTERLEUKINS CONCENTRATIONS IN BLOOD OF PATIENTS WITH PARKINSON'S DISEASE.

G. Stypuła*, H. Stępień, K. Żylińska, M. Pawlikowski, J. Kunert-Radek. Neurological Department of District Hospital Morawica-Kielce*, Institute of Endocrinology, University School of Medicine, 91-425 Łódź, Poland.

Parkinson's disease (PD) is characterized by markedly decreased number of nigrostriatal dopaminergic neurons. The pathogenesis of PD is still unknown. Among other etiological factors immunological abnormalities have also been suggested. Recently Lapchak (NeuroReport 3, 165, 1992) suggest that interleukin-2 (IL-2) may be an endogenous neurokine that regulates striatal dopaminergic function. We examined the concentrations of ILs: 1, 2, 6 and ACTH, cortisol, prolactin levels in blood of 21 new-registered (non-treated previously) patients with PD (7F, 14M, age 64 ± 9.2 years). An age- and sex-matched 25 person group without any neurological or immunological disease was used as control. ILs were measured using Amersham (England) RIA kits, sensitivity 2.5 fmol/ml. Significantly higher concentration of IL-2 in sera of the patients with PD was found (control - 9.6 ± 4.4, PD patients -$25{,}9 \pm 14{,}4$ fmol/ml, $p < 0.01$ - Aspin-Welch test). No differences of concentration of IL-1, IL-6 and examined hormonal parameters were detected. In PD patients treatment with L-dopa or amantadine reduced IL-2 concentrations. These findings suggest the functional relationship between central dopaminergic and immune systems.

Supported by University School of Medicine, Łódź, Poland, Grant No 502-11-008.

P1.71

DATA SUGGESTING THE PRETERM PARTURITION MAY ALTER THE BIOACTIVE PRL IN RAT MILK Veress Z., Majoros A., Oláh Z., Tóth E.B., Grosvenor C.E.. 2nd Dept. of Anatomy, Semmelweis Univ. Medical School, Budapest 1094 Hungary, Dept. of Molecular and Cell Biology Penn. State University PA 16802, USA

In case of preterm parturition the development of the mammary epithelium may be incomplete to produce milk proteins and biologically active compounds. In our experiments we investigated the altered forms of prolactin in milk obtained from lactating rats after an artificial preterm parturition induced by ovariectomy on the days 17-18 of pregnancy. The gel-filtration chromatography of day-2 milk samples resulted in differences in the number and amount of bioactive PRL variants. The preterm milk exhibited a wide range of bioactive weight variants between 7.3 and 95 kDa with maximal levels at less than 24 kDa, which is the approximate weight of monomeric PRL. In normal day-2 (term) milk the weight ranged between 14.3 and 95 kDa with maximal levels higher than 27 kDa. Neither serum prolactin levels, nor secreted PRL from pituitaries of ovariectomised and SHAM operated rats into DMEM medium during a 2- and 12-hour period in tissue culture did not show significant difference. The difference of extracted PRL of those pituitaries also were non significant. These data suggest that the concentrations of bioactive PRL forms of milk, like the levels of other milk components, are highly influenced by the developmental stage of mammary epithelium, regardless to the serum PRL levels. (Supported partly by NIH grant to C.E.G..)

P1.72

EFFECT OF MILK AND PROLACTIN ON MITOGEN INDUCED LYMPHOCYTE PROLIFERATION IN VITRO B.E.Toth, Z.Forrai, A.Szeghalmi, B.Kacsoh, B.Bour, C.E.Grosvenor, Dept.2. of Anatomy, Semmelweis University Med. School, Budapest 1094, Hungary; Dept. Molecular and Cell Biology, Penn State University, University Park, PA 16802 USA

Milk infranatant obtained from lactating rats on the days of 2 and 20 postpartum were tested in cell proliferation assays. Group of 100-120-day-old male, cycling- ovariectomised- and lactating female rats were used as a lymphocyte donor. Mitogen induced cell proliferation was measured by the H3-thymidine uptake after a 24+40 h assay and pulse period, while in the same type of assay the cells were counted by a cell counter on a consequent three days. The mitogen stimulated H3-thymidine incorporation, as well as the proliferation of the cells were inhibited in a dose-dependent manner by day 20 rat milk infranatant. Coincubation of day 2 milk resulted only stimulation over the levels of resulted by the mitogen alone. Prolactin in a concentration of 10-500 ng/ml administered to the mitogen assay had no significant effect in lymphocytes of male rats but stimulated in case of the OVX or early proestrus donors. Similar type of anti-proliferative effect were demonstrated in our previous reports when rat milk was tested on the PRL sensitive Nb2 (originally T-lymphoma) cells. These data suggest that the mitogen induced response of lymphocytes altered by the endocrine status of donors. Endocrine factors, present in serum and milk as well as their receptors may have an important role in the regulation of lymphocytes in adults and in the mother-neonate interaction. (In parts supported by NIH grant to CEG)

P2.1

Nitric oxide synthase in the anterior pituitary and the role of nitric oxide in regulation of hormone secretion from the anterior pituitary. A.L. Hulting, S. Ceccatelli, L. Gustafsson, E. Theodorsson, T. Hökfelt. Dept. of Molecular Medicine and Neuroscience, Karolinska Institute, S-171 77 Stockholm, Sweden.

Using immunohistochemistry and in situ hybridisation, the nitric oxide (NO)-synthesizing enzyme NOS has been demonstrated in rat gonadotrophs with a marked increase in NOS protein and mRNA levels after gonadectomy. In addition, NOS was also found in folliculo-stellate cells of rat anterior pituitary. In monkey anterior pituitary, NOS is present in corticotrophs.

Analysis of the effect of NO on rat LH secretion in vitro showed that the NOS inhibitor MeArg markedly potentiated GnRH induced LH secretion, and the NO donor SNP reduced the GnRH stimulated LH release. In cultivated monkey anterior pituitary cells, MeArg had no clear effect on ACTH secretion, whereas SNP significantly inhibited CRH stimulated ACTH release. In addition, Hb, which binds NO, markedly stimulated basal ACTH secretion.

These observations suggest that NO may be synthesized in the anterior pituitary playing a role in the control of anterior pituitary hormone secretion. The results also point at an autocrine action of NO, both in rats and monkeys, NO being produced in rat gonadotrophs and monkey corticotrophs influencing LH- and ACTH secretion, respectively.

P2.2

NEUROENDOCRINE RESPONSE TO HYPOGLYCEMIA: POTENTIATION BY INCREASED ENVIRONMENTAL TEMPERATURE. D. Ježová*, K. Nazar, R. Kvetňanský, M. Vigaš. Institute od Experimental Endocrinology, Slovak Academy of Sciences, Bratislava, Slovakia, 83306.

To evaluate the influence of a slight increase in body temperature on neuroendocrine response to stressful stimuli, healthy male volunteers participated in two randomized trials. In the first trial, insulin-induced hypoglycemia was performed at room temperature. In the second trial, the subjects were exposed to ambient temperature of 53 °C for 45 min before insulin injection and 45 min thereafter. Increased ambient temperature failed to modify basal hormone levels and only slight rise in body temperature occurred at the end of exposure. Under conditions of increased ambient temperature insulin injection induced less severe hypoglycemia. In spite of this, responses of most but not all hormones to hypoglycemia were exaggerated. Sympathetic-adrenomedullary system was significantly activated which was manifested particularly by enhanced norepinephrine release. The huge increase in ACTH and ß-endorphin release was not accompanied by concomitant increase of plasma cortisol response. Growth hormone response to hypoglycemia was not modified while that of prolactin was enhanced. Though the mechanisms involved are not known, it is clear that mild increase in environmental temperature results in increased sensitivity of neuroendocrine system to other stress stimuli.

P2.3

DISSOCIATION IN THE SITES AND MECHANISMS OF PITUITARY HORMONE SECRETORY ACTIONS OF ALPHA2-ADRENOCEPTOR ANTAGONISTS. Kiem D.T., Barna I., and Makara G.B. Institute of Experimental Medicine, Hungarian Academy of Sciences, Budapest (Hungary.)

We studied the effect of glucocorticoid pretreatment, mediobasal hypothalamus lesion (MBHL) and the clonidine-yohimbine interaction on the α2-antagonists-induced ACTH, ß-endorphin and PRL secretion in male Wistar rats to elucidate the sites, modes and/or mechanisms of actions of α2-antagonists. The pretreatment of 1 mg/kg s.c. dexamethasone for 4 days effectively prevented the stimulatory effect of α2-antagonists yohimbine (5 mg/kg i.p.) and CH-38083 (1 mg/kg i.p.) on ACTH secretion, while, PRL and ß-endorphin actions of these antagonists remained unchanged. The central pretreatment of 5 μg/rat clonidine failed to antagonize the PRL and ß-endorphin releasing effect of yohimbine. However, it prevented the ACTH action of this drug. MBH lesion resulted in a significant enhancement in basal plasma PRL levels. However, basal plasma ACTH levels have not been changed in MBH lesioned animals. Yohimbine failed to stimulate ACTH secretion in MBH lesioned animals, while PRL and ß-endorphin response to yohimbine was potentiated in these animals. We suggest that the α2-antagonists stimulate ACTH secretion by a corticosteroid-sensitive mechanism located at central level. They affect PRL and ß-endorphin secretion at peripheral level independently from central control.

P2.4

HORMONE SECRETION OF CULTURED HUMAN PITUITARY CELLS. I. Nagy, E. Bácsy, A. Gyévai, A. Kittel, M. Szabó, M. Kurcz. Heim Pál Pediatric Hospital and Inst. of Experimental Medicine, Budapest, Hungary

Mammotrophs and somatotrophs were originally described as two morphologically and immunocytochemically distinct cell types; a partial co-localization or co-secretion of the two hormones was later recognized in a number of species. The data on mammo-somatotrophs in the normal adult human pituitary are scarce and usually derived from para-adenomatous non-tumorous tissue. In order to define more closely the cell-biological status of the mammo-somatotrophs we developed primary cultures of dispersed human adenohypophyseal cells collected from the bodies of adult individuals within two hours after sudden death. The cells were responsive to 10^{-7} M somatostatin and bromocryptine but did not significantly react to 10^{-8} M somatoliberin as judged by GH and PRL immunoassays in the medium. The cultures were fixed, embedded in Epon, then GH and PRL were localized with a double immunogold procedure.

Our results show that adult human pituitary cells obtained from cadavers of individuals without known endocrine alterations preserve their morphological differentiation, their capacity to release GH and PRL, and to respond with decreased release to somatostatin and bromocriptine, respectively. Cells storing one of the two hormones alone belong to two morphologically consistent cell types. Some cells in each of them contains the other hormone as well, in the same storage granule. We think therefore that no separate and consistent mammo-somatotroph cell population exists but the cells differentiated as somatotrophs or mammotrophs preserve the ability to secrete the other hormone as well, depending on normal or pathological physiological circumstances.

Acknowledgement. This work was supported by the Hungarian national grants OTKA 2917 and ETK T-10 T337/1990.

P2.5

THE INFLUENCE OF αT3-1-CELL-CONDITIONED MEDIUM ON THE DEVELOPMENT OF LACTOTROPHS, CORTICOTROPHS AND SOMATOTROPHS IN NORMAL PITUITARY CELL AGGREGATES.

C. Bert*, M Andries, D. Tilemans, C. Denef.
Laboratory of Cell Pharmacology, University of Leuven, Medical School, Leuven, Belgium.

We have previously shown in rat pituitary reaggregated cell cultures that growth and differentiation of lactotrophs, corticotrophs and somatotrophs may be influenced during postnatal development by paracrine factors secreted by the gonadotrophs. Since αT3-1 cells are a gonadotrophic, α-subunit secreting, pituitary cell line, we tested whether α T3-1 cell conditioned medium could influence growth in the above mentioned anterior pituitary cell types.
We report that addition of αT3-1 cell-conditioned medium to reaggregate pituitary cell cultures of 14-day-old rats is capable of stimulating the number of ^{3}H-thymidine (^{3}H-T) incorporating lactotrophs and inhibiting the number of ^{3}H-T incorporating somatotrophs.
In contrast to gonadotroph-conditioned medium the αT3-1 cell-conditioned medium caused a dose dependent decrease in ^{3}H-T labeling of corticotrophs .
Culture medium with only 5% conditioned medium was already able to increase the number of ^{3}H-T labeled lactotrophs ($p<0.005$), whereas 20% conditioned medium was necessary to decrease the number of ^{3}H-T labeled somatotrophs ($p<0.05$). These observations suggest that αT3-1 cells emanate paracrine growth factors influencing the development of lactotrophs and somatotrophs in a similar way as normal gonadotrophs Since the αT3-1 cell line might be derived from a progenitor of the gonadotrophs, they may provide a good in vitro model for the putative influence of this gonadotroph precursor on the early development of the pituitary gland.

P2.6

EGF RELEASE FROM RAT GONADOTROPES IS ENHANCED BY LHRH. A. Mouihate*, D. Verrier, F. Valeins, J. Lestage. INSERM U 394. Laboratoire de Neurobiologie Intégrative. 33077 Bordeaux Cedex FRANCE

The anterior pituitary gland (AP) has been described as a site of synthesis and release of EGF. However, little was known until now about cellular origin of EGF. In this report, AP cells were dissociated from 14 day old female rats and EGF release was tested using reverse hemolytic plaque assay (RHPA). Small plaques were spontaneously formed by a large proportion of AP cells. The stimulation of EGF release by luteinizing hormone releasing hormone (LHRH) at 10 nM was evaluated by the hemolyse area formed around EGF secreting cells. A combination of RHPA and immunocytochemistry indicated that a high proportion of plaque forming cells are LH containing cells. These data demonstrate that EGF release is mainly produced by gonadotrophs and that EGF release is enhanced by LHRH. Thus, it can be suggested that one hypothalamic secretagogue is able to induce secretion of more than one polypeptide from its pituitary target cell. This study raises questions about the concept of specificity between hypothalamic secretagogues and their anterior pituitary target cells in terms of specific hormone induced release.

P2.7

SYNAPTIC CONTACTS BETWEEN SP-LIKE IMMUNOREACTIVE NERVE FIBERS AND THE GLAND CELLS IN THE ANTERIOR PITUITARY OF THE RAT. G. Ju*, Y-.Y. Liu. Dept. of Neurobiology, Institute of Neurosciences, 4th Military Medical University, Xi'an, PR China, 710032

Our previous studies have discovered substantial amounts of peptidergic nerve fibers in the anterior pituitary in several mammalian species. EM studies in the dog have further demonstrated that SP- and CGRP-LI nerve fibers make synaptic contacts with corticotropes and somatotropes. Moreover, the CGRP-LI nerve fibers of the anterior pituitary have been found to increase in amount following adrenalectomy in the rat. In the present study the synaptic relationship of SP-LI nerve fiber of the anterior pituitary were examined in the rat. The nerve fibers were unmyelinated and varicose. Direct contacts between the nerve fibers and every cell type of the gland, including folliculostellate cells, could be ascertained. Typical asymmetrical synapses were identified, with small clear vesicles and large dense cored vesicles. Prominent subsynaptic dense bodies were common, often merged into a plate. Most of the synapses were found on lactotropes. A few were also identified on somatotropes, gonadotropes, and corticotropes. This is quite different from our early findings in the dog, in which corticotropes and somatotropes were the only cell types bearing synapses, and more frequently the former. The results prove morphologically that direct neural factor may play a role in the regulation of the anterior pituitary in the rat. The difference between rat and dog in the type of synapse bearing gland cells may be related to the difference in the environment they confront with.

P2.8

EFFECTS OF INTRAVENOUS ADMINISTRATION OF INTERLEUKIN-1β ON THE RELEASE OF PROSTAGLANDIN E_2 , CORTICOTROPIN-RELEASING FACTOR , AND ARGININE VASOPRESSIN IN SEVERAL HYPOTHALAMIC AREAS OF FREELY MOVING RATS : ESTIMATION BY PUSH-PULL PERFUSION.

H. Watanobe*, S. Sasaki , K. Takebe. Third Department of Internal Medicine, Hirosaki University School of Medicine, Hirosaki, Japan, 036

Utilizing the push-pull perfusion technique, we examined the effect of iv bolus injection of recombinant human interleukin(IL)-1β on the release of prostaglandin E_2 (PGE_2), CRF, and AVP in several hypothalamic areas of freely moving rats, simultaneously monitoring plasma ACTH levels. Hypothalamic areas we perfused were the median eminence(ME), the paraventricular nucleus(PVN), and the medial preoptic area(MPOA). During the period of 12:00-15:00 h, perfusates and blood samples were collected every 10 min(between 13:00-13:40 h) or 20 min(between 12:00-13:00 h, and between 13:40-15:00 h). IL-1β (1.0 μg/rat) or vehicle only (in control groups) was injected at 13:00 h. In both the ME and the PVN but not in the MPOA, the outputs of CRF and AVP were significantly stimulated by IL-1β, prior to the rise in plasma ACTH. A significant stimulation of PGE_2 by IL-1β was observed only in the PVN, and its temporal profile was very similar to those of CRF and AVP in the PVN. These results suggest that PGE_2 increased in the PVN may be a trigger for the activation of CRF and AVP neurons, and thereby ACTH secretion, which follow IL-1β injection.

P2.9

MODULATION BY GONADAL STEROIDS OF INTERLEUKIN-1β-INDUCED ACTH RESPONSE IN MALE AND FEMALE RATS.

J. Anzai*, H. Watanobe, T. Nigawara, S. Habu, K. Takebe. Third Department of Internal Medicine, Hirosaki University School of Medicine, Hirosaki, Japan 036

Sexual dimorphism exists in both ACTH and corticosterone responses to stress, with females having higher levels than males. However, it has yet to be determined whether the immune-hypothalamo-pituitary-adrenal axis is also sexually diverse. Therefore, in this study we examined in the rat a possible sex difference in ACTH response to interleukin(IL)-1β, and also a possible role of endogenous gonadal steroids in determining the response. For comparison, we also examined whether immobilization stress-induced ACTH response can be affected by the gonadal steroid milieu. Human recombinant IL-1β (3μg/kg) was given as an iv bolus injection, and the duration of immobilization stress employed was 30 min. ACTH response to IL-1β was significantly higher in females than in males. Various treatments for both sexes which comprised gonadectomy alone and sex steroid replacement after gonadectomy provided data suggesting that roles of testosterone, estradiol, and progesterone in determining the ACTH response to IL-1β were inhibitory, stimulatory, and inhibitory, respectively. By contrast, neither a sexual difference nor a modulation by sex steroid milieu was demonstrated in the ACTH response to immobilization stress. These results suggest that physiological levels of gonadal steroids can significantly affect the CNS mechanism which governs the IL-1β-induced ACTH response in the rat.

P2.10

CLINICAL SIGNIFICANCE OF THE GROWTH HORMONE RESPONSE TO VASOACTIVE INTESTINAL PEPTIDE (VIP) AND GONADOTROPIN-RELEASING HORMONE (GnRH) IN ACROMEGALY

S.Habu*, H.Watanobe, T.Tamura, K.Takebe. Third Department of Internal Medicine, Hirosaki University School of Medicine (SH, HW, KT),Hirosaki, Japan, 036; and Department of Neurosurgery, Brain Research Institute, Niigata University(TT), Niigata Japan, 951

The pathophysiological significance of GH responses to TRH, GHRH, and bromocriptine (Br) in acromegaly is relatively well established. However, this is not the case with the GH responses to VIP and GnRH. Therefore, in this study we performed iv bolus injections of TRH (500μg), GHRH (100μg), VIP (100μg), and GnRH (100μg), and a peroral administration of Br (2.5mg) in 52 patients with active acromegaly, in order to determine possible relationships among the GH responses to these tests. There was a significant correlation that the higher was the GH response after TRH the greater was the GH decrease after Br. There was a trend that the higher was the GH response after GHRH the smaller was the GH decrease after Br. In addition, as novel findings, we observed that the GH responses to GHRH, VIP, and GnRH were in significant positive correlations to each other, and that the higher were the GH responses after VIP and GnRH the smaller was the GH decrease after Br. In agreement with this, we also found that a simultanous GH responsivity to VIP and/or GnRH in TRH-responsive acromegalics significantly enhanced the GH response to GHRH and lowered the Br responsiveness compared to the data of pure TRH-responders. From these results,we hypothesize that the positive GH responsiveness to VIP and GnRH, like that to GHRH, may be a feature of the somatotroph-like pituitary adenoma causing acromegaly.

P2.11

A REEVALUATION OF THE MECHANISM BY WHICH INTRAVENOUSLY ADMINISTERED INDOMETHACIN INHIBITS INTERLEUKIN-1-INDUCED ACTH RESPONSE IN THE RAT.

R.Nasushita*, H.Watanobe, K.Takebe. Third Department of Internal Medicine, Hirosaki University School of Medicine, Hirosaki, Japan, 036

It is now well established that interleukin(IL)-1 has a stimulatory effect on the hypothalamo-pituitary-adrenal axis in the rat. Several previous studies reporting that the IL-1-induced ACTH response was abolished or markedly suppressed by a prior iv injection of indomethacin(indo), a cyclooxygenase inhibitor, were construed as suggesting a pivotal role of prostaglandins(PGs) in the hormonal response. However, Rivier and Vale (Endocrinology 129: 384, 1991) reported that the inhibitory effect of indo was mediated principally by a fast negative feedback effect of corticosterone(B) which increases after indo, rather than by decreased PG synthesis. In the present study, we aimed to test this hypothesis. In agreement with earlier reports, iv bolus injection of indo(10 mg/kg) caused a significant rise in B levels 10-30 min postadministration without affecting ACTH secretion.ACTH response to iv injection of recombinant human IL-1β (3 μg/kg) was significantly suppressed by a prior injection of indo given at either 10 or 20 min before, and the latter protocol led to a more marked suppression of the ACTH response than the former. However, the initial rising slope of B after IL-1β was almost the same between the two treatments. These results suggest that the inhibitory effect of indo on IL-1β-induced ACTH response may be exerted primarily via PG synthesis inhibition rather than via negative feedback effect of B.

P2.12

A STUDY ON THE ROLE OF ARGININE VASOPRESSIN (AVP), OXYTOCIN (OT), ANGIOTENSIN Ⅱ (A Ⅱ), AND CHOLECYSTOKININ (CCK)-8 IN INTERLEUKIN (IL)-1β-INDUCED ACTH SECRETION IN THE RAT

S.Sasaki*, H.Watanobe, R.Nasushita, J.Anzai, K.Kageyama, S.Sakihara, T.Nigawara, K.Takebe. Third Department of Internal Medicine, Hirosaki University School of Medicine, Hirosaki, Japan, 036

It has been repeatedly shown that activation of hypothalamic CRH neurons at least partially mediates IL-1 stimulation of ACTH secretion in the rat. However, little is known about whether other neuropeptides in the brain possessing an ACTH-releasing activity are also involved in this response. Therefore, in this study we examined a possible role of AVP, OT, A Ⅱ, and CCK-8 in the IL-1β stimulation of ACTH secretion in the rat, utilizing immunoneutralization of these peptides. For comparison, we reexamined the effect of CRH immunoneutralization. Human recombinant IL-1β(50 ng/5μl) was administered into the third ventricle (icv) 15 min after an icv injection of normal rabbit serum(NRS), or specific antisera against CRH, AVP, OT, A Ⅱ, or CCK-8, respectively. NRS and all the antisera(undiluted) were given in a volume of 5μl. Blood was drawn through an indwelling jugular vein catheter at -15, 0, 10, 20, 30, 60, 90, and 120 min after the IL-1β injection, and plasma ACTH levels were determined. In NRS + IL-1β group, a significant stimulation of ACTH secretion was observed. Compared to the effect of NRS, a significant reduction of ACTH response was observed after anti-CRH, AVP, and A Ⅱ antisera but not after anti-OT and CCK-8 antisera. There results suggest that in addition to CRH, AVP and A Ⅱ may also mediate the IL-1β stimulation of ACTH secretion in the rat.

P2.13

TIME COURSE OF INDUCTION OF ACTH AND ACTIVATION OF FOS-EXPRESSION IN ENDOTOXIC SHOCK. Zs. Némethy and K.J. Kovács, Institute of Experimental Medicine Budapest, Hungary.

Infections result a big array of centrally mediated adaptive changes, including activation of hypothalamo-pituitary-adrenal axis. As a model of sepsis, rats were challenged by intraperitoneal or intravenous injection of bacterial lipopolysaccharide, (LPS). Plasma ACTH levels were measured by RIA, and activated neurons within the brain were visualized by FOS immunocytochemistry. Intraperitoneal injection of 2.5 mg/kg LPS significantly elevates plasma ACTH with a peak between 2-4 hours after the injection, while intravenous injection of 0.5 mg/kg LPS results more rapid induction of ACTH secretion (maximum between 30-90 min). Activation of Fos expression was detected 2 hours after LPS challenge in the preoptic and anterior hypothalamic areas as well as cells in the surrounding of the supraoptic and paraventricular (PVN) nuclei. 4 hours after ip LPS parvocellular neurons within the medial and dorsal subdivisions of the PVN were intensively labeled, Fos immunoreactive neurons were found in the arcuate nucleus. Scattered immunostaining was detected in the supraoptic nuclei, and in the central amygdala. Fos immunoreactivity disappeared by 8-24 hours from all regions.
Our data indicate in septic shock results activation of neurons involved in the regulation of pituitary ACTH secretion and induction of ACTH secretion preceeds the induction of immediate-early gene product Fos after immunologic challenge.

P2.14

MODULATION OF CORTICOTROPIN-RELEASING FACTOR AND INTERLEUKIN-1 RECEPTORS BY ETHER-LAPAROTOMY STRESS IN THE MOUSE BRAIN-ENDOCRINE-IMMUNE AXIS. T. Takao*, C. Tojo, T. Nishioka, H. Kurokawa, K. Hashimoto, E.B. De Souza. Second Dept of Internal Medicine, Kochi Medical School, Kochi, Japan 783 and Neurocrine Biosciences, Inc., San Diego, CA, USA 92121

Previous study demonstrated the upregulation of interleukin-1 (IL-1) receptors following treatment with corticotropin-releasing factor (CRF) in mouse AtT-20 pituitary tumor cells *in vitro*. In order to investigate whether the same upregulation can be observed *in vivo*, we utilized C57/BL6 mice with or without the treatment of ether-laparotomy. Ether-laparotomy stress resulted in a dramatic decrease in specific iodine-125-labeled ovine CRF binding ($[^{125}I]$oCRF) in the anterior lobe of the pituitary at 2 h after the onset of the stress. However, $[^{125}I]$oCRF binding was unchanged in the frontal cortex at 2 h after the stress. In contrast, iodine-125-labeled recombinant human IL-1α ($[^{125}I]$IL-1α) binding was increased in the anterior lobe of the pituitary at 2 h after the onset of the stress. $[^{125}I]$IL-1α binding in hippocampus, spleen and testis was unchanged at 2 h after the stress. Plasma adrenocorticotropic hormone (ACTH) and corticosterone were increased at 2 h after the onset of the stress. In summary, these data demonstrate complex interactions between CRF and IL-1 on ACTH secretion at the pituitary level and identify potential novel mechanisms for cytokines to alter neuroendocrine function.

P2.15

SYNERGISTIC EFFECTS OF INTERLEUKIN-1 AND TUMOR NECROSIS FACTOR ON THE ACTIVITY OF THE PITUITARY-ADRENAL AXIS. M. v.d. Meer*, C. Sweep, G. Pesman, A. Hermus. Dept. of Medicine, Div. of Endo and Dept. of Exp. & Chem. Endo, Univ. Hosp. Nijmegen, The Netherlands.

Interleukin-1ß (IL1) and tumor necrosis factor-α (TNF) are important mediators of biological effects of lipopolysaccharides (activation of the pituitary-adrenal axis and induction of fever, anorexia and hypotension). Both synergism (e.g. with respect to haemodynamic changes) and antagonism (e.g. induction of fever) between IL1 and TNF have been described. In the present study we examined the effects of continuous infusion (3 days) of rhIL1ß (2.0 μg/day) alone, rhTNFα (0.2, 2.0 or 10 μg/day) alone or IL1 combined with TNF on the activity of the pituitary-adrenal axis (plasma ACTH and B levels), daily food intake and rectal temperature in rats (6-9 rats per group). For daily blood sampling (10.00-12.00 h) rats were implanted with indwelling jugular cannulas. One week afterwards rats were implanted (ip) with osmotic pumps filled with IL1, TNF or IL1 in combination with TNF. Results are shown as areas under the curves (area units, day 1-3, mean ± SEM), corrected for preinfusion values (day -1 and 0).

	ACTH	B	FOOD INTAKE	TEMPERATURE
-saline	-	1.3±3.5	-3.1±0.8	-0.29±0.06
-IL1	3.5±6.7	34.6±17.4	-5.6±1.5	0.24±0.15[a]
-TNF 0.2	-6.4±4.6	-3.8±14.3	-1.6±0.7	-0.15±0.05
-TNF 2.0	-1.5±7.7	1.8±4.3	-4.3±1.5	-0.14±0.05
-TNF 10	-1.7±8.8	25.1±20.7	-4.8±1.1	-0.03±0.07[b]
-IL1+TNF 0.2	11.2±9.5	65.1±21.2	-9.9±1.5	0.41±0.12
-IL1+TNF 2.0	28.5±13.4	131.4±34.8[d]	-13.0±1.2[c]	0.75±0.05[c]
-IL1+TNF 10	53.6±14.3[c]	212.3±36.9[c]	-18.4±0.9[c]	0.93±0.08[c]

[a] $p<0.01$ vs. saline, [b] $p<0.05$ vs. saline, [c] $p<0.01$ vs. IL1, [d] $p<0.05$ vs. IL1.

Conclusion: Our data clearly shows that IL1 and TNF act synergistically in activating the pituitary-adrenal axis and in inducing anorexia and fever, when infused continuously in rats.

P2.16

LONG-TERM CHANGES IN PEPTIDE MAKE-UP OF HYPOTHALAMIC CRH NEURONS AFTER SINGLE ADMINISTRATION OF INTERLEUKIN-1ß. **E.D. Schmidt, A.W.J.W. Janszen, R. Binnenkade, J.H.A. Persons, F. Wouterlood*, F.J.H. Tilders. Research Institute Neurosciences Vrije Universiteit, Dept. of Pharmacology, *Dept. Anatomy, van der Boechorstraat 7, 1081 BT Amsterdam, The Netherlands.**

CRH neurons of the hypthalamus that have their secretory terminals in the outer zone of the median eminence (ZEME), control ACTH release from the adenohypophysis. Some CRH neurons coproduce vasopressin (AVP), a peptide that potentiates the ACTH releasing effect of CRH. The fraction of CRH terminals that costore AVP increases after adrenal extirpation or chronic stress. Here we report the long-term effects of a single dose of interleukin-1ß (IL-1), a cytokine that activates CRH neurons. Quantitative immunocytochemistry shows that a single injection of IL-1 (5μg/kg i.p.) induces a long-term increase (50-100 %) of the AVP content of the ZEME without affecting the CRH content. The increase in AVP is not present after 1 or 4 days, but first appears 7 days post-injection. The effect peaks at 11 days and is maintained till day 20, but has disappeared by day 40. Immunoelectronmicroscopy, using a post-embedding double labelling procedure, shows that the increased AVP content of the ZEME is accompained by an increase in the fraction of CRH neurons that contain AVP from 40.3±4.1 % to 63.3±4.6 % (X±SEM). We tested whether the IL-1 induced long-term increase of AVP expression in CRH neurons affects the response of the pituitary-adrenal axis by measuring plasma ACTH and corticosterone concentrations. Eleven days after IL-1 administration, a second IL-1 challenge or exposure to electric footshocks showed enhanced ACTH and corticosterone responses, consistent with an increased ACTH releasing potential of hypothalamic CRH neurons. We postulate that a short-term activation of CRH neurons by IL-1ß induces a slow developing but, long-term change of their secretory peptide make-up. (NWO grant: 900-543-101).

P2.17

A CRITICAL ROLE FOR CRH IN THE INTEGRATIVE CONTROL OF ACTH SECRETION.

M.J. Evans*, R.S. Mulligan, J.H. Livesey, R.A. Donald. Dept. of Endocrinology, Christchurch Hospital, Christchurch, New Zealand.

To mimic the pattern of cortisol, CRH and AVP secretion observed *in vivo* in the horse, dispersed horse anterior pituitary cells were perifused in a 15-column system with continuous cortisol (0 or 100nM from -100 min (start of perifusion) to +210 min (end of perifusion), continuous "background" CRH (0 or 20pM from 0 to +210 min), and 5-min pulses of AVP (10nM every 30 min from +30 min to +180 min). ACTH was measured in 5-min effluent fractions. Cortisol significantly ($p<0.001$) decreased the ACTH response to CRH at onset and during the experiment in pre-AVP pulse fractions ($p<0.01$). With 0pM CRH, cortisol significantly ($p=0.01$) decreased the ACTH response to AVP (measured as area above the baseline) but with continuous 20pM CRH, the ACTH response to AVP was not significantly altered by cortisol. CRH significantly ($p=0.02$) potentiated the ACTH response to AVP in the presence but not in the absence of cortisol. Cortisol significantly ($p=0.003$) decreased the AVP-ACTH dose-response in the absence but not in the presence of continuous 20pM CRH. These findings suggest that "background" CRH has a critical role to play in the physiological control of ACTH secretion by (i) allowing negative feedback control of ACTH via cortisol's suppression of the ACTH response to CRH, but (ii) ensuring an increased ACTH response to a new stress by both protecting the ACTH response to pulses of AVP from suppression by cortisol, and by potentiating the ACTH response to AVP.

P2.18

POSTNATAL DEVELOPMENT OF NEUROTENSIN IMMUNOREACTIVITY IN THE ADENOHYPOPHYSIAL CELLS OF THE RAT.

A.R.Bello(1), G. Hernández(2) and G. Tramu(3). UDI of Cell Biology(1) and Lab of Neuroendocrinology.(2),La Laguna University,Spain. Lab of Functional Neurocytochemistry(3),Burdeos I University,France.

Neurotensin (NT), a peptide localized in pituitary gonadotroph and thyrotroph cells in both male and female adult rats, modifies its expression after orchidectomy in adult male rats [1]. Our aim was to further investigate the role of NT in adenohypophysial function. We used male and female Sprague-Dawley rats since birth to 60 days old. Animals were perfused intracardially and their pituitary glands postfixed in picric acid paraformaldehyde. Cryostat sections of the hypophysis were processed to detect NT by means of indirect immunohistochemical method. The use of the elution restaining procedure allowed us to determine the nature of the cells expressing Neurotensin immunoreactivity (NT-IR). We used antibodies against thyroid stimulating hormone (TSH) and follicle stimulating hormone (FSH). Pituitary NT-IR was only observed after the first week of life, and only in TSH-IR cells, in animals from both sexes. Its expression was progressively higher between 15 and 25 days postnatally. NT-IR in the gonadotroph was also observed during this period,but not before day 15 postnatally. Maximum levels of NT expression were observed at day 25 postnatally in both types of cells. In male rats, NT-IR in FSH-positive cells increased progressively from postnatal day 25 to 60, whereas it diminished in TSH-positive cells. In female rat, NT-IR showed wide variations among all cell types, probably due to the estrous cycle phases. These results suggest that, in gonadotroph and thyrotroph pituitary cells, Neurotensin shows some plasticity in its expression depending on gonadal status. (Grants from Gob.Aut.Canarias 92/089,DGICYT PM92-0160,Spain, and URA CNRS 339,France).

[1]A.R. Bello et al. Neuroendocrinology 1992; 55: 714-723.

P2.19

Arginine vasopressin as the primary activator of the HPA axis during adjuvant-induced arthritis.

Chowdrey, H.S., Larsen, P.J[2]., Harbuz, M.S., Jessop, D.S., Aguilera, G[1]., and Lightman, S.L.

Department of Medicine, Bristol Royal Infirmary, Bristol BS2 8HW. U.K. [1]Section of Endocrine Physiology, NICHD, NIH, Bethesda, USA. [2]Institute of Medical Anatomy, University of Copenhagen, Denmark.

Adjuvant-induced arthritis (AA) is an immunologically mediated inflammatory disease that results in chronic activation of the hypothalamo-pituitary-adrenal (HPA) axis, as indicated by increased adrenal size, increased expression of anterior pituitary POMC mRNA, increased morning circulating ACTH and corticosterone and loss of the normal diurnal rhythm of these hormones. We have further characterised the role of corticotropin-releasing factor (CRF) and arginine vasopressin (AVP) in the regulation of the HPA axis during development of AA in PVG and SD rats. AA was associated with a significant increase in AVP mRNA levels in the medial parvocellular division of the hypothalamic paraventricular nucleus. CRF mRNA levels were either unchanged in the SD or decreased in the PVG rats. Coincident with the onset and the progression of inflammation, ir-AVP levels in the portal plasma of PVG rats markedly increased. In the SD arthritic rats maximum binding of [^{3}H]AVP to anterior pituitary membranes was increased whereas that of [^{125}I]-Tyr-oCRF was significantly decreased. However the ACTH secretory response to CRF and AVP in vitro was unchanged in both rat strains. The data are consistent with the view that activation of the parvocellular vasopressinergic system has an important role in the adaptation of the HPA axis to chronic stress.

P2.20

SEROTONIN (5-HT)$_3$, BUT NOT 5-HT$_4$, RECEPTORS ARE INVOLVED IN THE REGULATION OF ACTH RELEASE IN VITRO.

A.E. Calogero*, G. Bagdy[1], N. Burrello, M.L. Moncada, F. Bonaffini, R. D'Agata[2], Department. of Internal Medicine and [2]Chair of Andrology, University of Catania, Italy, 95123 and [1]Laboratory of Experimental Medicine, National Institute of Psychiatry and Neurology, Budapest, 1281 Hungary.

Although several 5-HT receptor types are capable of stimulating pituitary ACTH release, relatively little is known on the role of 5-HT$_3$ and 5-HT$_4$ receptors. In this study, we tested the effects of the 5-HT$_{3/4}$ receptor antagonist 3-tropanyl-indole-3-carboxylate (ICS 205-930) and of the 5-HT$_3$ receptor antagonist 3-tropanyl-3,5-dichlorobenzoate (MDL 72222) on 5-HT-stimulated ACTH release from rat pituitary cell cultures. We tested also the effects of the 5-HT$_3$ receptor agonist 1-(m-chlorophenyl)-biguanide (m-CPBG) and of the 5-HT$_4$ receptor agonist zacopride on basal, CRH- and AVP-stimulated ACTH release. The stimulatory effect of 5-HT (10^{-9} M) on basal ACTH release was antagonized by ICS 205-930 and by MDL 72222, suggesting an involvement of 5-HT$_3$ receptors on ACTH release. In addition, m-CPBG stimulated basal ACTH release, whereas in contrast to 5-HT, did not have any effect on CRH (10^{-9} M)-stimulated ACTH release, and inhibited the stimulatory effect of AVP (10^{-8} M). In contrast, zacopride did not have any effect on basal and CRH-stimulated ACTH release, whereas it inhibited AVP-stimulated ACTH release, but only at the dose of 10^{-8} M. These data suggest that activation of the 5-HT$_3$ increases basal and suppresses AVP-stimulated ACTH release in vitro, whereas the 5-HT$_4$ receptor is substantially devoid of effects. 5-HT receptors appear to mediate multiple and opposite, effects on pituitary ACTH release in vitro.

P2.21

ROLE OF MELANIN-CONCENTRATING HORMONE AND NEUROPEPTIDE-E-I IN BASAL AND STRESS-INDUCED RELEASE OF PITUITARY HORMONES IN THE RAT.

Mounier F, Presse F, Voko Z, Bluet-Pajot MT, Hoeger C, Epelbaum J, Nahon JL. INSERM U159 Paris, UPR 411 CNRS, Valbonne, France.

Cloning and sequence characterization of the rat MCH (rMCH) cDNA revealed the existence of additional peptides encoded into the MCH precursor. One, named neuropeptide-E-I(NEI) is co-processed and secreted with MCH in rat hypothalamus. rMCH mRNA levels are constant during daylight hours, but increase and reach a maximum four hours after the onset of darkness. Either alone or co-administered, rMCH and NEI do not modify basal secretion of GH and PRL at any times nor do they alter the stress-induced changes in these two hormonal secretions. During day time, when basal ACTH levels are high, administration of rMCH but not NEI leads to a decrease in ACTH levels while there is no significant effect during the dark phase of the cycle (i.e., when basal ACTH levels are already low). Using a moderate ether induced stress, ACTH levels were only stimulated during the dark, but not the light, phase of the cycle. rMCH dampened the rise in ACTH release while NEI had a tendency to increase the stress response. Co-administration of both peptides before stress resulted in an abolition of the rMCH induced inhibition of ACTH plasma levels. We also demonstrate that hypothalamic rMCH mRNA content is decreased following pro-MCH derived peptide injections. On the other hand, POMC mRNA expression is slightly enhanced under the same conditions. Thus, exogenous rMCH may act as a corticotropin inhibitory factor under basal condition during day time and following acute-stress during the active phase of the rat circadian cycle while NEI antagonize action of rMCH under those conditions. The decrease by rMCH or NEI of rMCH gene activity suggests the existence of a short feed-back regulation of these peptides.

P2.22

ANATOMICAL AND PHARMACOLOGICAL SUBSTRATES FOR NEUROTENSIN ACTION ON THE HYPOTHALAMIC-PITUITARY-ADRENAL AXIS (HPA) ACTIVITY.

A. Nicot, A. Bérod*, D. Gully[1], W. Rowe[2], E. Ron De Kloet[3] and W. Rostène. INSERM U339, Hôpital St-Antoine, Paris, France; [1]Sanofi Recherche, Toulouse, France; [2]Douglas Hospital Research Center, Mc Gill University, Quebec, Canada; [3]Center for Bio-Pharmaceutical Sciences, Leiden, The Netherlands.

Central administration of neurotensin (NT) has been shown to activate the HPA, an effect which seems to be mediated by corticotropin-releasing factor release. In this study, we described the distribution of NT binding sites in the hypothalamus using in vitro receptor autoradiography. Among the ^{125}I NT labeled hypothalamic nuclei, relative high densities of labeling were detected over the magnocellular and parvocellular parts of the paraventricular nucleus. Moreover, we showed that two newly developed NT receptor antagonists, SR 48692 and its analog SR 48450, competed for ^{125}I NT binding to hypothalamic tissue sections and membrane preparations with Ki values in the nanomolar range. The intracerebroventricular injection of SR 48450 was able to block the NT-induced HPA activation in freely moving rats, whereas its administration alone did not significantly affect basal plasma levels of ACTH and corticosterone.

These data provide anatomical substrate for a potential neurotensin action at the level of the hypothalamus in the HPA activation and highlight the use of new non-peptide NT receptor antagonists to characterize NT effects on neuroendocrine functions.

P2.23

IN VIVO AND IN VITRO PITUITARY-ADRENAL FUNCTION AFTER CHRONIC STRESS.

O. Martí*, A. Gavaldà, E. Soriano and A. Armario. Departament de Biologia Cel.lular i de Fisiologia, Universitat Autònoma de Barcelona, Ø8193 Bellaterra, Barcelona, Spain.

The influence of chronic immobilization stress (IMO) on pitutary-adrenal (PA) function was evaluated in male SD rats. Chronic IMO (14 days, 2 h/day) increased adrenal responsiveness to ACTH in vitro. At the pituitary level, this treatment increased the size and number of corticotropes in the adenohypophysis and caused a two-fold increase in basal ACTH release in vitro, but did not alter the percent ACTH response to CRF in vitro. Nontheless, in vivo, it was observed that the ACTH response to CRF, but not to AVP, was increased after chronic IMO. These results suggest that chronic IMO, rather than impairing the PA function, increases the adrenal response to ACTH and keeps intact or even exacerbates the capacity of the pituitary to secrete ACTH in response to CRF.

P2.24

EFFECT OF INTRAHIPPOCAMPAL GLUCOCORTICOIDS ON THE ACTH PLASMA LEVELS AND AMINO ACID NEUROTRANSMITTERS.

I. Ábráhám, K.J. Kovács, A.K. Kékesi* and G.Juhász* Institute of Experimental Medicine Budapest, Eötvös Loránd University, Dep. of Comparative Physiology*

Corticosteroid receptors of the hippocampus play important role in feed-back regulation of glucocorticoids. Our aim was to determine whether administration of type II corticoid receptor agonist dexamethasone into hippocampus has an effect on stress induced plasma ACTH level and on local GABAergic and glutaminergic system.

Dexamethasone was dialysed through microdialysis probe into the CA1 and CA2 region of the right hippocampus in freely moving animals after ether stress. ACTH plasma levels were measured by RIA from blood samples obtained from the jugular vein. The extracellular level of glutamate, GABA and relative release of dexamethasone was determined from dialysates by OPA derivatives of amino acid and by UV detection at 280 nm on a small bore chromatograph (SMART). After ether stress glutamate level in the hippocampus increased paralel with the increase of plasma ACTH while the GABA levels were unchanged in the dialysates. Ether stress induced glutamate release was higher after infusion of dexamethasone to the CA1 and CA2 regions although GABA and plasma ACTH levels were not different in artificial cerebrospinal fluid infused versus dexamethasone infused, stressed rats.

Unilateral administration of dexamethasone into CA1 and CA2 fields of the hippocampus has no influence on plasma ACTH level in ether stress. Corticosteroids may play a role in regulation of amino acid release. It could effect the intrinsic amino acidergic connections in the hippocampus and influences the hipothalamo-pituitary adrenal axis.

P2.25

HYPOTHALAMIC-PITUITARY-ADRENAL AXIS IN THE NON INSULIN DEPENDENT DIABETIC RATS. C. Tojo* T. Takao, T. Nishioka, H. Kurokawa, K. Hashimoto. Second Dept of Internal Medicine, Kochi Medical School, Nankoku, Japan, 783

Corticotropin-releasing factor (CRF) is a primary integrator of the organism's coordinating neuroendocrine, autonomic, behavioral, and immune responses to stress. In an attempt to define the regulation of hypothalamic-pituitary-adrenal axis in the non insulin dependent diabetic rats, we utilized Otsuka Long Evans Tokushima Fatty (OLETF) rats. We measured iodine-125-labeled ovine CRF ([^{125}I]oCRF) binding in the brain and pituitary and CRF concentrations in the median eminence (ME), remainder of the hypothalamus (rHY) and neurointermediate lobe of the pituitary (NIL) and plasma CRF, adrenocorticotropic hormone (ACTH) and corticosterone (B). Plasma ACTH levels were significantly increased in OLETF rats compared with control rats (Long Evans Tokushima Otsuka; LETO) In contrast to ACTH levels, no significant difference was observed in plasma CRF and corticosterone levels between OLETF and LETO rats. CRF concentration in the ME, rHY and NIL, and ACTH concentration in the anterior lobe of the pituitary were unchanged between OLETF and LETO rats. No significant difference of [^{125}I]oCRF binding was observed in the anterior pituitary and frontal cortex between OLETF and LETO rats. These findings demonstrate that differential pituitary-adrenal function may exist in the non insulin dependent diabetic rats.

P2.26

THE EFFECT OF PREVIOUS FEEDING WITH UNSATURATED FATTY ACIDS ON THE CORTICOTROPH AND MEMBRANE FUNCTIONS OF CULTURED RAT PITUITARIES. J. Julesz*, M. Gálfi, A. Juhász[1], M. Vecsernyés, J. Gardi, S. Karcsú. Endocrine Unit and [1]Dept. of Psychiatry, A. Szent-Györgyi Medical University, Szeged, Hungary, H-6720.

Earlier, we have demonstrated that in vitro treatment with unsaturated fatty acids (eicosapentaenoic acid, EPA; dodecahexaenoic acid, DHA) alters the growth hormone and prolactin release of rat pituitary cell cultures. The present study was scheduled to investigate the effects of a previous 14-day "Eskimo diet" (18 % EPA and 12 % DHA of total fat) on the ACTH/α-MSH release, membrane fluidity and Mg^{++}-dependent ATPase activity of 12-day-old pituitary cell cultures of Wistar rats. Hormones were measured by RIA, fluidity by fluorescent anisotropy and ATPase by photometry. No changes were observed in the hormone release, however, both membrane fluidity and Mg^{++}-ATPase activity decreased after previous in vivo treatment with EPA and DHA when compared with these parameters of normally fed control animals. After a further 24 h in vitro treatment with 10^{-6} mM EPA, the hormone release was found to be reduced and the ATPase values approached those of the controls. These changes suggest that unsaturated fatty acids, widely introduced for human consumption, may be worth checking for endocrine effects on a clinical scale, too. (Supported by ETT grant T-92/1990.)

P2.27

GONADOTROPIN-RELEASING HORMONE (GnRH)-INDUCED CALCIUM SIGNALS IN MALE RAT GONADOTROPES ARE ALTERED FOLLOWING CASTRATION.

V.A. Tobin and B.J. Canny, Dept. of Physiology, Monash University, Clayton VIC 3168 AUSTRALIA*

Hypothalamic and gonadal factors interact to regulate the secretion of gonadotropins from the anterior pituitary. GnRH generates a number of intracellular responses following receptor occupation; the changes in intracellular calcium ion concentration ($[Ca^{2+}]_i$) are believed to play an important role in exocytosis. The changes in $[Ca^{2+}]_i$ fall into two distinct categories:- repetitive oscillations, which are associated with low concentrations, and "spike-plateau" responses seen with high concentrations of GnRH. As *in vivo* and *in vitro* GnRH-induced gonadotropin secretion is elevated after castration, we have compared Ca^{2+} signals from intact and one- and eight-week castrate male rats. A single cell suspension of anterior pituitary cells was obtained by enzymatic dipsersion, the cells were subsequently loaded with fura-2/AM (1 μM), and an inverted microscope configured for fura-2 was used for $[Ca^{2+}]_i$ measurement. Single gonadotropes were identified, and Ca^{2+} signals in response to 1 and 100 nM GnRH recorded. Following eight weeks of castration 14 of 21 gonadotropes (67%) exhibited oscillations in response to 100 nM GnRH; this was significantly greater than the proportion seen in intact rats (9 of 32 (28%), $\chi^2=7.7$, $P<0.01$). A similar finding was observed in gonadotropes from one week castrate rats (castrate *vs.* intact, 16 of 23 (70%) oscillations *vs.* 9 of 32 (28%) oscillations, $\chi^2=9.3$, $P<0.005$). The same trend was observed in response to 1 nM GnRH, the differences between castrate and control groups, however, did not achieve statistical significance. These findings demonstrate that Ca^{2+} signalling in gonadotropes is influenced by gonadal status. Whether this effect is mediated directly at the pituitary, and which testicular factor(s) is involved in the feedback are currently being investigated. The relationships between altered Ca^{2+} signals and the secretory profile is yet to be determined.

P2.28

SUBSTANCE P DIRECTLY STIMULATES LH SYNTESIS AND RELEASE AND POTENTIATES GnRH EFFECT ON PORCINE PITUITARY CELLS.*

C. Hidalgo, J.L. González de Aguilar, S. García-Navarro and F. Gracia-Navarro. Dept. Cell Biology. Univ. of Cordoba. Spain.

Substance P (SP) is a peptide of 11 aminoacid residues belonging to the tachykinins family. Previous reports, most of them performed *in vivo* , have shown its influence on the release of several pituitary hormones. However, little is known about the effect of SP on LH secretion in vivo and in vitro. The aim of the present report as to investigate the role of SP on the release and syntesis of luteinizing hormone (LH), and its interaction with gonadotropin releasing hormone (GnRH), on isolated female pig pituitary cells. After enzimatic and mechanical dispersion, cells were incubated with increasing doses of SP in the range of 0.01 nM to 10 uM for 4 hours. Then, culture medium was collected to quantify LH release, using an enzyme immunoassay for porcine LH. The results showed a dose-dependent stimulatory effect on LH release being the optimal concentration 100 nM. In a second set of experiments, pituitary cells were treated with 10 nM GnRH, 100 nM SP, or 10 nM GnRH plus 100 nM SP. In GnRH-treated cells, LH release increased 155% compared to control cells whereas the increment produced by SP was 65%. When GnRH and SP were administered together, LH release was of 260% higher than that induced by GnRH alone. On the other hand, the quantification of LH content in cellular homogenates showed a decrease of 40% in GnRH-treated cells and an increase of 62% and 42% in SP and SP+GnRH treated cells, respectively. Taken together, these date demostrate that 1) SP acts directly on gonadotrope cells, inducing a stimulation of both release and syntesis of LH, and 2) SP potentiates GnRH action, increasing the GnRH-simulatory effect on LH release and producing a high accumulation of hormone. Thus, these experiments indicate that this peptide could play a physiological role in the regulation of the hypothalamo-pituitary-gonadal axis.

***Supported by Junta Andalucia (Group no. 3087) and DGICYT (Grant no. PB92-1102)**

P2.29

INVOLVEMENT OF CRH IN THE SUPPRESSION OF LH RELEASE INDUCED BY AN α-ADRENERGIC RECEPTOR ACTIVATION IN THE PVN IN RATS. *H.Tsukamura, S. Nagatani, F.R.A. Cagampang, S.-I. Kawakami, A. Yokoyama, K.-I. Maeda. Sch. Agricultural Sciences, Nagoya University, Nagoya, Japan, 464-01.

The present study examined the subtype of adrenergic receptors in the paraventricular nucleus (PVN) regulating pulsatile luteinizing hormone (LH) secretion, and involvement of the corticotropin-releasing hormone (CRH) in the suppression of LH release induced by norepinephrine (NE) injection into the PVN in ovariectomized (OVX) and ovariectomized estradiol (E_2)-treated (OVX+E_2) rats. Conscious animals were bled 3 h at 6-min intervals immediately after the micro-injection of α_1-, α_2-, β-adrenergic agonists or NE into the PVN. Some animals were injected with α-helical CRF, an antagonist of CRH, into 3rd ventricle 5 min prior to the NE injection to the PVN. NE and both α-receptor agonists inhibited pulsatile LH secretion throughout the 3-h sampling period in OVX+E_2 rats. On the other hand, LH secretion was inhibited transiently for the first 1-2 hours by an injection of NE or an α_2-receptor agonist into the PVN in OVX rats. Injection of a β-agonist did not affect pulsatile LH secretion in both OVX and OVX+E2 animals. Intracerebroventricular injection of α-helical CRF prior to NE injection to the PVN completely blocked the NE-induced suppression of pulsatile LH secretion in OVX+E_2 rats. These results suggest that 1) the noradrenergic system projecting to the PVN suppresses pulsatile LH secretion via the activation of α-adrenergic receptors, 2) this inhibition is mediated by CRH release, and 3) estrogen enhances this suppression. The *in vitro* effect of NE on CRF expression in the PVN is under investigation at present.

P2.30

IMMUNONEUTRALIZATION OF INTRACEREBRAL NPY IN CASTRATE EWES HASTENED ONSET OF ESTROGEN-INDUCED LH SURGE. P.V. Malven*, S.A. Haglof and H. Jiang. Purdue Univ., W. Lafayette, IN 47907, USA.

Administration of neuropeptide-Y (NPY) has been reported to have both stimulatory and inhibitory effects on release of LHRH and LH depending on species and level of steroid feedback. In vivo immunoneutralization of endogenous NPY using anti-NPY serum provides one method to determine the physiological role of endogenous NPY on LHRH/LH. Anti-NPY serum was generated in sheep against a conjugate of porcine NPY and bovine thyroglobulin. Five castrated ewes (7-8 mo. old) were stereotaxically implanted with an 18-gauge guide tube into the 3rd ventricle in the mediobasal hypothalamus. Each guide tube was fitted with a removable 22-gauge infusion cannula that extended about 0.8 mm beyond the end of the guide tube. Randomly selected ewes received 100 μl infusions of either anti-NPY (1:10 dilution in saline) or control serum diluted identically. During every 2-day trial, each ewe received five such infusions as follows: one each at 14 and 16 h before IM injection of 50 μg estradiol-17ß (E2 at midnight on day 1) and one each at 8, 10 and 12 h after E2. Serum LH concentrations were determined at 10-min intervals for 4 h on day 1 and at 1-h intervals on day 2 of the trial. Two weeks later, the trials were repeated with each ewe receiving the opposite type of infusion. A second replication of both treatments was conducted 2 and 4 weeks after the second trial of the first replicate. On day 1 of the trials, pulse frequency, pulse amplitude and mean concentration of LH did not differ between anti-NPY and control infusions. On day 2, E2-induced surges of LH occurred in 19 of 20 trials. The day-2 increase of serum LH above each ewe's day-1 mean occurred earlier in ewes infused with anti-NPY (12.6 ± 1.4 vs. 14.4 ± 2.1 h after E2; $P < .05$). The magnitude of the LH surge was not affected, and the total duration of the LH surge was not determined. In summary, immunoneutralization of endogenous NPY did not affect pulsatile discharges of LH in untreated castrates. Chronic immunoneutralization of NPY hastened the onset of the E2-induced surge of LH suggesting an inhibitory role for endogenous NPY in timing the onset of the LH surge presumably by inhibiting the onset of the LHRH surge. Supported in part by USDA grant 90-37240-5504.

P2.31

THE FEEDBACK ACTION OF ESTROGEN AT THE PVN OR A2 IS REQUIRED TO SUPPRESS THE PULSATILE LH RELEASE DURING FASTING IN FEMALE RATS. *S. Nagatani, H. Tsukamura, K-I. Maeda. School of Agricultural Sciences, Nagoya University, Nagoya, Japan, 464-01.

The feedback sites of estrogen within the hypothalamus and lower brainstem involved in the suppression of pulsatile LH secretion during 48-h· fasting were examined in female rats. Animals were ovariectomized and immediately implanted stereotaxically with stainless-steel cannula containing crystal estradiol (E_2) diluted 10 times by crystal cholesterol into the medial preoptic area (mPOA), pavaventriclar nucleus (PVN), arcuate nucleus (ARC), locus coeleus (LC), A1 or A2. Five days later, animals were deprived of food for 48 h and then blood samples were collected every 6 min for 3 h. They were immediately re-fed for 45 h and were bled again as described above. The fasted animals with E_2 implants in the A2 showed a significant decrease in mean LH concentrations compared with the cholesterol-implanted controls. The more potent suppression of LH pulses was found in fasted rats with E_2 implant in the PVN. E_2 implants in the mPOA, ARC, LC or A1, did not induce any significant changes in LH pulses during fasting compared to cholesterol-implanted controls. These results suggest that the feedback action of estrogen at the PVN and/or A2 is required for the fasting-induced suppression of pulsatile LH release.

P2.32

EFFECTS OF RU486 ON LHRH SECRETION AND ON LH AND FSH SURGES. G. Hernández*, M. Tébar, C. Bellido, D. González, A. Díaz-Cruz, R. Alonso, J.E. Sánchez-Criado. Depts. of Physiology, Faculties of Medicine, Universities of Córdoba (14004) and La Laguna (Tenerife) (38320), Spain.

The preovulatory surge of LH and FSH in the rat is enterely coupled to the LHRH surge in the afternoon of proestrus, while the secondary surge of FSH during early estrus is dependent on both the preovulatory surge of LH and the permissive absence of circulating inhibin. The antiprogestagen RU486 injected at proestrus morning blunts the preovulatory secretion of LH and FSH and abolishes the FSH secondary surge. In this work we have explored whether LHRH secretion is involved in these effects. So, the effects of RU486 (4 mg on proestrus) on the secretion of LHRH into the portal vessels and on serum concentrations of LH and FSH on proestrus and estrus were studied. Also we determinated the effects of an LHRH antagonist (1 mg on proestrus) and LHRH (100 ng on estrus) on serum concentrations of LH and FSH on estrus in oil- and RU486-treated rats. RU486 decreased preovulatory LHRH secretion coinciding with a reduction in both LH and FSH surges, and increased LHRH secretion on estrus which was only accompanied by an elevated concentration of LH. The injection of LHRH stimulated, and that of LHRHa inhibited, serum concentrations of LH in either oil- and RU486-treated rats. Exogenous LHRH only increased FSH levels in oil-treated rats, while LHRHa had no effect on FSH concentrations. These results indicate that, in the rat, progesterone secretion during the afternoon and evening of proestrus enhances preovulatory LHRH and supresses LHRH release during early estrus. While the secretion of LH on early estrus is blunted by progesterone and entirely coupled to LHRH secretion, the secondary FSH surge is not dependent on endogenous LHRH but completely dependent on the actions (direct and/or indirect) of progesterone. This work has been supported by DGICYT (PM92-0118 and PM92-0160). Spain.

P2.33

INHIBITORY EFFECT OF CORTICOSTERONE ON THE LH-IMMUNOREACTIVE ADENOHYPOPHYSEAL CELLS. A COMBINED IN VIVO-IN VITRO STUDY. M. Rubio*, F. Sánchez, J. Carretero, J.J. Cabo, J.M. Riesco, J.A. Juanes, E. Blanco and R. Vázquez. Dept. Human Anatomy. Faculty of Medicine. University of Salamanca. 37007. Salamanca. Spain.

To date, it is well-known that glucocorticoids exert an inhibitory effect upon the LH release in the male rat. However, most of these studies are biochemical and consequently there is less degree of knowledge at the morphological-morphometric level. Based upon the foregoing, a combined in vivo (adrenalectomy and adrenalectomy + corticosterone) and in vitro (adenohypophyseal cells in monolayer culture incubated with corticosterone) immunocytochemical study has been carried out. The morphological and morphometric changes found in the LH-immunorreactive cells, both in vivo and in vitro (especially the decrease in the cellular area following corticosterone administration) confirm the inhibitory effect of corticosterone upon the LH-adenohypophyseal cell.

P2.34

EFFECTS OF PENTOBARBITAL SODIUM ON THE PREOPTIC NORADRENALINE RELEASE AND LHRH PULSE GENERATOR ACTIVITY IN THE OVARIECTOMIZED RAT. F. Kimura*, E. Ito, A. Sano, T. Mizuno, K. Jinnai, H. Hiruma, Dept. of Physiology, Yokohama City University School of Medicine, Yokohama, Japan, 236.

CNS mechanism for ovulatory surge of luteinizing hormone (LH) secretion is sensitive to pentobarbital sodium (PB). In the present study, the sensitibity of CNS mechanism for tonic LH secretion to PB was studied using ovariectomized rats with or without estrogen priming. First, the effect of PB on noradrenaline (NA) release in the medial preoptic area was studied by means of a microdialysis method coupled to HPLC. Dialyzates were collected at 6-min intervals. Second, the effect of PB on the LH-releasing hormone (LHRH) pulse generator activity was studied electrophysiologically. The hypothalamic multiunit activity (MUA) with intermittent (15-30 min intervals) increases (volleys) was recorded, simultaneously with blood sampling at 6-min intervals to determine the LH pulse in association with each MUA volley In both experiments, PB was injected intraperitoneally at 32 or 35 mg/kg bw. The results were as follows. (1)PB caused a marked, approximately 40-60% decrease in NA release, which became evident 50 min after the injection and lasted for another 60 min during which the observation was performed. (2)The appearance of MUA volley immediately after PB injection was slightly delayed, but afterwards, the volley appeared at similar intervals to those before PB. No changes were seen in the amplitude of LH pulses. (3) When PB was injected the day after estradiol treatment, where MUA volleys had become unclear, MUA volleys became evident. The results suggest that LHRH pulse generator responsible for tonic LH secretion is insensitive to PB. Further, it appears that LHRH pulse generator fails to operate normally when NA release is acutely changed, but is able to operate normally if NA release is stable, eventhrough the level is very low.

P2.35

AMINO ACID RELEASE IN THE PREOPTIC AREA BUT NOT IN THE MEDIOBASAL HYPOTHALAMUS CHANGES DURING THE ESTROGEN INDUCED LH SURGE IN THE OVX RAT. H. Jarry*, S. Leonhardt, W. Wuttke. Dept. Clin. & Exptl. Endocrinology, University of Göttingen, 37075 Göttingen, Germany

Both, inhibitory and excitatory amino acid neurotransmitter (AAN) have been suggested to participate in the induction of the preovulatory like estrogen induced LH surge in the female rat. Little is known about the site of action within the hypothalamus but in vitro experiments with superfused fragments of the mediobasal hypothalamus (MBH) indicate that AAN affect LHRH release at the level of LHRH nerve terminals. However, in vivo experiments with push-pull cannula (PPC) in rats demonstrated that application of AAN into the preoptic area (POA) clearly affect LH release. To assess spontaneous release of AAN in either POA or MBH prior to and during an estrogen induced LH surge, ovx rats were implanted with PPC in either brain structure. Brain perfusates were collected at 30 min intervals and concentrations of AAN were determined by HPLC. In perfusates of both, POA and MBH the inhibitory AAN GABA, glycine, taurine and the excitatory AAN glutamate and aspartate were readily detectable. During the estrogen induced LH surge preoptic release rates of glutamate and asparte increased significantly ($p<0.01$). Taurine and glycine release in the POA remained constant throughout the experiment, wherease GABA secretion was significantly reduced ($p<0.01$). In the MBH, however, no changes of release rates of neither excitatory or inhibitory AAN were observed though in all animals a LH surge occurred. These data indicate that:I) the mechanisms inducing the estrogen induced LH surge reside in the POA and not in the MBH. Thus our data are in contrast to observations made in vitro II) it appears that LHRH release is increased by reducing preoptic release of the inhibitory AAN GABA and simultanously enhanced release of the excitatory AAN aspartate and glutamate.

P2.36

PULSATILE LH SECRETION IS REDUCED BY MICRO-INJECTION OF THE EXCITATORY AMINO ACID (EAA) ANTAGONISTS INTO THE ARCUATE NUCLEUS-MEDIAN EMINENCE REGION(ARC-ME) IN THE RAT. *H. Nagabukuro, S. Ohkura, H. Tsukamura, K.-I. Maeda. Shool of Agricultural Science, Nagoya University, Nagoya, Japan, 464-01

The role of endogenous EAA within or projecting to the ARC-ME in regulating pulsatile LH release was examined by antagonizing the EAA receptors located in the ARC-ME. Wistar-Imamichi strain rats ovariectomized for 2 weeks were stereotaxically implanted with a stainless-steel guide cannula (26G) into the ARC-ME. Five to ten days after the brain surgery, animals were recieved bilaterally micro-injection with NMDA (CPP, 2 nmol) or non-NMDA (DNQX, 1 nmol) antagonist through an internal cannula (31G) inserted to the guide cannula. Blood samples were collected every 6 min for 3 h through the indwelling atrial catheter immediately after the micro-injection. The injection of CPP or DNQX significantly lowered mean and SD of a series of plasma LH concentrations over the 3-h sampling period and the amplitude of LH pulses. The frequency of LH pulses was also reduced, but not significantly, by CPP or DNQX administration. These results suggest that LHRH pulses is regulated through both NMDA and non-NMDA receptors in the ARC-ME and that the endogenous EAA may be one of the neurotransmitters involved in the generation of LHRH pulses.

P2.37

GONADOTROPIN AND PROLACTIN SECRETION AFTER 3rd CEREBRAL VENTRICLE N-METHYL-D,L-ASPARTATE (NMDA) ADMINISTRATION IN CHRONIC OVARIECTOMIZED RABBITS AND WITH OESTRADIOL CAPSULES.

W.Z. Traczyk, B. Dziedzic, K.-Y.F. Pau[+], H.G.Spies[+] Dept. of Physiology, Inst. Physiol. Biochem., Medical University, Lodz, Poland, 90-131 and Reproductive Biology and Behavior, Oregon Regional Primate Research Center, Beaverton, Oregon, USA, 97006.

The influence of NMDA on gonadotropin secretion has been established but the role of oestrogen in it is still under investigation. The experiments were performed on five female ovariectomized rabbits with a 3rd cerebral ventricular cannula and jugular vein catheter. The surgery, intracerebroventricular injection (ICV), sequential 15-min blood samples collection during 6 hrs and the RIA blood plasma hormone determination were as described (W. Z. Traczyk et al. J Physiol Pharmacol. 1992; 43:279-298). The ICV injections at one-week intervals of normal saline, 1.47 µg (low dose) or 2.94 µg (higher dose) of NMDA failed to alter LH, FSH and PRL secretion. In the same animals with 17β oestradiol capsule implantation ICV administration of NMDA increased LH and PRL release 2 up to 10 times in one - after low dose, in two - after higher dose and in four of five animals after the highest dose (14.7 µg). The highest dose of NMDA was lethal in two of five animals after a latency of 40 - 70 min.

P2.38

NEUROSTEROIDS MODULATE THE RELEASE OF GnRH FROM GT1-1 IMMORTALIZED HYPOTHALAMIC NEURONS.

M. El-Etr, Y.Akwa, R.J. Fiddes, P. Robel, E.E. Baulieu. INSERM U.33, 80 rue du général Leclerc, Kremlin-Bicêtre, France, F 94276.

GT1-1 GnRH secreting neurons (kindly provided by R.I. Weiner) express $GABA_A$ receptors. RT-PCR analysis has shown that only α1 and β3 subunit mRNAs can be detected. The absence of a γ subunit explains the insensitivity of these neurons to benzodiazepines. [^{3}H]-muscimol binds to membranes of GT1-1 cells with a Kd of 10.9 ± 0.3 nM and a Bmax of 979 ± 12 fmol/mg protein. The binding of 4 nM [^{3}H]-muscimol is enhanced by 3α-5α-tetrahydroprogesterone (THPROG, 10 µM) and inhibited by pregnenolone sulfate (PS, 10 µM).
We have previously observed that muscimol dose-dependently stimulates the release of GnRH from GT1-1 neurons (Society for Neuroscience, Washington, 1993, abstract 632-13, p 1539). We now report that THPROG and PS both inhibit muscimol-induced release of GnRH. However, in the absence of muscimol, THPROG (but not PS) stimulates GnRH secretion. At a concentration of 1 µM, THPROG is as effective as 10 µM muscimol (180% over basal values). Thus THPROG exerts a dual effect on GnRH release both stimulating and counteracting the stimulating effect of muscimol. Interestingly, we have also observed that GT1-1 cells in culture synthesize THPROG from progesterone, suggesting an effect of progesterone on GnRH neurons through this metabolite.

P2.39

THE INFLUENCE OF NATRIUM VALPROATE ON GONADOTROPIN SECRETION IN MENOPAUSAL WOMEN

S.Spremović-Radjenović,V.Popović,S. Matijašević
Institut of Gynecology and Obstetrics, Institut of Endocrinology, Clinical Centre of Serbia, Belgrade,SR Yugoslavia.

The aim of the study was to investigate the effects of natrium valproate (GABA-A agonist) on gonadotropin secretion in steroid deprived state suchas menopause.
Patients and methods:acute dose dependent tests (300,600, 1200 mg of natrium valproate p.o.) were performed in thirty menopausa al women, aged 50-58 yrs and gonadotropins were measured hourly for 24 h. Eleven menopausal women received 1200 mg of valproate for five days. Basal gonadotropins were meassured before and after chronic valproate theapy. Thirty menopausal females substituted with Estroderm 100 ngr were tested as a control group with acute valproate in the same way. Results: astatistically significant and dose dependent suppression of LH levels was recorded in the 7th, and 10th hour after 300 mg of valproate, in the 7th,10th, 8th, 10ht, 11th, 12th and 23 rd hour after 1200 mg of valporate. Basal LH levels did nog differ significantly after chronic valproate therapy (34,1 ± 5,2 v.s. 39,1 ± 8 mIU/1). In substituted women LH levels did not change significantly during the acute valproate tests. In conclusion: in nonsubstituted menopause acute valproate suppressed LH secretion in a dose related manner, starting 6 h after ingestion and lasting for 5-6h on. Chronic valproate did not affect basal gonadotropin secretion.

P2.40

ANANDAMIDE (ANA)[arachidonylethanolamide, endogen cannabinoid] AFFECTS ANTERIOR PITUITARY HORMONE SECRETION IN ADULT OVARIECTOMIZED (OVX) AND MALE RAT.

T. Wenger*, H. Fragakiss, N. Yiannakakis. 2nd Dept. of Anatomy, Semmelweis Univ. Med. Sch., Budapest, Hungary

The delta^9-tetrahydrocannabinol (THC)is the main psychoactive component of the marihuana. Previous studies demonstrated that THC had mainly inhibitory effect on anterior pituitary (AP) hormone secretion. Recently a putative ligand for the cannabinoid receptor, the ANA has been discovered and purified. This provided us the opportunity to compare the effects of THC and ANA on AP LH, FSH, PRL and GH secretion in adult OVX and male rats. The animals were ovariectomized 3 weeks prior the experiments. Both OVX and male rats were given 0.02mg/kg b.w. ANA or THC i.p. for 14 consecutive days. By the end of the 2nd week after quick decapitation the trunk blood was collected and measured for the above mentioned AP hormones with RIA.
The results showed that in male ANA had no effect on serum LH level while it decreased this later in OVX rats. THC decreased more significantly LH content in both groups than ANA. Neither ANA, nor THC changed serum FSH level. ANA, like THC caused considerable decrease of serum PRL but a more pronounced level in male rats. Finally GH levels were decreased after ANA in both OVX and male rats, but increased slightly after THC in male animals.
It has been concluded that ANA has affected the PA hormone secretion and its effects in some cases have been different than that of THC.

P2.41

TUBEROINFUNDIBULAR DOPAMINE (TIDA) NEURONS RESPOND TO PRL FEEDBACK IN EARLY, BUT NOT MIDDLE, LACTATION. L.A. Arbogast*, J.L. Voogt, Physiology Dept., Univ. of Kansas, Kansas City, KS, USA 66160-7401

Lactation is a state of hyperprolactinemia associated with suppressed TIDA neuronal activity. The aims of this study were 1) to determine the responsiveness of TIDA neurons to PRL during early and midlactation and 2) to examine the effect of suppressing plasma PRL levels during lactation on TIDA neuronal activity. TH activity in the SME was assessed by the accumulation of 3,4-dihydroxyphenylalanine (DOPA) after inhibiting DOPA decarboxylase with m-hydroxybenyzlhydrazine (100 mg/kg,i.p.). Experiment 1: MMQ (cell line secreting PRL) cells were injected intracerebroventricularly (200,000cells/15µl), on day 3 or 10 of lactation and rats were killed on day 6 or 13, respectively. Some rats were injected with oPRL (4 mg/kg, s.c.) at 8 h intervals on days 5 and 6 of lactation. TH activity in the SME on day 6 of lactation was increased 1.3- or 2-fold by MMQ cells or oPRL, respectively. Separation from litters for 22h increased DOPA accumulation 70% above levels in suckled rats. MMQ cells or oPRL further increased TH activity 60% above the separated-induced rise on day 6. In contrast to early lactation, MMQ cells did not alter TH activity in the SME on day 13. MMQ cells suppressed plasma PRL to 40% of control levels on day 6, but did not alter plasma PRL levels on day 13. Experiment 2: Lactating rats were injected with bromocriptine (Bromo;3 mg/kg,s.c.) and were sacrificed after 4h or 12h on day 5 or after 12h on day 12. In some rats PRL was replaced by injecting oPRL (4 mg/kg, s.c.) simultaneously with and 8h after Bromo. Bromo reduced DOPA accumulation in the SME on day 5 by 40% or 65% within 4h or 12h, respectively. Bromo+oPRL restored TH activity to control levels. Bromo decreased TH activity by 40% within 12h on day 12, but co-treatment with oPRL did not restore levels to control. CONCLUSIONS: 1) The ability of TIDA neurons to respond to exogenous PRL is lost between day 6 and 12 of lactation. 2) The high endogenous PRL levels associated with the suckling stimulus may activate TH activity in the TIDA neurons during early lactation. Supported by NIH grant HD24190 and HD07368.

P2.42

ROL OF HYPOTHALAMIC SUBSTANCE P IN THE CONTROL OF PROLACTIN RELEASE. E. Isovich, M.C. Díaz, M. Lasaga, D. Pisera, C. Zambruno, M.S. Theas, A. Seilicovich, B.H. Duvilanski*. Centro de Investigaciones en Reproducción. Facultad de Medicina, Universidad de Buenos Aires, Paraguay 2155 (1121), Buenos Aires, Argentina.

Substance P (SP) acting on the anterior pituitary gland stimulates prolactin release. We investigated the effect of prolactin on the concentration of hypothalamic SP to determine if prolactin regulates it in a classical feedback loop. Hypothalamic fragments from male Wistar rats were incubated in KRB buffer in the presence of prolactin, dopamine or SP under basal and K^+ stimulated conditions. Prolactin (100 ng/ml) increased SP content (15.84±2.73 ng/mg protein vs control (C) 4.68±2.22; $p<0.05$) and release (3.93±0.72 vs C 0.27±0.06; $p<0.01$). Dopamine (10^{-7}M) decreased SP content (2.97±0.36 vs C 5.41±0.56; $p<0.01$) and release (0.10±0.02 vs C 0.24±0.02; $p<0.01$), while SP (10^{-7}M) stimulated dopamine release (23.19±2.42 ng/mg protein vs C 11.04±1.21; $p<0.01$). These results demonstrate an interaction of SP, dopamine and prolactin at the hypothalamic level and suggest that SP could mediate the feedback action of prolactin on dopamine release.

P2.43

THYROIDECTOMY (THX) INDUCES RECRUITMENT OF MORE AND ONLY MAMMOTROPES TO BECOME VIP IMMUNOREACTIVE. A.A. Léránt, K. Köves, Gy.M. Nagy. 2nd Department of Anatomy, Semmelweis University Medical School, Budapest, Hungary, H-1450

It is well known that vasoactive intestinal peptide (VIP) is synthetized in the anterior pituitary gland. VIP is supposed to play an autocrine or paracrine role in the secretion of prolactin (PRL), althuogh, hypothalamic influence on the pituitary VIP synthesis can not be excluded. It is also well documented that THX can increase the number of VIP immunoreactive cells in the anterior lobe (AL). This effect is at least partially mediated through the hypothalamus. The aims of our present studies were to determine the effect of THX on the VIP-immunoreactivity (IR) of the AL and the pituitary cell type(s) that contain VIP. Anterior pituitaries obtained from intact and thyroidectomized (3 weeks after surgery) male rats were monodispersed and subjected to the PRL reverse hemolytic placque assay (RHPA) and VIP and PRL immunocytochemisty (ICC) in order to determine PRL release and VIP-IR separately and in combination. In intact rats 6-8 % of all AL cells were found to be VIP-IR. In contrast, THX resulted an increase in the number of VIP-immunoreactive cells (10-15%). When PRL RHPA and VIP ICC were combined, all VIP-IR cells were found in PRL secretors in both intact and thyroidectomized animals. Our data suggest that VIP can only be synthetized in mammotropes and THX recruit more PRL secretors to synthetize VIP. THX-induced preferential recruitment of mammotropes to become VIP-IR and the role of hypothalamus in its organisation needs to be further clarified. (These studies were supported by OTKA T1024 to Gy.M.N and OTKA T5443 to K.K.)

P2.44

INHIBITION OF PROLACTIN (PRL) RELEASE IN LACTATING RATS WITH HIGHLY ELEVATED PLASMA ACTH LEVELS. Zs.Bánky*, G.M.Nagy, B. Halász, 2nd Dept. of Anatomy Semmelweis University Medical School, Budapest, Hungary, 1094

Recently it has been shown that pathways mediating the suckling- induced release as well as separation induced depletion of plasma prolactin (PRL) are extremely sensitive to a regulatory signal originating from the adrenal glands. Previously we have observed that separation results in an immediate depletion of plasma PRL with a concommitant increase in corticosterone. The aim of our present studies was to get more information about plasma level of ACTH after separation and about the effect of systemic administration of ACTH (4-days) on the suckling induced PRL release. There is a marked increase of ACTH after 15 min separation (48±6 fm/ml vs. 208±29 fm/ml). At the same time PRL decreases significantly (221±12 ug/ml vs. 32±4 ug/ml). Furthermore, suckling-induced PRL release is almost completely inhibited after 2-4 days of ACTH treatment (2 IU/rat/day im.). These data strongly suggest that separation of a mother from her pups is a severe stress that results in a classical pituitary-adrenal response. In addition, we conclude that highly elevated plasma ACTH levels may inhibit suckling-induced PRL release. The site and mechanism of this interaction needs to be investigated. **(This work was supported by OTKA 2616 B.H. and OTKA 5004 to G.M.N.)**

P2.45

MODULATION BY 17β ESTRADIOL OF ANGIOTENSIN II RECEPTOR SUBTYPES AND TRANSDUCTION MECHANISMS INVOLVED IN THE STIMULATION OF PROLACTIN SECRETION. C. Moreau, C. Llorens*, R. Rasolonjanahary , C. Kordon°, A. Enjalbert. UMR 9941, Marseille. *U36, Paris. °U159, Paris,FRANCE

We previously showed that the angiotensin II (AII) induced prolactin (PRL) release involved only one AII receptor type, the AT1, coupled to several transduction mechanisms: a positive coupling to PLC and, depending on PKC activation conditions, a negative or a positive coupling to AC. The AT2 receptors, also present in the antehypophysis are not involved in these pathways. The AT1 receptors are coupled to their effectors by distinct G proteins: AC inhibition, but not PLC stimulation is PTX sensitive. Two AT1 subtypes, AT1a and AT1b, encoded by distinct genes have been described. There is no specific antagonist able to differentiate between them. The 17β estradiol (17βE) is a peripheral hormone known to modify the expression of the AII receptors. We investigated whether this hormone differentially modulate the AII receptor subtypes and the different associated transduction mechanisms

The binding of AII to membranes of antehypophysis cells was decreased by 50% by the treatment of the cells with 10-9M17βE during 72H. In addition, incubation of the cells with 17βE decreased AII maximal inhibition of AC activity measured in membrane preparations (60%versus 80%) with no change in EC50. In this preparation,the basal level of cAMP was significatively increased by the 17βE and not by the 17αE. The Inositol Phosphates (IPs) basal level was not modified by the peripheral hormone when the stimulation of IPs formation by AII was decreased (200% versus 350%), with no change in EC50. The same treatment had no influence on the AII-induced cAMP accumulation in intact cells. In contrast, the cAMP basal level was clearly increased by 17βE, an effect partialy reversed by long term TPA treatment (10-6M). In 17βE pretreated cells, all AII effects were reversed by DuP753, an AT1 antagonist and not by the AT2 antagonist PD123319. Using PCR technique, the only approach that allows to differentiate between the two AT1 subtypes, we study the modulation by 17βE of expression of these receptors subtypes.

P2.46

INHIBITORY EFFECTS OF AMYLIN ON PROLACTIN AND GROWTH HORMONE SECRETION IN THE RAT. A. Pecile*, F. Guidobono, V. Sibilia, M. Coluzzi, N. Lattuada, C. Netti. Dept. of Pharmacol. Chemother.and Medical Toxicol., University of Milan, Italy.

Amylin, a peptide found in the pancreatic β–cells, is presently considered to have a potential role in the genesis of type-2 diabetes. Recently, amylin has also been detected in the CNS; the highest content of the peptide and specific binding sites were detected in the hypothalamus. We have studied in rats the effects of amylin given intracerebroventricularly (i.c.v.) on prolactin (PRL) and growth hormone (GH) release. Amylin (2.5; 5 μg/rat, i.c.v.) did not modify basal PRL and GH secretion but was able to inhibit the β-endorphin (0.5 μg/rat i.c.v) stimulated secretion of both hormones. The inhibitory activity of amylin was more pronounced on GH release rather than on PRL. The effect of amylin was examined also on GH secretion induced by GH-releasing hormone (GHRH, 2 μg/kg, intracarotid) a stimulus acting directly on the pituitary. Amylin (25, 250, 2500 ng/rat, i.c.v.) dose-dependently inhibited GH response to GHRH, but, when given peripherally, was ineffective. The involvement of somatostatin (SRIF) in the inhibitory activity of amylin on GH secretion seems to be ruled out since amylin was still effective in rats that were SRIF depleted by cysteamine.

Our results indicate a central site of action for amylin in the inhibitory effects on PRL and GH secretion and a possible role of the peptide as neuromodulator is suggested.

P2.47

INHIBITION OF GHRH RELEASE BY IGF-I AND -II FROM RAT HYPOTHALAMI *IN VITRO*. M. Korbonits*, P.J. Trainer, J.A. Little, I. Pull, G.M. Besser, A.B. Grossman. Dept. of Endocrinology, St. Bartholomew's Hospital, West Smithfield, London, EC1A 7EB, UK.

Insulin-like growth factors (IGFs) are involved in the feedback control of growth hormone (GH) secretion at both pituitary and hypothalamic levels, but the relative effects on GHRH and somatostatin (SS) release are unclear. We have therefore tested IGF-I and IGF-II alone and together on basal and potassium-stimulated GHRH and SS release in hypothalamic explants of male adult rats. Hypothalamic fragments were incubated with EBSS media containing 5 mM or 28 mM KCl alone and with (i) 33 ng/ml IGF-I or (ii) 33 ng/ml IGF-II or (iii) 33 ng/ml IGF-I+II. Results are expressed as the ratio of treated to basal release (mean ± SEM). One-way ANOVA and Student's t-tests were used to calculate significance ($p<0.05$). GHRH: basal or K^+-stimulated release was unaffected by 33 ng/ml IGF-I or IGF-II alone. However, IGF-I+II inhibited basal GHRH release, which was significant by 40 minutes (control [n=19] ratio to basal: 0.94±0.03 vs treated [n=23]: 0.79±0.03, p=0.006). K^+-stimulated GHRH release was blocked by IGF-I and IGF-II at 20 min (28 mM KCl ratio to basal [n=8]: 1.12±0.04 vs 28 mM KCl+IGF-I+II [n=8]: 0.9±0.04, p=0.002). Indeed, the effect of 28 mM KCl+IGF-I+II did not differ significantly from the control animals. SS: we were unable to demonstrate any consistent effect of 33 ng/ml IGF-I or IGF-II, alone or in combination, on basal or stimulated SS release; this was true also when the media glucose content was increased to 14 mM, a concentration known to inhibit basal SS release.

Conclusion: In rat hypothalamic explants IGF-I acts synergistically with IGF-II to inhibit GHRH release, while showing no consistent effect on SS. These results are in keeping with the *in vivo* data of Harel and Tannenbaum (*Endocrinology* 1992;131:758-64) who demonstrated synergy of intracerebroventricular IGF-I and -II in inhibiting GH secretion in rats. The molecular basis of this synergy requires further investigation.

P2.48

ENRICHED CULTURES OF PITUITARY RUMINANT CELLS: A NEW MODEL TO STUDY OF REGULATION OF GH SECRETION BY SEVERAL NEUROPEPTIDES. M. Rico, M.T. Lorenzo, I. Arnaiz, L. F. De La Cruz. Dept. de Fisiología. Fac. de Veterinaria. Univ. de Santiago de Compostela. Campus Universitario de Lugo. 27002. Lugo. España.

Growth hormone (GH) secretion is governed by the interplay between stimulatory GH-releasing factor (GHRH) and inhibitory (somatostatin, SS) hypothalamic peptides. In addition it has been shown the activity of synthetic hexapeptide GHRP 1-6, increase GH secretion both *in vivo* and *in vitro*. The most of these studies have been carried out in the rat. On the other hand, the role of SS in the control of GH appears to be more complex than it has been assumed so far. In our work we have compared the action of GHRH, GHRP and SS, as well as the action of SS on GH secretion-induced by GHRH and GHRP. All the studies were carried out in bovine somatotrophs obtained by centrifugal elutriation. After 96 h. in culture, cells were incubated during 4 h. with test substances. The supernatants were collected and assayed for GH content by EIA, using reagents and standards provided by NIDDK. In agreement with previous findings our data shows that incubation of cultured bovine somatotroph cells with GHRH 1-29 (10^{-7}M) and GHRP 1-6 (10^{-5}-10^{-7}M) stimulated GH secretion. The results shown that GH secretion is significatly greater in cells incubated with GHRH than in GHRP (10^{-7}M)-incubated cells. We did not find any inhibitory effect of SS on basal GH secretion from somatotrophs of cows. SS was only able to block GHRH and GHRP stimulatory effects on GH secretion at doses of 10^{-6} and 10^{-7}M, but not at 10^{-8}M.

P2.49

EFFECTS OF INTERLEUKINS ON RAT GH SECRETION *IN VITRO* AND *IN VIVO*. Y.Wada, M.Sato, M.Niimi, K.Murao, M.Tamaki, J.Takahara. Dept. of Internal Medicine, Kagawa Medical School, Kagawa, Japan.

Although the effect of interleukins (ILs) on CRF-ACTH axis has been extensively studied, the effect of ILs on GH secretion has not yet been elucidated especially *in vivo*. In the present study, we investigated the possible effect of ILs on rat GH secretion *in vitro* and *in vivo*. Eight-week-old male Wistar rats were used in all experiments. Reverse hemolytic plaque assay (RHPA) was performed to assess GH secretion from a single anterior pituitary cell *in vitro*. The RHPA allowed us to understand the subpopulations of somatotrophs which were sensitive to ILs. ILs were administered to conscious rats via femoral catheters or icv cannulas *in vivo* and sequential blood sampling was performed. The RHPA clearly showed that both IL1 and IL6 increased basal and GRF-stimulated GH secretion in a dose dependent manner *in vitro*. On the other hand, IL1 inhibited pulsatile GH secretion by the continuous iv infusion *in vivo*, though IL6 had no effect. Icv injection of IL1 at smaller doses also inhibited pulsatile GH secretion in the conscious rats. These results suggest that the major action of IL1 is an inhibition of GH secretion which primarily occurs at the hypothalamic site. The stimulatory effects of IL1 and IL6, which were found only *in vitro*, may reflect its autocrine or paracrine action in the pituitary.

P2.50

IN FASTED RATS WITH ANTEROLATERAL HYPOTHALAMIC DEAFFERENTATION (ALC), GROWTH HORMONE (GH) SECRETION AUGMENTS BY NUTRITIONAL INTAKE. K. Okada*, N. Suzuki, J. Kamegai, S. Minami, H. Sugihara, I. Wakabayashi. Dept. Med., Nippon Med. Sch. Tokyo 113, Japan

Fasting inhibits GH secretion in rats. Refeeding augments GH-releasing factor (GRF) secretion, but it remains unknown whether the process depends on a specific macronutrient. In the present study, the effect of macronutrients on GH secretion was tested in fasted ALC rats. ALC was made to remove somatostatin influence on GH secretion. Adult male Wistar rats were subjected to ALC or sham operation 2 weeks previously. They were deprived of food for 72 h. Serial blood samples were collected for 12 h beginning 6 h before food intake. Pulsatile GH secretion with low amplitude was observed in control rats, while in ALC rats, baseline GH levels tended to be higher compared to trough levels of control rats, and no pulsatile GH secretion was observed. Refeeding mixed meal, consisting of CHO 60%, P 25%, F 15% immediately increased pulsatility and the amplitude of GH pulse in control rats. Among fasted ALC rats, baseline GH levels significantly raised with small fluctuation following the ingestion of mixed meal, protein deficient meal consisting of CHO 85%, F 15% or protein meal. The data suggest that GRF stimulation does not depend on a specific macronutrient of refed meal in fasted rats.

P2.51

NALOXONE DOES NOT INHIBIT THE GH RESPONSE TO PYRIDOSTIGMINE IN NORMAL FEMALE SUBJECTS
A. Mancini*, C. Fiumara, G. Conte and L. De Marinis
Inst. of Endocrinology, Catholic University, Rome, Italy

The existence of a sex-related control of GH secretion in man is controversial. We have previously observed that the GH response to pyridostigmine (PYR) administration can be abolished by a naloxone (Nal) infusion in normal males, suggesting an interaction between opioids and cholinergic activity in the control of GH secretion.
We have now tested 6 normal females, aged 19-48 ys, at 1.00 p.m., administering PYR (60 mg p.o.) alone or during a Nal infusion (1.6 mg/h) started 30 min before.
We observed, after PYR alone, a peak (mean±SEM) of 11.8± 3.6 ng/ml and, after PYR during Nal, a peak of 4.5±1.9 ng/ml (p=n.s.). Areas under the curves (mean±SEM) were: 379.8±109.3 ng/ml/90 min (PYR alone) and 459.7±343.0 ng/ml/90 min (Nal+PYR, p=n.s.). A response to PYR administration was observed, under Nal infusion, in 50% of the subjects.
These data confirm the existence of an opioid modulation of the cholinergic control of GH secretion; however, it seems to be different in the two sexes and could explain the various results of the authors regarding the mechanisms of regulation of GH.

P2.52

Neurons expressing a non-mammalian form of LHRH originate from the olfactory placode and migrate into the brain prior to mammalian LHRH neurons in the rhesus monkey. C.D.Quanbeck, N.M.Sherwood*, R.P.Millar† and E.Terasawa. Wisconsin Regional Primate Research Center, Univ. of Wisconsin, Madison, WI 53715, U.S. A., *Dept. of Biology, Univ. of Victoria, Canada, and † Univ. of Cape Town Medical School, Cape Town, South Africa.

To examine the hypothesis that neurons expressing an evolutionarily ancient form of LHRH appear during early primate development, time-mated fetuses of the rhesus monkey at E30 to E40 days were immunocytochemically stained for 7 known forms of LHRH (mammalian, chicken I, chicken II, dogfish, catfish, salmon, and lamprey). We found a population of neurons expressing an LHRH-like peptide that was similar, but not identical to any of the known LHRH forms including mammalian LHRH (mLHRH). These non-mammalian LHRH (non-mLHRH) neurons originated in and migrated out of the olfactory placode, entering the brain several days earlier than mLHRH neurons. On E30 non-mLHRH cells, but not mLHRH cells, were found around the olfactory epithelia, in the nasal mesenchyme, and in the rostro-ventral edge of the telencephalon. On E34-E36 mLHRH cells seen in the olfactory placode and the terminal nerve region, were extending neurites toward non-mLHRH neurons which continued to migrate caudally and medially in the base of the telencephalon. On E38-E40, non-mLHRH cells were concentrated in the septal/preoptic area reaching the hypothalamus. At this stage large numbers of mLHRH neurons were located in the forebrain where the most advanced migrating neurons were in apposition to the lagging edge of the non-mLHRH population. Non-mLHRH cells (~10x7μm) were smaller than mLHRH cells (~15x7μm). Double staining studies further indicate that non-mLHRH cells, but not mLHRH cells, expressed a sialylated form of a neuronal cell adhesion molecule (N-CAM) in the migratory pathway. These data and the juxtaposition of mLHRH fibers to non-mLHRH cells in the brain on E34-E36 and the cell-cell contact between the two cell types at E38-E40 suggest that non-mLHRH neurons provide guidance cues for the migration of mLHRH neurons. The structure of the LHRH-like peptide remains to be determined. (Supports: NIH grants HD15433 & HD11355).

P2.53

PATTERNS OF IMMUNOSTAINING FOR GnRH IN NASAL EPITHELIUM OF ADULT MALES WITH AND WITHOUT KALLMANN'S SYNDROME, AND IN FETAL AND ADULT BRAINS.

*W Hasan[1], R Quinton[1], T Cowen[2], R E Quiney[3], V M Duke[1], P-M G Bouloux[1].
Departments of [1]Medicine, [2]Anatomy and [3]ENT Surgery, Royal Free Hospital School of Medicine, London NW3 2PF.

GnRH secreting neurones are known to originate in the epithelium of the medial olfactory placode, whence they migrate along the axons of the vomeronasal and terminalis nerves into the forebrain and from there to the hypothalamus. Schwanzel-Fukuda and Pfaff demonstrated the failure of GnRH positive neurones to penetrate the forebrain in a 19 week fetus with X-linked Kallmann's Syndrome (KS: anosmia and hypogonadotrophic hypogonadism). Whereas GnRH immunoreactivity was already demonstrable in the hypothalamus of a matched normal fetus it was confined to the nasal septum and cribriform plate area in the KS fetus.

GnRH positive neurones are thought to persist in the nasal epithelium of normal adults but we hypothesised that there might be a different pattern of GnRH immunoreactivity in the nasal epithelium of KS men as compared with normal controls. We utilised an immunofluorescent double immunostaining technique with anti-GnRH and anti-Neurofilament antibodies on biopsies of nasal mucosa obtained from a male with KS, a normal male cadaver and a normal, live male, and on sagittal sections of brain from a male cadaver and 13 week human fetus. Strongest GnRH immunoreactivity was seen in the median eminence of the cadaveric hypothalamus. In the 13 week fetus, GnRH positive neurones were largely located in the hypothalamus but could still be seen actively migrating towards it within the forebrain. We intend to continue the studies on fetuses of different gestational ages but our findings todate suggest that in the 13 week human fetus GnRH cell migration is close to completion. Isolated GnRH positive neurones were demonstrated in all 3 nasal biopsies, with no evident excess in the Kallmann specimen, but definitive confirmation will require further nasal biopsies performed endoscopically under direct vision from topographically homologous regions of epithelium.

P2.54

DEVELOPMENT OF FEEDBACK REGULATION IN CULTURED FETAL RAT PITUITARIES. **Á. Nemeskéri. 2nd Dept. of Anatomy, Semmelweis University Medical School, Budapest, Hungary, 1094.**

The present study was performed to test whether the feedback control of ACTH, FSH, TSH expression develops also in cultured fetal pituitary glands. For this purpose 13-day-old fetal pituitaries were maintained in organ culture for six days in the presence of adult pituitary, ovary and hypothalamus. Fetal pituitaries cultured alone or in the presence of non-endocrine tissues served as controls. The functional differentiation of pituitary primordia was evaluated by immunocytochemistry. The number of ACTH, FSH and TSH positive cells and the density of their immunostaining were significantly reduced in pituitary anlagen coincubated with adult pituitary when compared to those observed in fetal glands incubated alone or in the presence of non-endocrine tissue. Coincubation with adult ovary prevented the differentiation of FSH cells in the fetal pituitaries. Hypophyseal primordia incubated in close contact with adult mediobasal hypothalamus exhibited significantly higher number of ACTH, FSH and TSH cells and greater staining intensity comparing them to all other experimental groups. These results show that ACTH, FSH and TSH of adult pituitary origin exerted negative feedback effect on the biosynthesis and/or the accumulation of these hormones in the fetal glands. This fact might indicate the existence of autoregulation at the level of fetal corticotroph, gonadotroph and thyrotroph. Furthermore the gonadal feedback regulation of FSH synthesis also seems to be operational in the cultured fetal glands. **Supported by OTKA, grant no. 2616 and 1008.**

P2.55

FACTORS PRESENT IN MEDIUM CONDITIONED BY NORMAL GONADOTROPHS STIMULATE THE DIFFERENTIATION OF LACTOTROPHS IN THE PITUITARY IN VITRO. A.Van Bael* and C.Denef. Laboratory of Cell Pharmacology, K.U.Leuven, 3000 Leuven, Belgium.

As estimated by computer-image analysis, addition of LHRH to reaggregate cell cultures of 14-day- old female rat pituitaries resulted in a significant increase in the total cytoplasmic areas of cells containing PRL mRNA as measured by in situ hybridization and of PRL as measured by immunocytochemistry. Gonadotrophs, stimulated by LHRH, probably release paracrine growth factors promoting the postnatal development of lactotrophs. To define these growth factors, secretory products of a highly enriched population of gonadotrophs were collected in serum-free medium in the presence of LHRH. Biomolecules in this medium were concentrated and after ultrafiltration the material retained was run on a C18-reversed phase HPLC column. Several bioactive fractions wich mimicked the effect of LHRH were found. After further purification of one of these fractions on reversed phase HPLC and on a gel filtration column, we found a single fraction stimulating the recruitment of lactotrophs but having no mitogenic effect. Experiments are in progress in order to purify and characterize this factor. It is concluded that gonadotrophs may control the differentiation of lactotrophs from progenitor cells through a paracrine growth factor.

P2.56

EXPERIMENTAL EVIDENCE FOR THE VERY EARLY COMMITMENT OF GONADOTROPIC CELLS. A. ElAmraoui, P.M. Dubois. CNRS URA 1454, Claude Bernard University-Lyon I, Faculty of medicine Lyon-Sud, BP 12, F-69600 Oullins.

Whereas LH cell and GnRH neuron interactions are largely studied, data are still lacking at very early developmental stages. In the chick embryo, during early neurogenesis (2- to 4-somitic stages), GnRH precursor cells are distributed within the presumptive ectoderm of nasal cavity (ElAmraoui and Dubois, Neuroendocrinology, 1993, 57:991-1002) close to the presumptive adenohypophysis which is already committed (ElAmraoui and Dubois, Neuroendocrinology, 1993, 58:609-615). To investigate whether any interactions between these presumptive territories can influence the commitment and the differentiation of the gonadotropic cells, uni- and bilateral ablations of the whole nasal territory were performed from 2- to 4-somitic stages (28-30 hours of incubation) in the chick embryo. At later stages, the adenohypophysis was always present. By day 8 of incubation, the number of βLH cells did not vary in normal and operated embryos as well. These data suggest that gonadotropic cells could differentiate without any influence of GnRH neurons, which failed to develop in operated embryos. It can be also suggested that gonadotropic cells could be committed as early as 3-somitic stage and their differentiation could appear under the influence of other factor(S) than GnRH as suggested in rat. This should explain the occurence of gonadotropic cells in some pathologies related to GnRH deficiency.

P2.57

MIGRATION AND DEVELOPMENT OF GnRH NEURONS IN THE MIGRATORY SALMON. I. S. Parhar*[1], M. Iwata[1], D.W. Pfaff[2], M. Schwanzel-Fukuda[2]. [1]National Research Institute of Aquaculture, Nikko, Tochigi 321-16, Japan and [2]Lab. Neurobiology and Behavior, The Rockefeller University, N. Y., New York, USA, 10021.

Gonadotropin hormone-releasing hormone (GnRH, salmon type) was detected by immunocytochemistry in the brain and in the nervus terminalis of mature and embryonic sockeye salmon (*Onchorhynchus nerka*). GnRH was first detected at 19 days after fertilization in the medial part of the olfactory placode. By day 24 (eye pigmentation), GnRH neurons were seen in the apical, intermediate and basal layers of the olfactory placode. By day 30 GnRH neurons were seen emerging from the epithelium, along the olfactory nerve and at the rostral olfactory bulb (OB). By day 41 cords of GnRH neurons were seen on the nasal septum, immunoreactivity was lost in the nasal epithelium. By day 72 (hatching) a large noval GnRH ganglion was seen at the cribriform bone (gCB) and a small GnRH ganglion at the rostral olfactory bulb (gROB). These ganglions increased in size with age (83-253). On day 293 (downstream migration) an apparent decrease in GnRH neurons in the gCB and gROB was concomitant with an initial appearance of GnRH neurons and fibers along the caudoventral OB. At 2 1/2 years (start of maturation), GnRH neurons decreased to a stretch of scattered cells along the medial regions of the olfactory nerve, caudoventral OB and for the first time GnRH neurons were seen along the ventral telencephalon and the anterioventral preoptic area. Midbrain neurons were not immunoreactive. Prior to day 293, GnRH fibers were seen in the rostral OB, thereafter they also appeared in caudoventral OB, next to growth hormone and somatolactin cells.

P2.58

EFFECT OF CYSTEAMINE ON GHRH EXPRESSION IN FETAL HYPOTHALAMIC NEURONS IN CULTURE. C. Loudes, C. Viollet-Grenet, J. Epelbaum, C. Kordon and A. Faivre-Bauman. U 159 INSERM, 2ter rue d'Alésia, 75014 Paris France.

GHRH expression was measured in fetal hypothalamic cells grown in serum-free medium, in conditions in which somatostatin was depleted or not by the addition of 1 mM cysteamine for 24 h. By northern blotting quantification with specific oligonucleotide probes, at 14 days in vitro, GHRH mRNA levels (a single transcript of 0,75 kb) were increased while Somatostatin mRNAs (0,8 kb) did not change after cysteamine addition. GHRH and Somatostatin neurons were visualized by in situ hybridization with the same ^{33}P labelled oligoprobes after 7, 14, 21 and 28 days in vitro. Specificity of labelling was attested by the absence of signal when sense probes were used. GHRH neurons were detected only after 2 weeks in culture and represented less than 1% of the total neuronal population. Cysteamine treatments modified neither the number of GHRH neurons nor that of Somatostatin neurons. In conclusion, these data suggest that Somatostatin exerts a negative control on the developmental expression of GHRH neurons in culture by regulating the quantity of GHRH mRNAs per neuron as previously observed in vivo in the adult.

P2.59

INTERACTION OF GRF AND LHRH IN THE POSTNATAL DEVELOPMENT OF SOMATOTROPHS IN RAT PITUITARY CELL AGGREGATES. **M. Proesmans*, A. Van Bael and C. Denef. Laboratory of Cell Pharmacology, K.U. Leuven, 3000 Leuven, Belgium.**

In a previous investigation we showed that LHRH, presumably via a paracrine action of gonadotrophs, exerted a negative influence on the development of somatotrophs in pituitary reaggregate cell cultures from 14-day-old female rats as estimated by immunocytochemistry and (^{3}H)thymidine ([^{3}H])T) incorporation autoradiography. In the present study we studied the effect of LHRH on the number of cells expressing GH mRNA measured by in situ hybridization with a digoxigenin-labelled riboprobe. Both the total pituitary cell population and cells processing through the S-phase of the cell cycle ([^{3}H])T incorporating) and presumably mitosis were examined. Addition of 1 nm LHRH for 40 hours to aggregate cell cultures of 14-day-old rat pituitary did not affect the number of [^{3}H]T cells displaying a positive hybridization signal for GH mRNA but significantly decreased the number of [^{3}H]T cells immunostained for GH protein. Treatment of the cultures for 40 h with 0.1 nM GRF provoked a 47 % increase in the number of [^{3}H]T labelled cells containing GH mRNA and a 30% increase in the number of cells immunostained for GH protein. The effect of GRF on the number of [^{3}H]T labelled GH mRNA expressing cells was completely blocked by simultaneous addition of 1 nM LHRH to the cultures. LHRH had an inhibitory effect on the total number of cells containing GH mRNA and a comparable effect on the total number of cells stained for GH protein. The present data show that LHRH is capable of inhibiting the GRF-independent as well as the GRF-dependent development of somatotrophs in postnatal rat pituitary in culture.

P2.60

GABAergic EFFECTS ON GH SECRETION AND INTRACELLULAR CALCIUM IN SINGLE SOMATOTROPH CELLS FROM NEWBORN RAT PITUITARIES. Gy. Horváth*, Zs. Ács, A. Taupignon, Gy. Nagy, I. Nagy, B. Dufy, G.B. Makara. Heim Pál Ped. Hosp., Inst. of Exptl. Medicine, Acad. Sci., 2nd Dept. of Anatomy, Semmelweis Medical Scool, Budapest Hungary; Lab. of Neurophysiology, URA CNRS 1200, University of Bordeaux, France.

The effect of GABA on some characteristics of GH-secretion (proportion of secreting cells, distribution of secreted hormone amount) and the effect of the GABAergic agonists muscimol and baclofen on intracellular free calcium levels were studied in freshly dispersed neonatal (postnatal day 2-5) rat pituitary cells attached to microscopic slides (secretion experiments) or glass cover slisps (intracellular calcium measurement). Identification of GH secreting cells in both cases was performed by reverse haemolytic plaque assay. Secreted hormone amount was characterised by the plaque-area. Intracellular calcium levels of identified somatotrophs were analysed using fluorescent probes and micro-spectrofluorimetric techniques.
Approximately 10% of all pituitary cells (25% of GRF-responsive cells) showed spontaneous GH secretion. The number of secreting cells was doubled when cells were incubated in the presence of 10^{-5} M GABA for 30 or 60 min., but no difference could be seen in the distribution profile of plaque-sizes between the control and treated samples. This is clearly different from the response to GRF where a right-shift of the plaque-size profile was also observed. The effect of GABA in young animals seems to be a "turn-on" of silent GH-cells into secretion-state with no consequences on the secretion later on.
In the fluorimetric measurements, the majority of somatotrophs have a very stable basal $[Ca^{2+}]_i$. Only few cells show spontaneous Ca-transients. In this respect, there was no difference between spontaneously secreting (plaque-building) and GRF-responsive cells. GABA-like Ca-peaks could be elicited with the agonist muscimol but not with baclofen. (This work was supported by the grants OTKA 2925, ETK T-10 T-337/1990 and the EC's fellowship ERB3510PL924632/6655)

P2.61

ONTOGENY OF GROWTH HORMONE GENE EXPRESSION IN THE CHICKEN.

R. Józsa*[†], K. Reiprich, E. Mühlbauer, R. Grossmann. Inst. for Small Animal Res., Celle, Germany, 23223; [†]Dept. of Anatomy, Univ. Med. School, Pécs, Hungary, 7643.

Development and growth in birds, as in mammals, appears to be under an intricate control mechanism which involves several hormonal factors. In birds, GH is required for normal rate of growth. The question however, whether GH can stimulate growth in intact birds is enigmatic, since GH has relatively little direct effect on tissue growth in birds. The aim of the present study was to investigate the relationship between patterns of GH gene expression and body growth in growing chickens of different age, sex and breed by in situ hybridization histochemistry. Pituitaries of laying- and meat-type chickens and chicken embryos of both sexes were collected at different ages of embryonal (E) and posthatch (D) life (from E5 to D7) and frozen on dry ice. Subsequent coronal sections were hybridized with a ^{35}S-CTP radiolabeled riboprobe which was in vitro transcribed from a 760 bp cDNA fragment. Quantitative data were obtained from Northern blot analysis. During embryonic life, specific signals were first detectable in the region of the Rathke's pouch as early as E7. A slight increase in number of GH expressing cells was observed on the following days. The cellular content of GH mRNA elevated rapidly from E11 onward. Consistent and strong signals were observed in all specimens from E14 onward with a progressive increase between E14 to ~7. GH mRNA-containing cells were evenly distributed over the caudal lobe of the pituitary. Obvious strain differences were observed from E14 onward: higher levels of GH gene expression in meat-type specimens compared to laying types were observed. Highest GH mRNA content was found in D7 meat-type males.

P2.62

CONTROL OF GH SECRETION FROM PORCINE FETAL AND NEONATAL PITUITARY TISSUE IN VITRO BY GRF AND SRIF.

R. Torronteras*[1], F. Gracia-Navarro[2], F. Elsaesser[1]. 1. Institut für Tierzucht und Tierverhalten FAL, Mariensee, 31535-Neustadt, Germany. 2. Department of Cell Biology, Univ. of Cordoba, Spain.

The physiological mechanism underlying the enormously elevated plasma GH concentrations in the fetal pig is not well understood. We postulated that a decreased sensitivity to the inhibitory effects of SRIF at the pituitary level during fetal life might be one factor in the hypersecretion of GH. Therefore porcine anterior pituitary (AP) tissue pieces derived from male and female fetuses (95 days p.c.) and neonates (10-12 days p.p.) were perifused (6 replicates per treatment and sex) at a rate of 0.1 ml/min and fractions were collected at 10 min intervals. Tissue was subjected to various treatment in radom order: a 10-min GRF pulse (1 nM) with or without concomitant 40-min exposure to SRIF (1, 10 or 100 nM). None of treatments revealed sex differences, therefore data from males and females were pooled. Exposure to GRF resulted in a rapid stimulatory GH response both in fetuses (from 50.8 ± 2.3 to 100.1 ± 2.7 ng GH*60 min^{-1}*mg^{-1} AP) and neonates (from 38.1 ± 2.2 to 73.2 ± 3.2 ng GH*60 min^{-1}*mg^{-1} AP). Exposure to 1 nM SRIF during a GRF pulse inhibited the GH response in neonates to 34.4 ± 1.9 ng GH*60 min^{-1}*mg^{-1} AP but no in fetuses (98.8 ± 3.1 ng GH*60 min^{-1}*mg^{-1} AP). When 10 or 100 nM SRIF were used, the GH response to GRF was totally blocked in neonates (39.4 ± 4.8 and 47.1 ± 3.2 ng GH*60 min^{-1}*mg^{-1} AP, respectively). However, when using 10 nM or 100 nM SRIF in fetuses, the GH response was inhibited only during the first 30 min after GRF (26.4 ± 3.9 and 26.4 ± 5.1 ng GH*30 min^{-1}*mg^{-1} AP), and a rebound effect occured during the next minutes (63.9 ± 1.8 and 72.2 ± 3.7 ng GH*60 min^{-1}*mg^{-1} AP). In conclusion the grossly elevated plasma GH levels in the porcine fetus *in vivo* (compared to the neonates) may be explained, at least in part by decreased sensitivity to the inhibitory effects of SRIF at the pituitary level.

P2.63

OPIOID RECEPTORS IN N. SUPRAOPTICUS AND N. PARAVENTRICULARIS IN NORMAL AND OSMOTIC STIMULATED CHICKENS.

N. Örding, R. Großmann, N. Parvizi*. Insti. of Anim. Breeding & Behav.; Inst. of Small Anim. Science, 29223 Celle, Germany

Osmoregulation and ovipositin are controlled by neurohypophyseal hormone Arg-Vasotocin (AVT), which is synthesized in the nucleus opticus (SON) and n. paraventricularis (PVN) in birds. Opioids modulate AVT secretion induced by hypertonic saline, but exert no significant effect on AVT in normohydrate animals. We investigated the effect of osmotic stimulation on the opioid system at receptor level in PVN and SON. Groups of male and female chicken at embryonal (E) day 18, 1 day after hatching (D 1), at D 30 or adults were used. Osmotic stimulation was induced in half of the animals in each group by either i.p. injection of 0.3 ml, 10% NaCl (E 18 and D 1), 19 h (D 30) or 48 h (adult) of water deprivation. These stimuli cause significant enhancement of plasma osmolality and AVT concentration. Animals were decapitated, brains were removed immediately and frozen on dry ice. PVN and SON were punched out of serial brain slices. Scatchard assays were performed using [H^3]-diprenorphine (0.1-2.5 nM) in presence or absence of naloxone. In the PVN the highest receptor density was measured on day E 18 (B_{max} = 170±15 fM/mg protein (P). The levels fall significantly ($p < 0.01$) until D 30 (55±6.0 fM/mg P). In the SON the pattern was different, maximal levels were measured on D 1 (130±12 fM/mg P). There were no significant differences between E 18, D 30 and adult animals. Osmotic challenge reduced the number of active receptors in the PVN (98±5 fM/mg P) and enhanced it in the SON (90±6 fM/mg P) on E 18. The osmotic challenge attenuated the B_{max}-age differences were seen in PVN. In conclusion, opioidergic mediated AVT osmoregulation is modulated in parts by opioid receptors in PVN and SON.

P2.64

DAILY MEASUREMENTS OF TIBIAL GROWTH IN A GH DEFICIENT RAT MODEL.

A. Perez Romero, M.A. Rol de Lama, B. Granados, J.A.F. Tresguerres, M. Hermanussen, M.C. Ariznavarreta.
Dept. of Physiology. Medical School, Univ. Complutense. Madrid. Spain.

The daily accurate measurement of tibial growth in conscious rats using a mini knemometer, enables for the first time to establish long bone growth patterns under different experimental conditions in the young male rat. All animals showed oscilatory changes in growth velocity (GV) with a periodicity of about 5,5 days that were not affected by GH treatment. A GH deficient model was induced by the neonatal administration of Monosodium Glutamate (MSG). The effect of treatments with GH, Testosterone propionate (TP) or combination of both on the GV and weight patterns between days 22 and 60 of life was investigated both in castrated and non castrated MSG treated rats. Pituitary GH content and plasma GH levels were measured at the end of the experiment. MSG treatment induced a reduction in GV and in the oscilation pattern with the periodicity being of 4,4 days as compared with 5,5 days in normal rats. Castration induced a further reduction in GV that was partially restaured with the administration of T.P. Growth was similar in all groups until day 31st despite of the different treatments. From this day on, GH or TP treatments were able to induced increases in growth velocity in both castrated and non castrated MSG treated animals. No differences could be seen between GH and GH plus TP treated animals as compared to controls. GH pituitary contents were significantly reduced in all MSG treated animals as compared to controls. Contents were further reduced with exogenous hGH treatments. In conclusion, the method is valid for the estimation of long bone growth over very short time periods. Normal male rats seem to grow at a maximal GV that cannot be enhanced by very high doses of hGH. During the first 30 days of life, growth seem not to be dependent on GH or TP.

P2.65

NEURITOGENIC EFFECT OF ESTRADIOL ON VENTROMEDIAL HYPOTHALAMIC NEURONS CO-CULTURED WITH AUTOLOGOUS OR HETEROLOGOUS GLIA. M.J. Cambiasso, H. Diaz, A. Caceres and H.F. Carrer. Instituto de Investigación Médica M. y M. Ferreyra, Córdoba, Argentina, 5000.

Dissociated neurons from ventromedial hypothalamus of 16 gestational days (E16) rats, were co-cultured for 7 days with glial cells taken from fetal rat hypothalamus (autologous), amygdala (heterologous) or without glial monolayer. Each culture contained exclusively cells from either male or female fetuses. Identical cultures were grown in media containing 17-ß-estradiol (E2) 100 μM (experimental) or without estradiol (control). Neural processes were classified as axons or dendrites according to accepted morphological and immunocytochemical criteria and measured in a video analysis system. The length of axons was significantly different, with significant interactions due to sex X E2 treatment ($p<0.001$) and E2 treatment X coculture ($p=0.001$) factors. Post-hoc analysis revealed that axons of neurons taken from male fetuses cocultured with glial monolayer from amygdalar region in media containing E2 were significantly longer ($p<0.001$) than controls without E2. It is proposed that at E16 hypothalamic neurons from males are sensitive to neuritogenic factor(s) segregated by glia from target regions (i.e. amygdala) under the control of E2.

Supported by grant CI1*-CT92-0084 from the EEC

P2.66

CHANGES IN ADULTHOOD IN THE SIZE OF COMPONENTS OF THE MEDIAL PREOPTIC AREA AFTER PREPUBERTAL TESTOSTERONE (T). G.J. Bloch and R. Mills, Dept. of psychology, BYU, Provo, UT, USA, 84602.

We have shown that LH and FSH, estrous cyclicity, and sexual behaviors are defeminized or masculinized in adulthood by prepubertal T treatment of female and neonatally gonadectomized (NeoGx) male rats. The periventricular preoptic (PvPO), the anteroventral periventricular (AVPv), and the medial preoptic nucleus (MPN) and its central and medial divisions (MPNc and MPNm) were measured in adult-sacrificed NeoGx males with Silastic capsules containing 7 mm T or nothing (blank) between days 15-30 of age. Camera lucida tracings of 50um sections were quantified. The width of the PvPO in T-treated NeoGx males decreased 20% compared to blank NeoGx controls (4.3 ± 0.3 mmx10^{-2} vs. 5.2 ± 0.2, $p<0.04$), and the volume of the AVPv decreased 30% (14.1 ± 2.5 mm^{3}x 10^{-3} vs. 20.1 ± 0.6, $p<0.02$). The T treatment increased the size of the MPNm by 27% ($p<0.01$, T-treated NeoGx males vs. blank NeoGx controls). The sizes of the MPNc and MPN were not affected by the prepubertal T treatment. The results demonstrate that a prepubertal T treatment that defeminizes or masculinizes reproductive function in adulthood has analogous effects on several sexually dimorphic components of the MPOA. (Supported by HD 27334)

P2.67

ESTROGEN RECEPTOR, EXPRESSED IN THE FACIAL NUCLEUS OF THE NEWBORN BUT NOT IN THE ADULT RATS, SEEMS RELATED TO DEVELOPMENT OF MOTONEURONS. S.Hayashi*, C.Orikasa, H.Ueda. Dept. of Anatomy and Embryology, Tokyo Metropolitan Inst. for Neuroscience, 2-6 Musashidai, Fuchu, Tokyo 183, Japan.

We have already reported a transient expression of estrogen receptor (ER) in the ventromedial subnucleus of the facial nucleus in the newborn rat (Yokosuka and Hayashi, Neurosci.Res. 15:90–95, 1992). This was confirmed by using other antibodies, which detect distinct epitopes of the native ER (ER-21 and ER-715, generous gifts from Dr.G.L.Greene, Univ. of Chicago and NHPP, NIDDK, USA). This transient expression was also confirmed at gene expression level by *in situ* hybridization histochemistry. Electron microscopy revealed the neurons in this subnucleus with or without ER signals had similar ultrastructure. Microinjection of retrograde tracers into the posterior auricular muscles, where projections from the motoneurons in this subnucleus terminate, revealed that the majority of motoneurons which were marked with the tracer did not contain ER in the cell nucleus. However, on the other hand, all the cells which contained ER in their nuclei contained immunoreactivity of choline acetyl transferase in their cytoplasm. These observations suggest that only the immature motoneurons in this subnucleus retain ER. Thus, ER, and probably together with its ligand, seems to be related to development and determination of the motoneurons of this subnucleus.

P2.68

NEUROTRANSMITTERS TURNOVER IN THE DEVELOPING BRAIN: SEXUAL DIMORPHISM AND MODULATION BY TESTOSTERONE. N.D.Nosenko. Res. Institute of Endocrinology and Metabolism, Kiev, Ukraine

Testosterone-induced changes in sexual differences on catecholamine and serotonin (5-HT) turnover in preoptic area (POA) and mediobasal hypothalamus (MBH) in rats on postnatal day IO were studied. Noradrenaline (NA) and dopamine (DA) turnover was measured by changes catecholamine contents after synthesis blockade with α-methyl-p-tyrosine. 5-Hydroxyindolacetic acid (5-HIAA) and 5-HT ratio was calculated as an estimate of turnover. Distinct sex differences in POA NA and 5-HT turnover on day IO after birth have been revealed. NA turnover rate and the ratio of 5-HIAA to 5-HT in males were higher than in females. It correlates with decreased POA NA content and hypothalamic 5-HT level in males. Neonatal androgenization in females eliminated the male-female differences in 5-HT turnover in POA. No significant androgen effect on NA turnover in POA was observed, while DA turnover in POA and MBH was accelerated. These results indicate that the target for androgen damaging effect on sex differentiation of NA-5-HT metabolism is POA that controls sexual behavior in males and ovulation in females.

P2.69

TESTOSTERONE METABOLISM IN HYPOTHALAMUS OF PRENATALLY STRESSED DEVELOPING RATS. L.Tarasenko. Res. Institute of Endocrinology and Metabolism, Kiev, Ukraine, 254II4.

The influence of maternal immobilization stress on hypothalamic testosterone metabolism in postnatal, immature, and mature male and female offsprings was studied. Aromatase (AA) and 5α-reductase (RA) activities were measured by product isolation assay. Sexual dimorphism in AA was found both in IO- and 20-day-old intact rats being significantly higher in males. The highest AA was demonstrated in IO-day-old males lowering twice by the 20th day and almost I4 times in 90-day-old males. Prenatal stress significantly decreased AA in 20-day-old males while postnatal males only tended to AA lowering. On the contrary, in the females stress resulted in AA increase on the IOth day of life. RA was not modified by the prenatal stress either in IO- or 20-day-old males while mature ones were shown to have increased RA. Stressed IO-day-old females had lower RA than controls. The data obtained suggests that prenatal stress-induced alterations of sexual brain differentiation and gonadotropin secretion control come through developmental changes in brain steroid aromatase activity.

P2.70

CONTENT OF ANDROGEN-BINDING PROTEIN IN IMMATURE RATS EXPOSED TO STRESS DURING INTRAUTERINE DEVELOPMENT. S.V.Varga, Dept. of Endocrinology of Reproduction and Adaptation, Inst. of Endocrinology and Metabolism, Kiev, Ukraine, 254114.

Content of androgen-binding protein (ABP) was studied in 20 day-old male rats, stress-exposed in the prenatal period (pregnant females were immobilized in dorsal position for 1 hour on days 17-21 of pregnancy). ABP content was measured by incubation of testicular cytosol (105000 g) with saturating ^{3}H-5α-dihydrotestosterone concentrations in the absence or presence of excessive non-labeled hormone with further removal of unbound ligand with activated carbon. It was established that stress-exposed males lagged behind in their development (body weight: stress-33.0±1.8, control - 39.4±1.7g, $P < 0.05$; testicular weight: stress-154.8±6.6, control - 185.4±10.4 mg, $P < 0.05$). Testicular ABP content was decreased (stress-151.8±8.8, control-193.0±8.0 fmol ^{3}H-DHT/mg DNA, $P < 0.01$). These changes in ABP content are supposed to effect harmfully reproductive function of stressed animals.

P2.71

PITUITARY GLAND MAY BE AN IMPORTANT TARGET IN THE MECHANISM OF GROWTH INHIBITION AFTER NEONATAL TREATMENT OF RATS BY GLUCOCORTICOID HORMONE. V.I.Goudochnikov*, Silvana F.Vaccari, S.L.Dalmora Depto. de Farmácia Industrial, Centro de Ciências da Saúde, Universidade Federal de Santa Maria, Santa Maria, RS, Brasil, 97 II9.900

The mechanisms of glucocorticoid-induced growth inhibition are not well understood. In our present work on rats three neonatal (but not prepubertal) injections of dexamethasone phosphate (2 mg/kg b.w., s/c) resulted in distinct suppression of growth. In adult state the rats treated neonatally by glucocorticoid hormone exhibited significant decrease in body weight (by 36.0 and 25.6% in males and females respectively). However, the absolute weight of pituitary gland diminished much more in such animals (by 66.7 and 44.3% in males and females respectively). In contrast, the weights of mature liver, heart and kidneys, i.e. the organs known to be glucocorticoid-sensitive (J.N.Loeb, I976), showed less changes after neonatal treatment by dexamethasone phosphate than the weight of pituitary gland. Our results permit to suggest that glucocorticoid-induced growth inhibition may be mediated in part by decrease in proliferative and/or functional activity of pituitary cells.

P2.72

PITUITARY-ADRENOCORTICAL FUNCTION AND BRAIN CATECHOLAMINES IN THE ONTOGENY OF RATS WITH INHERITED STRESS-INDUCED ARTERIAL HYPERTENSION. L.Maslova*, V.Bulygina, A.Markel, E.Naumenko. Institute of Cytology and Genetics, Siberian Branch of Russian Academy of Sciences, Novosibirsk, Russia, 630090.

Central catecholaminergic mechanisms regulating pituitary-adrenocortical system and arterial blood pressure are closely related. Age-dependent changes and interstrain differences in basal and stress-induced plasma corticosterone levels and brain noradrenaline (NA) and dopamine contents were studied at the age from 2 up to 18 weeks in rats with inherited stress-induced arterial hypertension (ISIAH) and normotensive Wistar rats. It was found that the 4th week of life in the ISIAH rats is a critical period in the development of inherited hypertension. At this time fast forming of the hypertension is accompanied by an increase in adrenocortical stress responsivity and a fall in the medulla and hypothalamic NA contents. A short-term augmentation of the brain NA synthesis on the 4th week of life by L-DOPA treatment was followed by a normalization of the arterial pressure and pituitary-adrenocortical function in adult animals as a result of restoration of the brain NA level and the number of alpha-1-adrenoceptors taking part in their regulation.

P2.73

VARIABILITY IN ADRENOCORTICAL STRESS REACTION AND IN THE FUNCTION OF THE BRAIN NORADRENERGIC SYSTEM. N.N. Dygalo, G.T. Shishkina. Institute of Cytology and Genetics, Siberian Branch of the RAS, Novosibirsk, Russia, 630090.

Magnitude of an increase of corticosterone level in the blood of rats and mice under restriction depends on animals genotype and life history. This increase positively correlated with the hormone response to i.c.v. norepinephrine injection in 7 genetic groups of rats. Reactions to stress and norepinephrine simultaneously decreased in adult rats after prenatal glucocorticoid treatment. Prenatal stress or corticosterone treatment have a lasting effect on tyrosine hydroxylase (TH) activity in the brain. The best concordance was found between the changes in stress response and alterations in TH activity in the hippocampus among the studied brain regions: brain stem, substantia nigra, hypothalamus, striatum and cortex. Prenatal treatment increased TH activity in hippocampus and decreased binding of radiolabelled prazosine, clonidine and dihydroalprenolol in some brain regions as well as stress reaction in mice. Thus, individual variations in adrenocortical stress reactivity may be related to the differences in the function of the brain noradrenergic system.

P2.74

SEX-DEPENDENT VIOLATION OF KATECHOLAMINERGIC NEURONS DIFFERENTATION IN BRAIN STEM RAT FOETUSES DEVELOPING IN DIABETIC FEMALES. V.G.Sergeyev. Medical Institute, Izhevsk, Russia

It has been known that while early ontogenesis steps katecholaminergic (KA) neurons of brain stem take part through their terminals in maturation processes of peptidergic neurons in hypothalamus, and they are involved in neuroendocrine regulation in adults. It has been also established that hormonal environment exerts significant influence to KA neurons differentiation. In this paper we investigated the influence of hormonal disbalance in foetus of diabetic female to the differentiation processes.
Autoradiographic analysis of synthetic activity in A1 and A2 KA neuron groups and morphometric analysis of branching extent of their dendrites in 20-days foetuses of both sexes testify about decreased synthetic activity and decreased quantity of cellular terminals in diabetic female rats in comparison with male rats, as well as in with the control foetuses from non-diabetic females. It can testify about delay in differentiation processes of KA neurons under conditions of high insulin and corticosteroids concentrations in blood of female foetuses.

P2.75

EARLY ONTOGENY OF MELANOTROPIN (MSH) BINDING SITES IN RAT CENTRAL AND PERIPHERAL NERVOUS SYSTEM. W. Lichtensteiger*, B. Hanimann, M. Schlumpf, W. Siegrist[b] and A. Eberle[b]. Inst. of Pharmacology, University of Zürich, CH-8057 Zürich, and [b]Research Dept., University Hospital, CH-4031 Basel, Switzerland.

Developmental changes in CNS function after manipulation of α-MSH levels suggest a role for MSH peptides in ontogeny. We studied the ontogeny of binding sites for the analog $[^{125}I]Nle^4$,D-Phe^7-α-MSH (^{125}I-NDP, Kd = 0.37 nM on diencephalic membranes) by in vitro autoradiography. Serial cryostat sections of fetuses and offspring from time-pregnant LE rats were incubated with 0.4 nM ^{125}I-NDP; non-specific binding was assessed in every second section by coincubation with 200 nM cold NDP. At the transition from embryonic to fetal life, specific binding is detected at gestational day (GD) 13 in the sympathetic chain and in the anterior roof of mesencephalon. From GD 15, prominent locations include spinal cord, inferior olive, solitary tract nucleus, spinal trigeminal tract nucleus and ventral mesencephalon, at GD 17 cerebellum, and certain brain nerve ganglia. The perinatal period is characterized by a marked peak of receptor density in striatum and by transient receptor expression in some cortical areas. In the region of the main POMC neuron group in mediobasal hypothalamus, binding sites increase slowly during postnatal life. Region-specific ontogenetic patterns and transient expression in areas virtually devoid of receptors in adulthood support a role of MSH-type peptides in ontogeny.

P2.76

STUDIES OF THE BIOSYNTHESIS OF SUBSTANCE P AND NEUROKININ A BY THE DEVELOPING RAT ENDOCRINE PANCREAS AND INSULINOMA CELLS. G.P. McGregor, R. Hartel, R. Haberberger, W. Kummer and K. Voigt. Institutes of Physiology and Anatomy, Philipps University of Marburg, 35033 Marburg, Germany.

The neuropeptides, substance P and neurokinin A are derived from the PPT-A gene. Using specific radioimmunoassays, reversed-phase HPLC, northern blot analysis and immunohistochemistry, we have found that the two rat insulin-producing cell-lines, RINm5F and RINr1046-38, express the preprotachykinin-A gene. Our analyses indicate that normal biosynthetic processes are involved and that products of the gene, substance P and neurokinin A, enter the regulated secretory pathway. These cell-lines are first the stable, clonal cell-lines to be identified that express this gene and provide a good "in vitro" model with which to investigate the biosynthetic processes and the regulatory factors involved in its expression. Slot-blot quantitation of PPT-A mRNA levels indicate that PPT-A transcription in the RIN cell may be up-regulated following protein kinase C activation and down-regulated by glucocorticosteroids. We have also shown that interleukin 1ß may up-regulate PPT-A gene transcription. These tumor cell-lines are derived from pancreatic endocrine cells, are well differentiated and are popular models for studying insulin biosynthesis. However, it is known that mature islet endocrine cells do not express the PPT-A gene. But RIN cells have phar-macological and morphological properties of foetal or neonatal beta cells rather that of mature beta cells. We have used immunohistochemical to show that the during development pancreatic endocrine cells express the PPT-A gene and following approximately post-natal day 20 expression cases. Our studies so far indicate RIN cells may be a useful model for studying the mechanisms and factors involved in PPT-A gene expression and, more specifically, serve as models for studying the transition expression of this regulatory peptide gene during pancreatic endocrine ontogenesis.

P2.77

EFFECT OF AGING ON HYPOTHALAMIC GnRH AND PITUITARY GONADOTROPIN CONTENT IN OVARIECTOMIZED AND SHORT TERM ESTRADIOL PRETREATED RATS. A. Gajewska*, K. Kochman. The Kielanowski Institute of Animal Physiology and Nutrition, 05-110 Jabłonna, Poland

Release of the anterior pituitary hormones after ovariectomy and estradiol treatment in young and old animals was widely investigated. However, there is a lack of information concerning the influence of these factors on the GnRH content in hypothalamus and LH/FSH in the anterior pituitary. In the present work we studied the effect of ovariectomy and exogenous estradiol on GnRH content in medial basal hypothalamus (MBH), in hypothalamus without MBH (H) and gonadotropins in the pituitaries of 3 and 22 month old female rats. Estimation of GnRH and gonadotropins were performed by RIA method. In 3 month old rats ovariectomy caused a significant decrease of GnRH both in MBH and in H. In their pituitaries great increase of LH and FSH was observed. In 22 month old ovariectomized rats GnRH levels in MBH and H were not changed, but in their pituitaries a significant increase of LH and FSH took place. However, this increase was lower than in parallel group of young rats. We observed the increased level of GnRH in MBH and decreased in H after estradiol injections, but only in 3 month old females; while in the old rats GnRH content either in MBH and in H was unchanged. After short term treatment of estradiol there were no significant changes in LH and FSH content in the pituitaries both in 3 and 22 month old female rats.

P2.78

PHEROMONAL MALE-INDUCED RELEASE OF HYPOTHALAMIC GnRH IN AGING FEMALE RATS. M. M. Cabrera, O.A. Mora*. Dep. de Fisiología, Facultad de Medicina. UCM. Ciudad Universitaria. 28040 Madrid. Spain.

Aging female rats show irregular estrus cycles and anovulatory persistent vaginal estrus. A male urinary pheromone restores normal estrus cycles in such rats (Mora & Cabrera: Biol. Reprod. 50, 1994, in press). This study shows the effect of male urine on hypothalamic content of GnRH in anovulatory persistent estrus (PE) and irregularly cycling (IC) aging 8-11 mo. old Wistar rats maintained in a light-dark-temperature controlled room. Estrus cycle was controlled by daily examination of fresh vaginal smears. Rats were considered PE when vaginal estrus was visualized for 15 consecutive days. To determine basal levels (controls) of hypothalamic GnRH, 8 IC (4 in estrus -E- and 4 in diestrus -D- -proestrus could not be affirmed in IC rats-) as well as 8 PE rats were decapitated before treatment. A sample of 4 IC (2 in E and 2 in D) and 3 PE rats were treated by spraying in the nostrils 50 μL of male urine every 10 minutes for one hour, on only one day, and 2 hours later the hypothalami were obtained by decapitation. GnRH was determined by a double antibody RIA method. Neither IC nor PE showed cyclic variations of hypothalamic GnRH. The treatment induced the reduction by 88.9% of the GnRH, as compared with controls. This means that GnRH had been released and accounts for an almost simultaneous increase of plasma LH and FSH. It seems that the hypothalamic impairment of aging rats does not affect the synthesis but does affect the release of GnRH, since PE and IC levels are higher than the highest levels during a normal four-day estrus cycle at 7 mo. old (data from our laboratory). These results support the idea that the male urinary pheromones which induce regular cyclicity in aging IC and PE females, act on the hypothalamic GnRH release mechamisms through a pheromone-activated olfactory pathway. Thanks to DGICYT grant no. PM92/0030.

P2.79

GROWTH HORMONE (GH) RESPONSE IN ELDERLY SUBJECTS AFTER THE COMBINED ADMINISTRATION OF GHRP-6 AND GHRH: EVIDENCE FOR SYNERGISTIC ACTION. D.Micić*, A.Kendereški, V.Popović, Dj.Macut, M.Šumarac, S.Zorić, D.Manojlović, C.Dieguez**, F.Casanueva**. Institute of Endocrinology, 11000 Beograd, Yugoslavia and **Endocrine Section, Faculty of Medicine, Santiago de Compostela, Spain

His-dTrp-Ala-Trp-dPhe-Lys-NH2 (GHRP-6) is a synthetic compound that releases GH in a dose-related and specific manner in man. To further characterize the effects of GHRP-6 on GH secretion in normal human subjects, we assessed plasma GH response in 10 healthy elderly people (7 female, 3 male, age: 59.60+/-1.56 years; BMI: 23.58+/-1.02 kg/m2) following a) GHRH-6 (100 mcg i.v.); b) GHRH (100 mcg i.v.) and c) combined GHRP-6 + GHRH administration. GH (DELFIA hGH kit, mU/l) was measured in -30;-15;0;15;30;45;60;90 and 120 min. There were no difference between basal GH in all three tests. Significantly higher increase in plasma GH levels was found after the administration of GHRP-6 than after GHRH (Peaks : 68.13+/-19.40 vs 13.85+/-3.92; $p<0.05$); the areas under curve (AUC: 3828.76 +/-1255.86 vs 1054.04+/-259.63, $p<0.05$, respectively). The peak GH response to GHRP-6 and GHRH were not correlated ($r=-0.03$; $p=0.91$). Combined GHRH-6 and GHRH induced a much greater increase in plasma GH levels (Peak: 108.51+/-24.61; AUC: 7130.03+/-1578.29) than GHRP-6 alone (Peak: 68.13+/-19.40; $p>0.05$; AUC: 3828.76+/-1255.86,$p>0.05$) or GHRH alone (Peak: 13.85+/-3.92; $p<0.05$; AUC: 1054.04+/-259.63, $p<0.05$). In conclusion, our results gave evidence that combined administration of GHRP-6 and GHRH exibit synergistic effect on GH discharge in elderly people.

P2.80

INFLUENCE OF TESTOSTERONE DECLINING ON GROWTH HORMONE DEFICIENCY IN AGING RATS. J.López-Fernández, L.Cacicedo, R.M.Tolón, M.J. Lorenzo, B.Vega and *F.Sánchez-Franco. Endocrinology Dpt. Hospital Ramón y Cajal and C.N.I.C. Instituto Carlos III. MADRID. SPAIN. 28034.

Growth hormone (GH) and testosterone (T) secretion decline in elderly people and rats. Moreover, it is well known that sex steroid hormones have dramatic effects on GH-axis in neonatal and peripubertal ages although the mechanisms by which sex steroids influence GH secretion are uncertain. The aim of this work was to study the possible influence of T declining on the aging GH-axis. Bilateral orchidectomy (Cx), sham operation (C) or Cx plus T-treatment (0.5 mg/Kg/day) were performed in 90-day-old and 2-year-old male Wistar rats. After sacrifice, pituitaries and hypothalami were processed for peptide and RNA extraction. Peptides were quantified by RIA and mRNA by Northern-blot. Aging rats had lower pituitary IR-GH and mRNA levels and higher IR-IGF-I content than adult rats. In these animals Cx altered neither pituitary parameters nor IR-SS or IR-GRF content. T-treatment significantly increased pituitary GH mRNA and content. In adult rats Cx diminished pituitary GH mRNA and IR-GH, and increased pituitary IR-IGF-I. T-treatment restored the GH alterations. In adult rats Cx decreased IR-SS and mRNA without altering GRF.

This study shows that androgens may influence the GH-axis in the adulthood and aging by causing a stimulatory effect at pituitary level. The increment on pituitary IGF-I content observed in aging rats and in T deficiency situations might partly contribute to the suppression of GH-axis through a paracrine/autocrine mechanisms.

P2.81

INCREASED CARDIOVASCULAR REACTIVITY TO CAFFEINE IN MENOPAUSE. *R. Menozzi, G. Del Rio, G. Zizzo, M.G. Venneri, M. Bonati, E. Toschi, M. Pantaleoni, A. Velardo. Cattedra di Endocrinologia, Universitá di Modena, 41100 Modena,Italia.

Cardiovascular disease is more frequent in menopausal than fertile women, and may be due to the increased catecholaminergic tone observed in menopause . The elevated turnover of catecholamines may be secondary to an increased sympathoadrenal response to physiological stimuli. We studied the catecholamine and cardiovascular responses to caffeine (250 mg per os) in 8 menopausal women (MW) and in 5 fertile women (FW) Blood samples were drawn at 0,15,30,45,60, 90,120 min. after caffeine administration for determination of catecholamines.Systolic, diastolic blood pressure (SBP, DBP) and heart rate (HR) were also measured. Basal levels of SBP, DBP and HR did not differ between FW (104 ± 3 and 65± 2 mmHg; 67± 4 pulse/min) and MW (110± 5 and 66± 4 mmHg; 58±5 pulse/min) (P=NS). Caffeine administration increased SBP and DBP values both in FW (111±2 and 72±2 mmHg) and MW (130±10 and 78±6 mmHg) (P<0.01 vs basal), but this increase was higher in MW (P<0,05). HR after caffeine did not change both in FW and in MW (70±8 and 64±7 pulse/min; P=NS vs basal). Resting levels of both epinephrine (E) and norepinephrine (NE) were not different in FW and in MW (E= 30±7 vs 24±5 pg/ml; P=NS) (NE=146±43 vs 160±22 pg/ml; P=NS). We observed a significant increase in plasma E after caffeine both in MW (47±6 pg/ml;P<0,01 vs basal) and in FW (65±19 pg/ml; P<0.05 vs basal) No difference was found in NE levels after caffeine both in MW (241±23 pg/ml; P=NS vs basal) and in FW (240±68 pg/ml; P=NS vs basal). This study demostrate that MW showed a greater cardiovascular response to caffeine than FW in presence of similar levels of catecholamines. The higher pressor response to caffeine in MW could be secondary to increased adrenergic sensitivity or to other factors like plasma renin activity and calcium influenced by caffeine per se.

P2.82

A SUB-ACUTE HYPOTHALAMIC ORGAN CULTURE SYSTEM SHOWS ORGANOTYPIC CELLULAR STRUCTURE AND MAINTAINED SECRETION AND RESPONSIVENESS OF CORTICOTROPIN RELEASING HORMONE NEURONS
Ehud Ur, Angela Tittle, Garry Chernenko, [1]Giacomo Pozzoli, [1]Pierluigi Navarra, *Ashley Grossman: Memorial University, St John's, NF, Canada, [1]Catholic University, Rome, Italy and *St Bartholomew's Hospital, London, UK

Extensive studies of the regulation of hypothalamic CRH release have been carried out using an acute explant *in vitro* system. This system is viable for a few hours after removal from the rat and cannot be used to study chronic neurohumoral phenomena. We have adapted an *in vitro* culture system using rat neonatal tissue. Slices of hypothalamus are cultured for several weeks using a roller-tube method, a technique that preserves cellular and connective organization of the parent tissue. Five-day-old rat pups were killed by decapitation and tissue was aseptically removed. Hypothalami were cut into 400 µm-thick slices which were placed on separate coverslips and cultured in plastic test tubes at 36°C in dry air, in medium consisting of a combination of basal medium, Hanks' BSS, supplemented with glucose and horse serum. Cultures were incubated for up to 6 weeks. Medium was changed weekly. Immunohistochemical staining was carried out after 20 days of culturing using the peroxidase/antiperoxidase (PAP) technique, with an in-house highly-sensitized rat CRH antibody at a dilution of 1:2000. *In situ* hybridization was performed using a cDNA probe for CRH message. CRH release experiments were conducted on 8 to 34 day old cultures by incubating slices in medium with or without 56 mM KCl for two hours at 37°C. Supernatant was assayed by RIA for CRH. Large numbers of CRH-immunopositive cells were seen in paraventricular areas, in a distribution similar to that seen in fresh explanted tissue. Similar results were obtained with *in situ* hybridization studies. Basal release of CRH into the medium was 24.19 ± 6 pg CRH/ml; this significantly increased (P<0.001) to 166.28 ± 28 pg CRH/ml in the presence of KCl. Thus, we have generated an organ culture system in which CRH neurons retain anatomical relationships and physiological release mechanisms.

P2.83

PULSDETEKT, A NEW METHOD FOR PULSE DETECTION IN HORMONE DATA. *M.Žarković, J.Ćirić, B.Trbojević, M.Stojanović, N.Tasić, M.Nešović, Institute of Endocrinology, Dr Subotića 13, 11000 Belgrade, Yugoslavia

We developed a new method for pulse detection in hormone data, based on the deconvolution of secretory and metabolic events. The algorithm is based on the following premises: 1. the secretory function is unknown, 2. the eliminatory (metabolic clearance) function follows single negative exponential time-curve, 3. the hormone clearance rate is unknown, 4. the noise in the system has a normal distribution. Hormone quantity at any time can be expressed as: $H_t = S_t + H_{(t-1)} \cdot e^{k \cdot \text{int}}$ where H_t is measured hormone quantity at time t, S_t is a quantity of hormone secreted at time t, $H_{(t-1)}$ is a measured hormone quantity at the previous sampling time, e is a natural logarithm, k is a metabolic clearance rate and *int* is a sampling interval. Method was evaluated on synthetic and real hormonal data, and compared with data obtained with *Pulsar* program. In 10 synthetic series composed of random numbers no one program detected any pulse. Analysis of synthetic series composed of defined pulse signals with different amounts of noise (5, 10 or 20% of signal value) and with different sampling rates, proved that program *PulsDetekt* is resistant both to noise and low sampling rates (actual number of pulses 9, detected at noise level 5% 9 ± 0, at noise level 10% 9 ± 0.8, at noise level 20% 7.3 ± 0.8 pulses). Analyses of real hormonal data (LH, ACTH, cortisol, insulin) showed good correlation with published data obtained by other programs, or pharmacokinetic data. *PulsDetekt* is simple to use, and is not computing intensive.

P2.84

IMMUNOCYTOLOGY WITH MICROWAVE FIXATION SHOWS CALCITRIOL INDUCED RAPID CYCLIC GMP ACCUMULATION AROUND REORGANIZING VITAMIN D RECEPTORS IN CULTURED CELLS. J. Barsony, I. Renyi, W. McKoy. Metabolic Diseases Branch, NIDDK, National Institutes of Health, Bethesda, MD, 20892 U.S.A. .

Signal transduction often involves intracellular redistribution of cAMP or cGMP after it is synthesized in response to agonists and these changes were not detectable with conventional fixation techniques. We developed a new immunocytology technique based on microwave fixation. Exposure of cells to high microwave energy for milliseconds arrests enzyme activity, preventing cyclic nucleotide degradation or redistribution. The small molecules are fixed to the surrounding proteins without decreasing their immunoreactivity. It provides sufficient preservation of cell structure and permeabilize the cell membrane, making the use of detergents unnecessary. Studies with fluorescent cAMP and cGMP derivatives showed that they are retained at their original location in proportion to their original concentration. This method enabled us to detect rapid, dose- and time-dependent changes in cGMP and cAMP accumulation patterns. Microwave fixation also allowed superior detection of receptor localization. In human dermal fibroblasts we found that a portion of vitamin D receptors (VDRs) reside in the cytoplasm. Calcitriol induced rapid and sequential changes in VDRs: clumping, alignment along microtubules, translocation into the nucleus through the nuclear pores, and intranuclear clustering. Cyclic GMP accumulated around clumped VDRs within 15 sec after hormone exposure in normal cells, but not in cells with defects in the VDR gene. Recent reports indicated the presence of high affinity binding sites for calcitriol and gene regulation by calcitriol in C6 rat glioma cells. We used this new technique to study VDR localization and the nongenomic effect of calcitriol to induce cGMP accumulation in C6 cell. Our result show that immunocytology with microwave fixation provides a poweful tool to study signal tranduction for steroids and for other agonists.

P3.1

NEUROPEPTIDE Y IN MAGNOCELLULAR NEURONS OF THE HYPOTHALAMO-NEUROHYPOHYSIAL SYSTEM: POSSIBLE ROLES ON THE RELEASE OF VASOPRESSIN.

P.J. LARSEN[1], J.D. MIKKELSEN, H.S. CHOWDREY[2], S.L. LIGHTMAN[2] AND D.S. JESSOP[2].
[1]Department of Anatomy, University of Copenhagen, Denmark, [2]Department of Medicine, University of Bristol, Bristol, U.K.

Neuropeptide Y (NPY) is co-localized with vasopressin and oxytocin in magnocellular neurons of the hypothalamo-neurohypophysial system, and a very high density of NPY binding sites of the Y_2 type is present within the neurohypophysis. Levels of NPY mRNA in magnocellular neurons of the paraventricular and supraoptic nuclei increase dramatically in response to the chronic osmotic stimulation. We have studied the actions of NPY on potassium evoked release of vasopressin and oxytocin from the rat neurointermediate lobe in vitro. NPY dose dependently potentiated vasopressin release evoked by high extracellular potassium (56 mM) with a maximal enhancement of 223% (10^{-7} M NPY) and a similar effect was obtained with the Y_2 selective agonist NPY^{13-36}. In contrast, no effect upon the evoked release of oxytocin was observed at this concentration. In addition it was seen that the effect of NPY upon potassium evoked secretion of neurohypophysial vasopressin is critically dependent on extracellular Ca^{++} ions. Finally, it was confirmed that stimulation by high K^+ significantly evoked the release of endogenous NPY from neurointermediate lobes of the pituitary gland. The present results provide evidence that NPY selectively and potently enhances evoked vasopressin secretion, and hence NPY may be an important component in the mechanisms associated with the control of body fluid homeostasis. Considering the co-existence of the two neuropeptides in magnocellular hypothalamo-neurohypophysial neurons this action is likely to be part of an autostimulatory feed-forward loop.

P3.2

THE EFFECT OF SOME HYPOPHYSIOTROPIC HORMONES ON VASOPRESSIN RELEASE FROM THE HYPOTHALAMO--NEUROHYPOPHYSIAL SYSTEM IN HAEMORRHAGED RATS.

E.Bojanowska[1*], J.Ciosek[1], A.Lewandowska[1], M.Orłowska–Majdak[2]. 1-Dept. of Pathophysiology, 2-Dept. of Physiology, University School of Medicine, Łódź, Poland, 90-136.

The influence of intracerebroventricularly injected thyroliberin (TRH) and luliberin (LH-RH) on vasopressin content in the hypothalamo-neurohypophysial system was investigated both in the intact and haemorrhaged rats.

A single TRH injection (200 ng per rat) to intact animals resulted in a significant increase in neurohypophysial and in a decrease of hypothalamic vasopressin content as determined by radio-immunoassay. On the other hand, similarly injected LHRH (100 ng per animal) markedly diminished the neurohypophysial vasopressin level.

In haemorrhaged animals (1ml per 100 g b.w.), the injection of TRH or LHRH 0.5h prior to the bleeding significantly diminished vasopressin depletion in the neurohypophysis as compared with haemorrhaged and saline-treated rats.

The present results indicate that TRH and LH-RH may be involved in functional control of hypothalamo-neurohypophysial system.

P3.3

IN VITRO EVIDENCE OF ENDOTHELIN-INDUCED STIMULATION OF VASOPRESSIN AND OXYTOCIN RELEASE VIA ET_A RECEPTORS

A. Costa, S. Yasin*, P. Navarra**, G. Pozzoli**, M.L. Forsling*, A. Grossman.
Dept. of Endocrinology, St. Bartholomew's Hospital, London (UK);
* Dept. of Gynaecology, UMDS, St. Thomas's Hospital, London (UK);
** Dept. of Pharmacology, Catholic University, Rome (Italy).

Endothelins (ET), a family of related peptides (ET-1, ET-2 and ET-3), are amongst the most potent vasoconstrictors known. While there is evidence to suggest that all three isoforms and their receptors are located in the central nervous system, including the hypothalamus, it is presently unclear whether ETs may function as central neuromodulators. Both in vivo and in vitro studies have suggested effects of ETs on vasopressin (AVP) release, and thereby a role in the control of blood pressure and possibly pituitary-adrenal function. To elucidate the precise isoform responsible for such actions, as well as the possible direct effects of ETs on hypothalamic oxytocin and corticotrophin-releasing hormone (CRH), we have utilised a previously validated system of rat hypothalamic explants maintained in vitro. Tissues were incubated for 20 mins in EBSS containing graded concentrations of ET-1 and ET-3. Hormones were measured by RIA. ET-1 was found to stimulate AVP release significantly at doses of 10^{-8}M and 10^{-10}M ($p \leq 0.01$ and $p < 0.05$ vs control, respectively) as well as oxytocin release at the dose of 10^{-8} M ($p < 0.05$ vs control). By contrast, ET-3 was entirely without effect on AVP and oxytocin secretion in the dose range 10^{-6}M-10^{-10}M. CRH release was found to be unaffected by either ET-1 or ET-3 in the dose range 10^{-6}M- 10^{-10}M, even with addition of nitric oxide (NO) synthase antagonists in order to exclude possible inhibitory modulation by NO. These data are consistent with the reported excitatory effects of circulating ET-1 on vasopressinergic neurons in the supraoptic and paraventricular nuclei of the hypothalamus, and suggest that the release of oxytocin is also stimulated by ET-1. The lack of effect of ET-3 further indicates that the ET receptor subtype involved in modulation of neurohypophyseal hormone secretion may be of the ET_A suptype. Stimulation of AVP release may thus represent a mechanism by which ET-1 controls blood pressure and possibly ACTH release, whereas CRH does not appear to be involved in these effects. ET-1 may also act in a paracrine and/or autocrine fashion, as it appears to be co-localised with neurohypophyseal hormones in the rat.

P3.4

HISTAMINE STIMULATES MAGNOCELLULAR OXYTOCIN NEURONS IN THE PARAVENTRICULAR AND SUPRAOPTIC NUCLEI OF CONSCIOUS RATS.

Andreas Kjær[1*], Ulrich Knigge[1], Philip J. Larsen[2] and Jørgen Warberg[1].
Departments of [1]Medical Physiology and [2]Anatomy, The Panum Institute, University of Copenhagen, Denmark.

Histamine (HA) acts as a neurotransmitter in the central nervous system. Histaminergic neurons in the tuberomammillary nucleus project within the hypothalamus to the paraventricular (PVN) and supraoptic nuclei (SON) where magnocellular oxytocin (OT) neurons are located. Therefore, the possibility exists that HA activates hypothalamic OT neurons. We investigated **1)** the effect of HA on OT mRNA levels in the PVN and SON, and **2)** the effect of HA or HA agonists on peripheral plasma levels of OT in conscious male rats.

Intracerebroventricular (icv) HA infusion (270 nmol) increased the OT mRNA levels 4-fold in the PVN and SON compared to saline treated animals. HA infusion increased the plasma OT level approximately 3-fold. Icv infusion of the H_1-receptor agonist 2-thiazolylethylamine (2180 nmol) or the H_2-receptor agonist 4-methylHA (790 nmol) increased the OT levels in peripheral plasma 2 to 3-fold and 10-fold, respectively.

We conclude that central HA activates magnocellular OT neurons in both the PVN and SON and causes release of OT to peripheral plasma. The latter effect is primarily mediated via H_2-receptor activation.

P3.5

CENTRAL OXYTOCIN (OXT) AND PARTURITION IN RATS. *J.A.Russell, I.Neumann†, R.Landgraf‡ & A.J.Douglas. Dept. Physiology, University Medical School, Edinburgh, EH8 9AG, U.K. †Dept. Physiology, University of Calgary, Calgary, Canada. ‡MPI of Psychiatry, Clinical Institute, Munich, Germany.

OXT secretion during suckling involves a central positive feedback action of OXT in the magnocellular nuclei and in the bed nucleus of the stria terminalis. OXT release within the supraoptic (SON) and paraventricular nuclei is increased in parturition. We have examined a role for OXT in the brain in the progress of parturition and in exciting the release of OXT within the SON. Under halothane or pentobarbitone anaesthesia, 14 day or 20 day pregnant rats were stereotaxically implanted with an injection cannula in a lateral cerebral ventricle or with a microdialysis/injection probe in the SON respectively. On the birth of pup 2 either 1) in rats with an icv cannula, an injection was given of either 4μl vehicle or OXT (1mU) or OXT antagonist (1μg, desGlyd(CH2) [Tyr(Me)2,Thr4] OVT=OTA) followed by infusion at 0.5μl/min for 15min; or 2) in rats with a microdialysis probe in the SON, either 50ng OTA in 0.5μl or vehicle was infused adjacent to the probe, and a 30min microdialysis sample was collected for OXT measurement by RIA. The results show: icv injection of OXT speeded up parturition transiently but icv OTA had no effect (birth interval for pups 2-3 was 10.8±2.6, n=6 and 20.9±3.9 min, n=6 respectively and 27±5.9 min, n=7 in icv vehicle group, $P<0.05$, t-test). Injection of OTA into both SON slowed parturition (e.g. interval between pups 4-5 was 13.1±3.2 min vs. 6.1±1.0 min in vehicle group, $p<0.05$ t-test) and the OTA reduced OXT release in the SON (1.25±0.26 pg, n=8 vs. 4.15±1.12 pg, n=7 in the vehicle group, $p<0.05$ t-test). The results indicate that OXT may act within the SON during parturition to facilitate the excitation of OXT neurones, and thus to regulate parturition; icv OTA may not reach this site, while icv OXT could act on an input to OXT neurones or in the magnocellular nuclei.
Supported by AFRC, ARC, HFSOP & VW.

P3.6

PARTURITION AND OXYTOCIN NEURONE ACTIVITY IN ANAESTHETISED RATS. *A.J.Douglas, I.Antonijevic‡, L.E.Johnstone, G.Leng‡ & J.A.Russell. Dept. Physiology, University Medical School, Edinburgh, EH8 9AG ‡Dept. Neurobiology, AFRC Babraham Institute, Cambridge CB2 4AT, U.K.

Parturition in rats normally occurs on day 21 of pregnancy and induces Fos gene expression in the brainstem and in oxytocin neurones of the supraoptic nucleus (SON). Parturition can be induced by pulsatile injections of oxytocin into conscious 21 day pregnant rats, and this treatment also induces Fos protein, even if no pups are born, indicating that uterine activity without birth induces positive feedback to oxytocin neurones. Unlike the milk-ejection reflex parturition in the rat will not occur spontaneously under anaesthesia. We have investigated whether parturition can be induced under anaesthesia and whether SON oxytocin neurones are activated at this time. 21 day pregnant rats were anaesthetised with pentobarbitone and vehicle or oxytocin (10mU per pulse for 2h then 20 mU for 2h, the regime shown to induce parturition in conscious rats) was administered intravenously in 30μl pulses every 10 min for 4 h. Rats were observed for signs of labour, uterine activity was monitored using an intrauterine balloon connected to a force transducer and any pups born were noted. Each oxytocin pulse transiently increased uterine contractile activity but vehicle had no effect. Oxytocin treatment induced the birth of at least 1 pup in 7/15 rats but 0/10 vehicle-treated rats showed signs of labour ($p<0.05$, Chi-square). The rats were killed 30 to 60 min after the end of injections and their brains removed, frozen, sectioned through the SON and processed for Fos immunocytochemistry. There were significantly more Fos-positive neurones per unit area SON in oxytocin than vehicle treated rats (3.22±0.93 per 10^4 μm^2 SON, n=6; 0.59±0.27 per 10^4 μm^2 SON, n=7, respectively; $p<0.04$, t-test). Results show that pup births can occur under pentobarbitone anaesthesia and suggest that oxytocin neurones become activated, with or without pup births, in a similar manner to that in normal parturition, by reflex activation following uterine contractions. [Supported by the AFRC]

P3.7

EXPRESSION OF C-FOS AND C-JUN PROTEINS IN THE SUPRAOPTIC NUCLEUS (SON) FOLLOWING PARAVENTRICULAR NUCLEUS (PVN) LESION. J. Dohanics, G. E. Hoffman, J. G. Verbalis, University of Pittsburgh, Pittsburgh, PA 15261

Expression of the c-Fos and c-Jun proteins is thought to be an indicator of neuronal activation in response to various stimuli. Injuries to many neurons also cause expression of these proteins, especially c-Jun, which often persist many weeks after the injury. Recent studies in our laboratory have shown that magnocellular OT neurons also express c-Jun following pituitary stalk damage. To determine whether these proteins were expressed during axonal regeneration in uninjured neurons, we studied adult male SD rats after PVN lesions or sham surgery. At 1 or 6 wks after the lesion rats received an iv injection of 2M NaCl or 0.15M Nacl (2 ml). Seventy-five min after the injection rats were anesthetized and perfused, and brain sections (40 μm) were double-immunostained for vasopressin (AVP) or oxytocin (OT), and c-Fos or c-Jun. Expression of c-Fos in SON neurons was virtually absent in sham-operated and PVN-lesioned rats injected with 0.15M NaCl. Similarly, only very weak c-Jun staining was present in SON AVP and OT neurons of sham-operated and 6 wks PVN-lesioned rats. However, many SON OT neurons in the 1 wk PVN-lesioned rats exhibited very strong c-Jun staining. Osmotic stimulation caused strong expression of c-Fos in SON AVP and OT neurons in both sham-operated and PVN-lesioned rats. These results indicate that 1) PVN lesions do not interfere with hyperosmolality-induced c-Fos and c-Jun expression in SON magnocellular neurons, and 2) a proportion of SON OT neurons in PVN-lesioned rats that are neither osmotically stimulated, nor injured, express intense c-Jun staining 1 week after the PVN lesions. These results raise the possibility that the SON OT neurons that express c-Jun may be the same OT neurons whose axons are known to sprout into the external zone of the median eminence in PVN-lesioned rats. This therefore suggests that c-Jun expression may reflect structural remodeling activity even in uninjured magnocellular neurons.

P3.8

DIFFERENT PATTERNS OF PLASMA AND CSF OXYTOCIN SECRETION IN RESPONSE TO HYPERTONIC SALINE OR MANNITOL. T. Iványi*, R. E. Blackburn, L. Rinaman, G. E. Hoffman, E. M. Stricker, J. G. Verbalis. University of Pittsburgh, Pittsburgh, PA 15261, USA.
To evaluate the effects of hyperosmolality on oxytocin (OT) secretion independently of concurrent increases in plasma Na^+ levels, the present study compared the peripheral OT and vasopressin (VP), and central OT, responses after injection of equiosmotic doses of NaCl (1M; HS) or mannitol (2M; M). Both HS and M caused significant increases in plasma OT and VP concentrations, as well as elevations in cisternal CSF OT concentrations. However, the relative increases in plasma and CSF OT concentrations, shown below, were significantly greater 30 min after HS compared to M, despite identical increases in plasma osmolality and CSF Na^+ levels (number of rats in each group in parentheses; $^*p<0.05$ compared to HS):

	1 M NaCl (3 ml iv)		**2 M Mannitol** (3 ml iv)	
Plasma	30 min	60 min	30 min	60 min
Na^+ (mmol/L)	10.0±1.0 (17)	6.0±1.0	-3.0±1.0 (13)*	0±1.0*
Osm (mOsm/kg)	14.0±1.0 (17)	10.0±1.0	16.0±1.0 (13)	11.0±1.0
VP (pg/ml)	8.8±2.7 (9)	10.8±2.5	12.4±4.2 (8)	15.5±5.8
OT (pg/ml)	41.9±5.8 (12)	10.5±1.5	23.0±4.5 (11)*	11.9±2.9
CSF				
Na^+ (mmol/L)	7.0±1.0 (10)	3.0±1.0	8.0±1.0 (10)	5.0±1.0
OT (pg/ml)	55.4±18.4 (14)	32.1±8.1	12.7±7.6 (9)*	17.0±3.7

Examination of neuronal cFos expression following ip injection of HS or M (n=9,9) showed identical patterns of activation in the hypothalamic paraventricular and supraoptic nuclei, but in the brainstem more pronounced cFos expression was observed in the nucleus of the solitary tract and area postrema after HS compared to M. These results show that OT secretion is more sensitive to stimulation with HS than M in the rat. The cFos expression studies suggest that this may occur because HS activates excitatory inputs to the hypothalamus arising from the brainstem, in addition to the activation of hypothalamic osmoreceptors which is produced by both stimuli. Whether the increased brainstem activation after HS treatment is due to elevated plasma Na^+ levels or visceral aversive signals remains to be determined.

P3.9

DAHL SALT SENSITIVE RATS SHOW INCREASED PLASMA OXYTOCIN (OT) AND VASOPRESSIN (VP) RESPONSES TO DEHYDRATION. M.F. Callahan*, M. Ludwig, G. Tsai, M. Morris. Department of Physiology and Pharmacology, Wake Forest University Medical Center, Winston Salem, NC 27157-1083, USA.

A high salt diet causes a greater elevation of plasma VP in Dahl salt sensitive (SS) rats than in salt resistant (SR) rats. The current study examined tissue and plasma peptide responses in male SS/Jr and SR/Jr rats during another chronic osmotic challenge, 3 days of dehydration. Plasma sodium and osmolality were also determined.

Dehydration increased plasma OT and VP and SS/Jr rats showed a significantly greater increase in OT than did the SR/Jr rats. OT increased from 3.7 to 8.2 pg/ml in SR/Jr and from 3.7 to 13.8 pg/ml in SS/Jr rats. Plasma VP increased 7 and 34 fold in SR/Jr and SS/Jr strains respectively. While SS/Jr rats had higher pituitary VP levels, dehydration caused a similiar decrease in pituitary peptides in the groups. Dehydration caused increases in plasma sodium and osmolality, however the SR/Jr group showed a greater increase in osmolality. There were no differences between the groups in peptide levels in the median eminence, paraventricular or supraoptic nuclei, and brainstem. These results suggest that peptide secretion is elevated in the face of a diminished osmotic challenge. Experiments are in progress to examine peptide mRNA in the hypothalamic nuclei. (Supported by NIH HL 43178).

P3.10

Dehydration during embryonic development modulates arginine vasotocin secretion in the chicken

Kisliuk S.M.,Grossmann R.*, Institute for Small Animal Research, Federal Research Center of Agriculture, 29223 Celle, Germany

The influence of low humidity during incubation (LHI) on arginine vasotocin (AVT) secretion in male and female White Leghorn chicken embryos and chicks was investigated. LHI embryos were incubated from day 8 (E8) to E18 at a relative humidity of 32-35%, while control embryos were incubated at 58-62%. In the control groups plasma AVT gradually increased from E15 to E18, increased sharply during hatching and returned to the E18 level within 4 h. LHI did not alter the level of AVT until E18. LHI E19 males had concentrations of AVT twice as high as those of control males (39 ± 3.9 *vs* 15 ± 1.6 pmol/l, $P<0.001$). Augmentation persisted during hatching and 4 h afterwords. In LHI females additional elevation reached significant level only at 4 h after hatching (58 ± 13 *vs* 16 ± 1.7 pmol/l, $P<0.01$). Deprivation of water caused an increase in plasma sodium concentrations in the 2-day-old chicks of the control groups, while no significant changes were observed in the LHI group. Deprivation of water together with a high environmental temperature caused an additional increase in AVT only in the LHI groups (42 ± 5.2 *vs* 22 ± 3.9pmol/l, $P<0.01$ for males; 32 ± 3.4 *vs* 19 ± 2.8pmol/l, $P<0.01$ for females). The results clearly showed that LHI leads to a more pronounced response of the AVT system on subsequent osmotic and non-osmotic challenges, especially in males. Embryonal activation of the AVT system probably helps the organism to cope with hatching and posthatching stresses.

P3.11

ROLE OF CENTRAL VASOPRESSIN IN THE REGULATION OF BLOOD PRESSURE IN SPONTANEOUSLY HYPERTENSIVE RAT. *K. Honda, S. Ishikawa and T. Saito, Department of Medicine. Jichi Medical School, Tochigi, JAPAN, 329-04.

By repetitive crossbreeding, we have developed a vasopressin (AVP)-deficient strain (SHR-DI) of spontaneously hypertensive rat (SHR) and another SHR strain (SHR-Het) which has a partial defect in AVP synthesis in hypothalamus. In an attempt to clarify the role of central AVP in the regulation of blood pressure in SHR, we measured mean arterial pressure (MAP) of each 12-week old animal under unanesthetized resting conditions and after stress with pressure transducer via the intra-arterial catheter. Furthermore, we examined the effects of intra-cerebroventricular (ICV) administration of d(CH2)5Tyr(Me)AVP, AVP V1-receptor antagonist. Basal MAP (mmHg, Mean±SD) of SHR-DI was significantly ($p<0.01$) higher than that of SHR (167.3±3.3 vs. 160.3±3.9), whereas basal MAP of SHR-Het (139.3±7.0) was significantly ($p<0.05$) lower than that of SHR. Increment of MAP by 2-minute immobilization of SHR-DI and SHR-Het were significantly ($p<0.05$, $p<0.01$) smaller than that of SHR (23.7±2.9, 15.0±3.7 vs. 42.3±15.7, respectively). In SHR, ICV administration of 15ng of d(CH2)5Tyr(Me)AVP raised MAP significantly (158.7±2.7 vs. 164.3±5.6, $p<0.05$) and diminished the rise of MAP by immobilization significantly (36.3+5.4 vs. 20.7+2.7, $p<0.01$) in comparison to ICV administration of artificial cerebrospinal fluid. These results suggest that endogenous AVP acts not only on the pressor system but also on the depressor system in the central nervous system in SHR. The pressor action of AVP may need intact hypothalamic AVP synthesizing ability, while the depressor action of AVP can be elicited in the animals having a partial AVP-deficiency.

P3.12

EXCITATORY AMINO ACIDS INDUCE *IN VITRO* LHRH RELEASE FROM THE MEDIAN EMINENCE (ME) FRAGMENT OF OVARIECTOMIZED (OVX) AND OVX ESTRADIOL (E_2)-PRIMED RATS. *S.-I. Kawakami, K. Murahashi, H. Tsukamura, K-I. Maeda. School of Agricultural Sciences, Nagoya University, Nagoya 464-01, Japan

We examined the effect of various neurotransmitters on *in vitro* LHRH release from the ME fragments. First, ME tissues taken from chronically (>2 weeks) OVX rats were incubated for 30 min in the medium containing various neurotransmitters following 30-min preincubation. Norepinephrine (60 µM), dopamine (60 µM), serotonin (600 µM), and histamine (1 µM) induced no significant increase in *in vitro* LHRH release. Glutamate (10 mM) significantly increased *in vitro* LHRH release from the ME tissue. Higher dose of monoamines, 20 mM of norepinephrine, dopamine, or histamine had no significant effect on LHRH release except for 20 mM of serotonin. Second, glutamate or a excitatory amino acid agonist, NMDA, AMPA or kainate, was added to the incubated median eminence of OVX rats at a dose from 0.1 to 20mM. All of these 4 drugs induced a dose-dependent increase in *in vitro* LHRH release with the maximum effect of NMDA and kainate, while AMPA had the minimum effect. Third, the effect of these agonists on *in vitro* LHRH release from OVX rat ME was compared with OVX E_2-primed rats. The responses to glutamate, NMDA or AMPA in OVX E_2-primed rats were similar to those in OVX rats. Only the response to kainate was significantly lower in OVX E_2-primed rats than that in OVX animals. These results indicate that the excitatory amino acids are the neurotransmitters which act at the ME and induce LHRH release with or without the presence of steroid hormones.

P3.13

ESTROGEN ENHANCES EXCITATORY AMINO ACIDS (EAAs)-INDUCED *IN VITRO* LHRH RELEASE FROM THE ARCUATE NUCLEUS-MEDIAN EMINENCE (ARC-ME) FRAGMENTS OF THE RAT.

*K. Murahashi, S.-I. Kawakami, H. Tsukamura, K.-I. Maeda. School of Agricultural Sciences, Nagoya University, Nagoya, Japan, 464-01

The effect of estrogen on *in vitro* LHRH release induced by EAAs from the ARC-ME fragments was studied to determine whether estrogen modulates the EAAs effect on LHRH release by acting on the ARC-ME. *In vitro* LHRH release from the fragments taken from ovariectomized (OVX) rats was increased only by glutamate (Glu) and kainate (KA). On the other hand, *in vitro* LHRH release from those from OVX estradiol-primed (OVX+E2) rats was increased by Glu and all of the selective agonists, i.e., NMDA, KA, AMPA. The amount of LHRH released by EAAs from the fragments of OVX+E2 rats was significantly higher compared with that of OVX rats. We previously confirmed that E2 priming did not enhance *in vitro* LHRH release from the ME fragments, and that the amount of LHRH release from the ARC-ME was much less than that from the ME. These results indicate that estrogen may enhance LHRH release induced by EAAs by removing the effect of the inhibitory input to the ME originating in the ARC. The effects of several neurotransmitter receptor antagonists, i.e., naloxone (opioidergic), bicuculline (GABAergic), SCH-23390 (dopaminergic) and strychnine (glycinergic) on NMDA-induced LHRH release from the ARC-ME fragments of OVX rats were also determined. All of the antagonists significantly enhanced the LHRH release induced by NMDA. These results suggest that the inhibitory input to the ME are probably the opioidergic, GABAergic, dopaminergic and glycinergic neurons.

P3.14

A CENTRAL 5-HYDROXYTRYPTAMINE$_2$ (5-HT$_2$) RECEPTOR MECHANISM AND ITS EFFECT ON THE LUTEINIZING HORMONE PROESTROUS SURGE IN THE RAT.

R.C. Dow*, B.C. Williams+, J. Bennie, S. Carroll, G. Fink. MRC Brain Metabolism Unit, 1 George Square, Edinburgh, EH8 9JZ, Scotland and Dept. of Medicine, Western General Hospital, Edinburgh, EH4 2XU, Scotland.

The role of 5-hydroxytryptamine (5-HT) in generating the pre-ovulatory surge of luteinizing hormone (LH) has been investigated by studying the effects of the selective 5-HT$_2$ receptor antagonist ritanserin, the selective α_1 adrenergic antagonist prazosin and ketanserin (a mixed 5-HT$_2$/α_1 adrenergic agonist) on the plasma concentrations of LH during the afternoon of proestrus in conscious female Wistar rats.

Serial blood samples were taken for hormone estimation through intra-atrial cannulae previously implanted under halothane anaesthesia. Both ketanserin and ritanserin administered i.p. blocked the LH surge as did prazosin given i.v. Ketanserin, but not ritanserin or prazosin alone or combined, also blocked basal LH release. These results provide the first robust evidence for the fact that a 5-HT$_2$ receptor as well as an α_1 adrenoreceptor mechanism is involved in the LH surge generator. This may be linked with our finding that oestradiol-17ß, in its positive feedback mode for LH release, stimulates a massive increase in the amount of 5-HT$_2$ receptor mRNA in the dorsal raphe nucleus in female rats (Sumner & Fink, 1993).

Sumner, B.E.H. & Fink, G. (1993) *Mol. Cell. Neurosci.* **4**: 83-92.

P3.15

POTENTIATION BY NEUROPEPTIDE Y (NPY) OF LH RESPONSE TO LHRH IN MAN.

T. Nigawara*, H. Watanobe, J. Anzai, S. Sakihara, K. Kageyama, R. Nasushita, S. Sasaki, S. Habu, Y. Kakizaki, A. Kohsaka, K. Takebe. Third Department of Internal Medicine, Hirosaki University School of Medicine, Hirosaki, Japan 036

It is well established that NPY exerts a stimulatory effect on LH secretion in rodents. In humans, however, it has yet to be determined whether NPY on its own stimulates LH secretion, and whether NPY modulates the effect of LHRH on LH secretion. Therefore, in this study we performed iv bolus injections of normal saline(control), NPY, LHRH, and NPY plus LHRH, in 6 normal males(24-31 yrs). Both peptides were given in a dose of 100 μg, and plasma levels of the 6 classical anterior pituitary hormones and cortisol were determined before and at intervals 120 min after the injection. In the samples from LHRH and NPY plus LHRH tests, only LH and FSH were measured. NPY alone did not significantly affect the secretion of any hormone examined. However, the coadministration of NPY with LHRH was able to significantly potentiate the LH response to LHRH. These results suggest that NPY has a stimulatory role in LH secretion also in humans, even though its effect appears to be complementary to LHRH.

P3.16

INFLUENCE OF β-ADRENERGIC STIMULATION ON THE DIFFERENTIATION OF THE CYCLIC GONADOTROPIN SECRETION PATTERN IN THE FEMALE RATS.

E.Gubała*, B. Jarząb[1], W. Achtelik, Döhler K.D[2]
University School of Medicine, Katowice, [1] Center of Oncology — Maria Skłodowska-Curie Memorial Institute, Gliwice, Poland and [2] Bissendorf Peptide, Hanover, Germany

Sexual differentiation of the brain is influenced by postnatal interaction of gonadal steroids with neurotransmitter system , particularly with the adrenergic system. In the present study we investigate the effect of the β-adrenergic agonist isoprenaline (Iso) of the differentiation of neural control of luteinizing hormone (LH) secretion in female rats. Cyclic secretion of LH was evaluated by a positive feedback test. Mean LH secretory response after EB+P was 31,9±5,7 ng/ml in control females. Iso given to rat neonates in doses of 2,5; 5; and 10 mg/kg significantly lowered the LH response observed in adult females.

In order to ivestigate the mechanisms of the lowered LH secretory response in the postnatally Iso-treated rats we repeated the positive feedback tests after clonidine (0,03mg/kg) and naloxon+clonidine pretreatment (naloxon - 2mg/kg). Clonidine reduced the LH secretory response ($p<0.01$): from 37,9±5,0 ng/ml in control females to 12,1±4,6 ng/ml. Naloxon pretreatment did not reverse the clonidine-induced inhibition of the positive feedback LH secretion in control rats. In postnatally Iso-treated rats there was a significant increase of LH response after naloxon + clonidine pretreatment: from 3,5±0,6 to 35,5±8,4 ng/ml ($p< 0,01$).

Conclusions : The inhibition of the positive feedback LH secretory response observed in adult female rats after postnatal isoprenaline treatment is due to the changed neuroendocrine opioid-adrenergic intractions controlling LH secretion.

P3.17

NORADRENERGIC MEDIATION OF GLUTAMATE-INDUCED LHRH/LH RELEASE.

A.O. Donoso*, C. Navarro, R.J. Cabrera. Laboratorio de Investigaciones Cerebrales. Mendoza, 5500 Argentina.

Recent evidence implicates excitatory amino acids in regulation of LHRH/LH release. Glutamate apparently exerts this effect by stimulating LHRH release at two key areas, the preoptic area (POA) and the mediobasal hypothalamus (MBH). This study characterizes the responses of LHRH neurons, indirectly by the measurement of plasma LH levels, to the effects of local administration of the glutamate agonist N-methyl-D-aspartic acid (NMDA) in the POA in unrestrained estradiol-progesterone-primed, ovariectomized rats.

LH release was stimulated in a dose-dependent manner with increasing concentrations of NMDA. These responses were blocked by both AP-7, a competitive NMDA antagonist, and prazosin, a selective α_1 adrenergic antagonist. Neither the GABA agonists muscimol or baclofen, nor morphine influenced the NMDA evoked response.

To determine whether noradrenaline (NA) would mediate NMDA action, as indicated by the results with prazosin, POA and MBH slices were loaded with ^{3}H-NA and superfused *in vitro*. Exposure of both areas to NMDA increased concentration-dependently ^{3}H-NA release from the slices. GABA-B receptor activation with baclofen prevented the NMDA effects.

Present studies suggest that a complex interaction between glutamate and GABA at noradrenergic nerve terminals in both POA and MBH may regulate LHRH/LH release.

P3.18

POSSIBLE RELATIONSHIP BETWEEN NMDA RECEPTOR-MEDIATED STIMULATORY AND OPIOIDERGIC INHIBITORY SYSTEMS IN THE CONTROL OF LH SECRETION.

A. Chiba*, T. Akema, F. Kimura[1], J. Toyoda. Dept. Physiol., St. Marianna Univ. Sch. Med., Kawasaki 216, [1]Dept. Physiol., Yokohama City Univ. Sch. Med., Yokohama 236, Japan.

The present study examined the functional relationship between the N-methyl-D-aspartate (NMDA) receptor-mediated stimulatory system and the opioidergic inhibitory one in the control of luteinizing hormone (LH) secretion in the ovariectomized estrogen-primed rat. Experiments were performed in unanesthetized animals bearing chronic intracerebroventricular (icv) cannulae. Prior icv injection of beta-endorphin inhibited the stimulatory effect of naloxone, a mu opioid receptor antagonist, injected icv on LH secretion, but did not interfere with the stimulatory effect of NMDA. On the other hand, prior icv administration of AP-5, a specific NMDA receptor blocker, markedly attenuated the LH secretory response to the subsequent icv injection of naloxone. It was concluded that the beta-endorphin neuronal system inhibits LH secretion at least partly via inhibition of NMDA receptor-mediated stimulatory system in female rats.

P3.19

LHRH RELEASE IS TONICALLY INHIBITED BY GABA NEURONS BEFORE THE ONSET OF PUBERTY IN PRIMATES.

Ei Terasawa. Wisconsin Regional Primate Research Center, University of Wisconsin, Madison, WI 53715, USA

The mechanism of the onset of puberty was investigated in female rhesus monkeys. Using a push-pull perfusion method, developmental changes in LHRH release in the stalk-median eminence (S-ME) were directly measured in prepubertal and pubertal monkeys. It was found that LHRH release was low in prepubertal monkeys and an increase in pulsatile LHRH release occurred at the onset of puberty. However, this increase was not due to a decrease in negative feedback sensitivity to ovarian steroids at the onset of puberty. Further studies with electrical stimulation and NMDA challenge indicate that LHRH neurosecretory neurons are functionally mature prior to puberty, but that the neuronal systems regulating pulsatile LHRH release may still be immature. Moreover, a series of studies suggests that γ-amino butyric acid (GABA) is an inhibitory neurotransmitter responsible for suppressing pulsatile LHRH release before puberty. 1) Bicuculline, a $GABA_A$ receptor antagonist at 10^{-7} and 10^{-5} M, greatly facilitated LHRH release in prepubertal monkeys, while bicuculline at only the higher dose slightly stimulated LHRH release in midpubertal monkeys, and 2) while GABA infusion did not cause any changes in prepubertal monkeys, GABA suppressed LHRH release in midpubertal monkeys, indicating a tonic inhibition of LHRH release by GABA neurons during the prepubertal period. Indeed, it was found that GABA release in the S-ME was much higher in prepubertal monkeys than in midpubertal monkeys. Moreover, infusion of antisense oligodeoxynucleotides for glutamic acid decarboxylase (GAD) mRNAs (GAD is the synthetic enzyme forming GABA from glutamate and is derived from 2 different genes) into the S-ME drastically increased LHRH release in prepubertal monkeys, suggesting that the reduction of GABA synthesis may be important for puberty. Therefore, the removal of GABA inhibition onto LHRH neurons, before facilitatory neural inputs such as those from norepinephrine neurons and NPY neurons are established, appears to be the critical factor for the onset of puberty in the nonhuman primate. (Supported by NIH grants HD11355, HD15433 & RR00167).

P3.20

RELEASE OF LUTEINIZING HORMONE - RELEASING HORMONE (LHRH) AND DOPAMINE (DA) BY THE NUCLEUS INFUNDIBULARIS/MEDIAN EMINENCE (NI/ME) DURING SEASONAL ANOESTRUS IN EWES.

L.K.Chomicka*, A.Gajewska, F.Przekop. The Kielanowski Institute of Animal Physiology and Nutrition, Polish Academy of Sciences, 05-110 Jabłonna near Warsaw, Poland.

Pharmacological evidence has been accumulated to indicate that in ewes, seasonal suppression of the release of luteinizing hormone results from an inhibitory action of dopamine on hypothalamic LHRH release. In order to address if the NI/ME may be a site of DA action, we undertook a study on the relationships between DA and LHRH release by the NI/ME during anoestrus in ewes. The study was performed on ewes during the mid and late periods of anoestrus. The in vivo release of DA and LHRH was assayed in perfusates collected from the NI/ME via push-pull cannulae. DA and LHRH were detected using HPLC-EC and RIA, respectively. It was found that LHRH release by the NI/ME markedly increased at the end of anoestrus, and that this rise in LHRH release was preceeded by a significant attenuation of DA release in the NI/ME. The obtained data revealed that in ewes, the termination of seasonal anoestrus coincides with marked changes in the release of LHRH and DA by the NI/ME. The results of the present study suggest that in ewes, the termination of seasonal anoestrus may result, at least partly, from a withdrawal of dopaminergic inhibition of LHRH neurons in the NI/ME.

This work was supported by KBN grant 500579101.

P3.21

EFFECT OF SUBSTANCE P ON GONADOTROPIN RELEASING HORMONE (GnRH) CONCENTRATION IN PITUITARY PORTAL BLOOD OF MALE RAT. A. Walczewska, U. Szkudlarek, B.Dziedzic, B.Jakubowska-Naziembło, W.Z.Traczyk Dept. of Physiology, Inst. Physiol. Biochem., Medical University, Lodz, Poland, 90-131.

The present study was designated to evaluate influence of SP on GnRH release into pituitary portal blood of male rat in the different hormonal states. Experiments were carry out four groups of male rat: intact, 30 days orchidectomized (ORCX), ORCX with s.c. testosterone (T) implants ORCX with s.c. 17β-oestradiol (E_2) implants. Pituitary portal vessels were exposed by transpharyngeal approach and cut. Then three 30 min portal blood samples were taken. First sample of blood was treated as a control. At the beginning of each the second sample the animals were injected 200 µl of 0.9% NaCl or 5, 25 µg SP in 200 µl 0.9% NaCl into internal carotid artery. Our results indicate that injection of substance P into internal carotid artery stimulate release of GnRH into pituitary portal vessels in intact male rat. It seems that castration or long-term action of testosterone and oestradiol abolish this effect.

P3.22

GONADOTROPIN-RELEASING HORMONE (GnRH) AND SUBSTANCE P (SP) RELEASED INTO THE CEREBRAL VENTRICULAR FLUID IN INTACT, ORCHIDECTOMIZED AND SEX STEROID TREATED MALE RATS.
B. Jakubowska-Naziembło, B. Dziedzic, A. Walczewska, E. Potargowicz, W.Z. Traczyk. Dept. of Physiology, Inst. Physiol. Biochem., Medical University of Lodz, Lodz, Poland, 90-131.

Previous evidence obtained in several species indicated that GnRH and SP are released into the cerebral ventricular fluid. The goal of the reported experiments was to prove that castration or sex steroids can modify this release. The experiments with lateral ventricles - cerebellomedullary cistern perfusion were performed in urethane anaesthesia in four group of male rats: intact, orchidectomized, with s.c. implants of 17β oestradiol or testosterone. GnRH and SP concentration in the perfusing fluid was measured by RIA. It was found that GnRH and SP were continuously released into the perfusion fluid but fluctuation in GnRH concentration in individual animals indicated that it was released in pulsatile manner. In this fluid GnRH content (pg/sample) was higher than SP. Orchidectomy or sex steroid implants failed to change significantly the amount of GnRH release into the fluid perfusing cerebral ventricles but there was a tendency towards its modification.

P3.23

GONADOTROPIN-RELEASING HORMONE (GnRH) AND SUBSTANCE P (SP) CONCENTRATION IN THE 3rd CEREBRAL VENTRICLE FLUID FROM CHRONIC RABBITS WITH INTACT OVARIES, OVARIECTOMIZED AND WITH OESTROGEN CAPSULE. B. Dziedzic, W.Z. Traczyk. Dept. of Physiology, Inst. Physiol. Biochem., Medical University of Lodz, Lodz, Poland, 90-131.

The aim of the present study was to find the correlation between the concentrations of GnRH and SP in the 3rd cerebral ventricle fluid (CVF). CVF was collected through an implanted cannula in ovarian intact does, ovariectomized (OVX) and ovariectomized with 17β oestradiol capsules (OVX + E_2). CVF GnRH and CVF SP concentrations were determined by radioimmunoassay. OVX caused increase of CVF GnRH and OVX + E_2, in turn, decreased CVF GnRH concentration. In OVX and OVX + E_2 does CVF SP concentration was significantly lower as compared with intact animals.
A significant correlation between CVF SP and CVF GnRH concentrations was observed between individual OVX and OVX + E_2 does. No linear relationship was found in intact does. These findings suggest that SP can be regarded as an oestrogen-dependent modulator of GnRH release into CVF.

P3.24

NEWLY SYNTHESIZED ANALOGUES OF SOMATOSTATIN INHIBIT PROLACTIN RELEASE. B. Baranowska, M. Radzikowska, E. Wasilewska-Dziubińska, A. Płonowski, K.Roguski*, A. Łęgowska[#], J. Przybylski[#].
Department of Neuroendocrinology, Medical Center of Postgraduate Education, Warsaw, Poland and [#]Department of Chemistry, Gdańsk University, Poland.

Since the isolation and characterisation of somatostatin considerable progress has been made in recent years in the synthesis of highly potent and selective analogues of somatostatin. Our previous studies demonstrate that analogues synthesized in Department of Chemistry (Gdańsk, Poland) ASS-52 and ASS-53 selectively inhibit GH release. In order to evaluate the effects of newly synthesized analogues of somatostatin on PRL and gonadotrophins release in WKY rats, serum PRL, LH, FSH, GH, IGF-1, insulin, glucagon concentrations as well as the content of PRL, LH, FSH in pituitary tissue and LH-RH in MBH (medial basal hypothalamus) were measured with RIA and EIA methods (bioMerieux). In the present paper we present the relationship between chemical structure and biological activity and five new somatostatin analogues which were synthesized. Differences in chemical structure in these analogues as compared with SS-14-S (SMS 201-995)-octreotide concerned reduction of amino-acids number and changes in N- and C-terminal. Analogues ASS-71(Arg) and ASS-71(Orn) contain the hydrazide group with 2 hydroxyl groups in C-terminal. In analogue ASS-71(Arg) Arg was substituted in position 5 in place of Lys and in analogue ASS-71(Orn) Orn was introduced in position 5 in place of Lys. ASS-71(Arg) and ASS-71(Orn) demonstrated a great activity for PRL inhibition. These analogues were more potent than octreotide. The maximal inhibition was observed at 60 mins after infusion of 0.05 µg. The inhibiting effects remained during 180 mins. Administration of higher doses produced opposite (stimulating) effects on PRL release. Inhibiting effects of these analogues on LH release were observed at 10 mins after infusion. The biphasic response of FSH to injection of analogues was found. Serum FSH dropped at 10 mins and after transient increase the renewal of the decrease was observed after 60 mins. ASS-71(Arg) and ASS-71(Orn) decreased markedly the content of PRL and gonadotrophin in pituitary tissue and significantly changed the LH-RH content in MBH. These analogues demonstrated the minimal inhibiting effects for GH, IGF-1, insulin and glucagon release. **Conclusions.** Newly synthesized analogues ASS-71(Arg) and ASS-71(Orn) appear to be very potent, long acting and selective analogues of somatostatin for inhibition of PRL release.

P3.25

CH-38083, A SELECTIVE ALPHA-2 ADRENOCEPTOR ANTAGONIST, INHIBITS THE PREOVULATORY PROLACTIN SECRETION IN RATS.

I. Kun*[1], E.S. Vizi[2], B. Tóth[3], [1] Dept. of Endocrinol. Univ of Medicine & Pharm. Tg. Mures, Romania, [2] Inst. of Exp. Medicine Hung. Acad. of Sciences, [3] 2nd Dept. of Anatomy, Semmelweis Univ. Medical School, Budapest, Hungary

CH-38083, a new, selective alpha-2 adrenoceptor antagonist was administered in doses of 5 and 10 mg/kg s.c. to young female rats in proestrus between 10.30-12 h a.m. A second group of rats was treated in the same period with morphine hydrochloride 10 mg/kg s.c., a third group received a combined treatment and the fourth saline only. The animals were sacrified between 3-4 h p.m. and blood collected for gonadotropin and PRL measurements by RIA.

CH-38083, injected alone or in combination with morphine, did not change significantly the FSH and LH plasma concentrations vs. the control saline group. However, it reduced the plasma PRL level and this effect was potentiated evidently by morphine. This result, taking together with similar effect of idazoxan (seen by others), pleads for the stimulatory role of the alpha-2 adrenoceptors on the PRL surge, possibly by reducing the inhibitory activity of the tuberoinfundibular dopaminergic neurons.

P3.26

PITUITARY ADENYLATE CYCLASE -ACTIVATING POLYPEPTIDE (PACAP) INCREASES PRL RELEASE AND TUBEROINFUNDIBULAR DOPAMINERGIC (TIDA) NEURONAL ACTIVITY. L.A. Arbogast, J.L. Voogt*, Dept. of Physiology, Univ. of Kansas Med. Ctr. , Kansas City, KS, USA 66160-7401

PACAP is a hypothalamic peptide that affects anterior pituitary cell function. The aims of this study were to determine the effects of PACAP on PRL release and on TIDA neurons by assessing tyrosine hydroxylase (TH) activity in the stalk-median eminence (SME). TH activity was evaluated by the accumulation of 3,4-dihydroxyphenylalanine (DOPA) after inhibiting DOPA decarboxylase with m-hydroxybenzylhydrazine (25 mg/kg i.v.) *in vivo* or 100 μM brocresine *in vitro*. Experiment 1: Both jugular veins were cannulated 2 weeks after ovariectomy. PACAP (20 μg/rat, i.v.) increased plasma PRL levels 3-fold and TH activity in the SME by 30%. Incubation of the SME with 1 μM PACAP *in vitro* increased TH activity 2-fold. The right cannula of some rats were connected to osmotic minipumps containing oPRL (2 mg/200 μl) infused at a rate of 1 μl/h. After 2 days, circulating levels of endogenous rat PRL were reduced to 20% of levels in control rats and TH activity in the SME was increased 1.7-fold. PACAP induced a 4-fold rise in endogenous PRL levels in oPRL-treated rats and a 30% increase in TH activity that was additive to the elevation caused by hyperprolactinemia. Experiment 2: PACAP via a jugular vein did not alter circulating PRL levels or TH activity in the SME of suckled lactating rats on postpartum days 5 and 6. When pups were removed from the dams for 4-5 h, systemic injection of PACAP stimulated PRL release 8-fold without altering TH activity. *In vitro* PACAP increased TH activity 2-fold in the SME of lactating rats. Conclusions: 1) PACAP has a role in controlling PRL release in female rats, but its PRL-releasing ability is dependent on the endocrine state. 2) The PACAP-induced rise in PRL release is modest and not due to a decrease in TIDA neuronal activity. 3) PACAP increases TH activity in the TIDA neurons, possibly by a direct action on nerve terminals within the SME. Supported by NIH grants HD24190 and HD07368.

P3.27

EXPERIMENTALLY-INDUCED HYPERPROLACTINEMIA CAUSES THE DE NOVO SYNTHESIS OF PROENKEPHALIN IN TUBEROINFUNDIBULAR DOPAMINERGIC (TIDA) NEURONS. I. Merchenthaler, LMIN, NIEHS, Research Triangle Park, NC 27709, USA

In contrast to male or cycling female rats, TIDA neurons of lactating animals express pro-enkephalin (ENK) (Endocrinology 133:2645, 1993). The present experiments were designed to determine the role of prolactin (PRL) in inducing ENK gene expression within TIDA neurons. Hyperprolactinemia was achieved by either implanting pituitaries under the kidney capsule of intact or hypophysectomized female rats or treating intact female animals with the dopamine receptor antagonists haloperidol or domperidone. The role of PRL was also studied by hypophysectomizing lactating dams. ENK gene expression was investigated using immunocytochemistry and in situ hybridization histochemistry. Vibratome sections were immunostained for leu-ENK using monoclonal antibodies and the ABC technique. Pro-ENK mRNA was detected on cryostat and vibratome sections using oligo- and riboprobes. The results show that chronically elevated levels of PRL are essential for inducing ENK gene expression in TIDA neurons. Sex steroids do not play a crucial role in this phenomenon; however, progesterone potentiates the action of PRL. Hyperprolactinemia, among other mechanisms, may maintain its own elevated plasma levels and increased milk secretion via stimulating the synthesis and release of ENK, which in turn, may stimulate the synthesis and/or release of PRL. In addition, ENK may inhibit the release of LHRH via axo-axonal synapses in the median eminence and, therefore, suppress ovulation during lactation or other endocrine states characterized by hyperprolactinemia, such as pregnancy, pseudopregnancy, and aging.

P3.28

EFFECT OF 5-HT2 RECEPTOR AGONISTS ON THE CONTROL OF PITUITARY SECRETION OF FSH, LH AND PROLACTIN IN MALE RATS. L.Pinilla, M.Tena-Sempere, E.Aguilar. Dept. of Physiology.Faculty of Medicine. Córdoba University.Córdoba.Spain.14004.

To analyse the role of 5-HT2 receptors in the control of FSH, LH and prolactin secretion, intact adult male rats (10-12 per group) were ip injected with different doses (10,20 or 30 mg/kg) of the agonists α methyl-serotonin maleate (α-CH_3-HT) and (±)-DOI hydrochloride (DOI) or vehicle and sacrificed 60 or 120 min later. Serum concentrations of FSH, LH and prolactin were measured by specific RIAs. We found that: (1) prolactin secretion was stimulated by the two agonists; (2) FSH secretion was significantly inhibited by α-CH_3-HT and DOI; and (3)LH secretion was only stimulated by α-CH_3-HT. These results suggested that: (a) activation of 5-HT2 receptors stimulated prolactin release; (b) FSH and LH secretion was differently modulated by agonists of 5-HT2 receptors, which suggests a multiple action mechanism; and (c) the agonists α-CH_3-HT and DOI elicited different responses, indicating the possible activation of different subsets of 5-HT2 receptors.

This work was subsidized by grant PM92-0754.

P3.29

ROLE OF GABAERGIC INNERVATION OF OXYTOCIN (OT) NEURONS DURING LACTATION IN RATS. F.C. Moos* & Ph. Richard. Laboratoire de Neurobiologie Endocrinologique, URA 1197 CNRS, Université de Montpellier II, Place Eugène Bataillon, 34095 Montpellier Cedex 5, France.

During parturition and lactation, the number of GABAergic terminals making synaptic contact onto the hypothalamic OT neurons increases (Theodosis, 1993). This synaptic remodelling, which occurs when the OT neurons have to display the rythmic high frequency bursts of spikes leading to pulsatile OT releases, could play a determinant role in the expression of this particular activity.
In vitro electrophysiological studies performed on magnocellular neurons of the supraoptic nuclei (SON) have shown that all IPSCs are due to activation of GABA-A receptors (Wuarin & Dudek, 1993). Thus, we tested the effect of GABA or GABA-A antagonists on the bursting pattern of OT neurons during suckling. Drugs were injected into one SON while simultaneously recording the electrical activity of an OT neuron within the injected nucleus (via a double-barelled micropipette) and/or in the contralateral SON. During the milk-ejection reflex, injection of GABA (10^{-4}M) decreased the delay between the next bursts (7 tests). Gabazine or picrotoxin (10^{-6}-10^{-4}M) induced a slight tonic increase in the basal activity of the OT neurons and significantly delayed the occurrence of the next burst(s) (n=11 tests). These effects, though slighter, could be compared to that obtained after an i.p. injection of hypertonic saline: a rapid, strong and sustained increase in basal activity (Negoro *et. al.*, 1987) accompanied by a large delay of the next burst following the stimulus (n=12 tests).
The role of GABA innervation on OT neurons could be to favour periodic bursting over tonic activation. The fact that responses to hyperosmotic stimuli or to stress are smaller in lactating than in cyclic female rats favours this hypothesis. Thus, simultaneous expression of both responses (burst or tonic activation leading respectively to pulsatile or sustained OT release) does not seem fully compatible.

P3.30

THE ACTION OF $GABA_A$ *VERSUS* $GABA_B$ RECEPTORS ON INTRACELLULAR CALCIUM AND MEMBRANE POTENTIAL OF MELANOTROPE CELLS OF *XENOPUS LAEVIS* B.G. Jenks*, W.J.J.M. Scheenen and E.W. Roubos, Dept. Animal Physiology, University of Nijmegen, 6525 ED Nijmegen, The Netherlands.

Both $GABA_A$ and $GABA_B$ receptors are involved in GABA-induced inhibition of α-MSH secretion from the melanotrope cell of *Xenopus laevis*. One of our aims is to determine the functional significance of two GABAergic mechanisms operating on this cell. The present study concerns the action of these receptors on intracellular calcium ($[Ca^{2+}]_i$) and membrane potential, analyzed by microfluorescence techniques. Melanotropes displayed spontaneous Ca^{2+} oscillations which were eliminated by treatment with either the $GABA_B$ receptor agonist baclofen or the $GABA_A$ receptor agonist isoguvacine. Baclofen had no effect on baseline $[Ca^{2+}]_i$ while isoguvacine treatment raised baseline $[Ca^{2+}]_i$. These results suggest that the Ca^{2+} oscillations, and not baseline Ca^{2+}, are the driving force for secretion. Activation of $GABA_B$ receptors led to hyperpolarization of melanotropes while activation of $GABA_A$ receptors gave depolarizations. These contrasting actions on membrane potential allowed us to examine the relative contribution of the two receptor types when the endogenous neurotransmitter GABA was applied to the cells. Low concentrations of GABA gave hyperpolarizations, indicative of $GABA_B$ receptor function, and high GABA concentrations gave depolarizations, indicative of $GABA_A$ receptor action. Thus, differential activation of ionotropic ($GABA_A$) and metabotropic ($GABA_B$) mechanisms on *Xenopus* melanotropes can be achieved through the different sensitivity thresholds of these mechanisms to GABA.

P3.31

GLUTAMIC ACID DECARBOXYLASE ACTIVITY RESPONSE OF THE OLFACTORY BULB AND HYPOTALAMUS TO DIVERSE PHEROMONAL STIMULI. C. Grigorjev, N. Navarro, N. I. Munaro*. Cat. de Farmacología, Fac. de C. Médicas, Univ. Nac. de Córdoba, 5000 Córdoba, Argentina.

We have studied the influence of pheromones on glutamic acid decarboxylase activity (GAD) in the main (MOB) and accessory (AOB) olfactory bulb (OB) and in the hypothalamus of proestrous rats odor deprived. The rats were exposed for 1 and 2 hr to the pheromonal stimuli of intact and castrated males and ovariectomized rats. As controls odor deprived proestrous rats were used. The exposure to 1 and 2 hr to an intact or a castrated male odor, increased MOB-GAD activity, while in the AOB the increase was induced only after 1 hr exposure to the castrated male odor. On the contrary, 1 hr exposure to an ovariectomized rat odor induced a decrease of GAD activity in both parts of the bulb. Two hr exposure to a castrated male and female odor enhanced GAD activity in the hypothalamic preoptic area, while a similar reduction was induced by the three pheromones in the median eminence and lateral hypothalamus during the first hr of exposure. These results indicate that in BO and preoptic area, GAD activity is influenced by the pheromone quality which depends on the rat hormonal state.

P3.32

DISTRIBUTION AND PHARMACOLOGICAL CHARACTERIZATION OF SOMATOSTATIN RECEPTOR BINDING SITES IN THE DIENCEPHALON, LOWER BRAINSTEM AND CEREBELLUM IN THE SHEEP. A. Slama, V. Guillaume*, M. Fodor, C. Videau, Zs. Csaba, C. Kordon, Ch. Oliver* J. Epelbaum. INSERM U159 Paris, France, 75014 and (*) U297 Marseille, France, 13015.

Somatostatin receptor binding sites were described in the diencephalon, lower brainstem and cerebellum of the sheep brain using ^{125}I-Tyr_0-$DTrp_8$-somatostatin, by quantitative high resolution light microscopic radioautography. Radiolabeled sections were analysed, on radioautographic film and on sections coated with photoemulsion, by densitometry using a Biocom image analysis system. Film analysis. Highest density was recorded in the superficial layer of the superior colliculus, mesencephalic periaqueductal gray, dorsal motor nucleus of the vagus nerve, inferior olive, superficial layer of the spinal trigeminal nucleus, and the ganglionar and granular layers of the cerebellum. Moderate to low receptor density could be measured in the medial habenula, thalamic periventricular nucleus, interpeduncular nucleus, pontine tegmentum, parabrachial nuclei, nucleus of the solitary tract. Section analysis. In most of the labeled areas somatostatin receptor binding was evenly distributed between both neuropil and perikarya. Furthermore perikarya bearing somatostatin receptors were detected in areas, which did not show detectable binding sites on film, like in the hypothalamic preoptic area, arcuate nucleus, medial hypothalamus, anterior thalamic nuclei, deeper layers of the colliculus superior, median raphe and locus coeruleus. In cerebellum as in temporal cortex, somatostatin 28 and somatostatin 14 were equipotent to displace ^{125}I-Tyr somatostatin binding. Octreotide displaced 70 % of specific binding with a nanomolar affinity. It is concluded for these data that in the sheep, brain somatostatin receptors represent a mixed population of the recently cloned subtypes $SSTR_2$, $SSTR_3$, and/or $SSTR_5$.

P3.33

INFLUENCES OF HYPOPHYSECTOMY ON HYPOTHALAMIC-SOMATOSTATINERGIC SYSTEM: MORPHOMETRIC VARIATIONS OF NEURONS AND DENSITOMETRIC CHANGES IN FIBERS OF MEDIAN EMINENCE. R. Vázquez, J. Carretero, T. González, F. Sánchez, M. Rubio, J.M. Riesco, E. Blanco, J.A. Juanes. Dept. of Human Anatomy and Histology, Faculty of Medicine, University of Salamanca, Spain.

In order to determine the influences of hypophysectomy on hypothalamic-somatostatinergic system, a morphometric and immunohistochemical study of periventricular somatostatin-immunoreactive neurons and a densitometric analysis of distribution of immunoreactive fibers in the median eminence were performed in male rats following 20, 40 or 60 days after hypophysectomy. Hypophysectomy induces the appearance of immunoreactive fibers in the retrochiasmatic region, a significant increase of these fibers in the internal zone (fibrillar and ependimary layers) and an increase of immunoreaction in external layer in the infundibular region of median eminence. These changes are related to morphometric variations of the size of immunoreactive periventricular neurons and a significant increase of immunoreactive fibers in the arquate nucleus.

P3.34

HEXARELIN STIMULATES GH SYNTHESIS IN A RAT MODEL OF IMPAIRED HYPOTHALAMIC CONTROL.

A. Torsello*, V. Locatelli, M. Luoni, M.C. Ghigo, R. Grilli, °R. Deghenghi, and E.E. Müller, Department of Pharmacology, University of Milan, Milan, Italy 20129 and °Europeptides, Argenteuil, France 95108.

The hexapeptide Hexarelin (His-D-2-Me-Trp-Ala-Trp-D-Phe-Lys-NH2) is a new synthetic growth hormone(GH)-releasing peptide. Recently, we have characterized it as capable to stimulate GH secretion and synthesis in GHRH-deprived infant rats. Our aim was to study its mechanism(s) of action by using rat models with functionally or anatomically impaired hypothalamic control. In 10-day old pups passively immunized against GHRH from the day of birth, a 5-day treatment with Hexarelin (80 μg/kg, sc) completely counteracted the inhibition of GH gene expression induced by the antibody; however, Hexarelin did not stimulate GH synthesis in control pups. To verify if Hexarelin can stimulate GH synthesis by acting on the pituitary site, we studied the effects of 3 and 72 hours stimulation with Hexarelin (10^{-6}M) on adult male rat pituitary cell monolayers. Both treatment schedules failed to stimulate GH gene expression in pituitary cells. The effects of a 5-day-Hexarelin treatment (150 μg/kg, sc, twice daily) was then studied in adult rats with surgical ablation of the medio-basal hypothalamus (MBH). Hexarelin did not stimulate GH gene expression in the pituitary gland of either MBH-ablated rats or normal controls. Similarly, 3 and 5 days of Hexarelin (150 μg/kg, sc, twice daily) treatment failed to or only marginally stimulated GH gene expression in pituitaries transplanted under the kidney capsule of intact rats. In all, our results demonstrate that Hexarelin is capable to stimulate GH gene expression in a model of functionally impaired GHRH function, but it is ineffective when the pituitary is anatomically disconnected from the hypothalamus. This suggests that Hexarelin may promote GH gene expression by stimulating a still unknown hypothalamic factor.

P3.35

THE EFFECT OF CONTINUOUS LIGHT ON THE CONCENTRATIONS OF CATECHOLAMINES OF THE HYPOTHALAMUS AND ADRENAL GLANDS AND PLASMA ACTH. **O. Ivanovisevic-Milovanovic, M. Demajo, A. Karakasevic, *V. Pantic. Inst. "Vinca", POB 522, 11001 Beograd, Yugoslavia.**

Female rats aged 4 months were exposed to continuous light for weeks. The concentrations of hypothalamic dopamine (DA) (10.23±0.94 nmol/g) and norepinephrine (NE) (33.33±2.91 nmol/g) were in controls significantly higher than in experimental animals (DA 6.48±0.36 nmol/g, NE 25.18±1.14 nmol/g). There was no difference in the content of adrenal DA (contr. 20.42±3.4 nmol/g, exp. 20.84±1.55 nmol/g) and NE (contr. 863±77.24, exp. 776.67±40.48 nmol/g) between control and experimental rats. The concentration of epinephrine (E) in the adrenals of the controls (2587±327.44 nmol/g) was significantly lower compared to experimental animals (2982±54.63 nmol/g). Continuous light induced a significant rise in plasma ACTH concentration (48.30±3.29 pg/ml) compared to the controls (39.10±3.09 pg/ml). These results indicate that: (1) there is an inverse relationship between hypothalamic CA content and plasma ACTH concentration; (2) the initiation of E synthesis in adult rat adrenal glands is controlled by the pituitary-adrenocortical system.

P3.36

EFFECTS OF DYNORPHIN ON NORADRENALINE RELEASE IN THE RAT MEDIAL PREOPTIC AREA. E. Ito*, T. Mizuno, F. Kimura. Dept. of Physiology, Yokohama City University School of Medicine, Yokohama, Japan, 236.

We investigated the effect of Dynorphin A (1–13) on the release of noradrenaline (NA) in the medial preoptic area (MPOA) by intracranial microdialysis method in the conscious male rat. Basal levels of NA release in MPOA began to decrease with the addition of Dynorphin to the perfusion medium, and the NA release was about 65% of the basal release after 30 min. We also examined the influence of Dynorphin on the stress-induced NA increase in MPOA. In control rats, a 30-min immobilization evoked a marked increase in the NA release, attaining its peak, about 770% of the basal release, at 30 min after the onset of stress. However, in rats given Dynorphin in the perfusion medium, immobilization produced a significantly less marked increase (about 580% of the basal release). These data indicate that kappa-opioid receptors play part of role in the inhibitory control of endogenous opioids over the NA release in MPOA.

P3.37

THE INFLUENCE OF DEXAMETHASONE ON THE ACTIVITY OF MONOAMINE OXIDASE AND CATALASE IN THE RAT HYPOTHALAMUS

V. Davidović, G. Cvijić, R. Radojičić, Ž. Matijašević, J. Dordević. Institute of Physiology and Biochemistry, Faculty of Biology, Belgrade, Yugoslavia, Akademski trg 16. Fax: 11-638-500

It is well known that in the processes of catecholamine demination H_2O_2 is produced in the central nervous system. Therefore, the effect of different doses (0.2 and 1.0 mg/kg b.m.i.p., for 2 days) of dexamethasone on the activity of both MAO forms (A and B) and catalase, peroxide catabolizing enzyme, in the rat hypothalamus were studied. The low dose of dexamethasone had no effect either on the activity of the two MAO forms or catalase. In contrast, the high dose of dexamethasone significantly decreased the activity of both forms of MAO, but remained without effect on catalase activity. These result suggest that the effect of synthetic glucocorticids, such as dexamethasone, on the activity of catecholamine degrading enzyme, is dose-dependent. Besides, they are indicative that this hormone probably controls the catecholamine metabolism in the hypothalamus by inhibiting MAO.

P3.38

ALTERNATIONS IN EXTRACELLULAR LEVELS OF MONOAMINES AND THEIR METABOLITES IN THE MBH-ME OF ESTROUS EWES DURING β-ENDORPHIN TREATMENT.

D. Tomaszewska, K. Mateusiak, F. Przekop.* Polish Academy of Sciences. The Kielanowski Institute of Animal Physiology and Nutrition, Jabłonna, Poland.

The aim of the present study was to analyse the effect of β-END applied locally into the MBH-ME of the estrous ewes on the NA, DA and 5-HT systems activity in this structure. The activity of monoaminergic systems was evaluated on the basis of extracellular concentration of monoamines and their metabolites (NA and MN, MHPG; DA and DOPAC, HVA; 5-HT and 5-HIAA) quantified in perfusates obtained by "push-pull" cannulae method, using HPLC with electrochemical detection. Ringer solution with 25 μg β-END/ml was infused at the rate flow of 5 μl/min for 5 hrs. In the animals, prior to preovulatory LH surge the monoamines in perfusates were detectable occasionally. During preovulatory LH surge NA appeared in most samples. The metabolites of monoamines of both groups remained essentially in different concentrations with a visible fluctuation. The increase of DA with concomitant decrease of metabolites of monoamines was apparent in all animals treated with β-END during preovulatory LH surge as well as prior to preovulatory LH release.
In conclusion, these results indicate that β-END induces an increase of DA release from MBH-ME and changes in metabolic activity of monoaminergic systems in this structure. It is suggested that β-END, at least in part, might affect gonadotropin secretion indirectly through monoaminergic systems in the MBH-ME.

P3.39

EVIDENCE FOR SUBSTANCE P AS A CENTRAL INHIBITOR OF CRF-41 DURING CHRONIC STRESS.

D.S. Jessop*, P.J. Larsen, S.L. Lightman, H.S. Chowdrey. Department of Medicine, University of Bristol, Bristol BS2 8HW, U.K. and Institute of Medical Anatomy B, University of Copenhagen, Denmark (PJL).

Substance P (SP) is an important central inhibitor of the stress hormone CRF-41. We have further investigated the inhibitory role of SP in a model of chronic stress following adjuvant-induced arthritis (AA) in rats in which the pituitary-adrenal axis is activated but hypothalamic CRF-41 mRNA and hypophysial portal blood concentrations of CRF-41 are decreased. To determine if SP is responsible for this inhibition of CRF-41, we measured SP peptide by specific RIA and the SP precursor preprotachykinin (PPT) mRNA by *in situ* hybridisation in areas of the hypothalamus where CRF-41 is synthesised and released. Fourteen days after injection, when all rats had developed the disease, SP levels in the paraventricular nucleus (PVN) were significantly increased (10.6 ± 1.3ng/mg protein) compared to the control group (6.6 ± 1.3ng/mg). In AA rats subjected to adrenalectomy (AA/ADX), SP in the PVN rose to 18.4 ± 3.3ng/mg. In the median eminence/arcuate nucleus area (ME/AN), SP concentrations in AA and AA/ADX groups were significantly elevated (4.6 ± 0.9 and 11.8 ± 2.4ng/mg respectively) compared to controls (2.8 ± 0.4ng/mg). PPT mRNA in the AN was not significantly altered in the AA groups. Tissue contents of ACTH, another potential CRF-41 inhibitor, were unchanged in the ME/AN, while ACTH in the PVN was decreased in AA and AA/ADX groups (22.2 ± 4.0 and 17.6 ± 3.5ng/mg respectively) compared to controls (41.3 ± 6.6ng/mg). POMC mRNA in the AN was significantly decreased in AA animals. We therefore conclude that hypothalamic SP is a prime candidate for the inhibition of CRF-41 during the chronic stress of arthritis, while ACTH does not appear to be involved.

P3.40

THE EFFECT OF DEHYDRATION ON PLASMA ENDOTHELIN LEVELS IN NORMOTENSIVE AND SPONTANEOUSLY HYPERTENSIVE RATS.

A.Płonowski*, M. Radzikowska, K. Roguski, E. Wasilewska-Dziubińska and B. Baranowska. Department of Neuroendocrinology, Medical Center of Postgraduate Education, Warsaw, Poland.

Endothelin (ET), 21 residue vasoconstrictive peptide, was originally discovered in endothelial cells. The presence of ET has been demonstrated in the paraventricular and supraoptical nuclear neurons and their terminal in posterior pituitary. The recent studies indicate that ET is colocalized with vasopressin in secretory granularity within neurohypophysis. Moreover, it has been found that prolonged water deprivation leeds to complete depletion of ET content in neural lobe of pituitary.
The aim of the present study was to investigate the effect of dehydration on plasma ET levels in normotensive (WKY) and spontaneously hypertensive (SHR) rats. Adult female WKY and SHR rats were used in the experiments. Dehydration was attained by withdrawal of drinking water for 22 hours before the experiments. In both - intact and dehydrated rats ET concentrations were measured at 15 mins after i.v. injection of clonidine (α_2-adrenergic agonist) in a dose of 25 μg or 0,3 ml saline. Trunk blood was collected to chilled tubes containing 7,5 mM EDTA (10 μl/ml) and aprotinine (500 U/ml). The ET levels were determined with RIA method using kits provided by Amersham Int, UK (RPA-535). **Results.** In both strains of rats 22-hour water deprivation produced a significant increase in plasma ET concentration (WKY: $p<0,01$; SHR: $p< 0,05$). Clonidine injection resulted in elevation of ET levels in intact WKY and SHR rats ($p<0,005$ and $p<0,05$, respectively). However, this effect was not observed in dehydrated animals (WKY and SHR).
Conclusion: 1. 22-hour water deprivation resulted in elevation of circulating ET level in WKY and SHR rats. 2. The inhibition of adrenergic activity was associated with significant increase of ET levels in intact rats. The water deprivation has abolished the influence of clonidine on plasma ET.

P3.41

OXYTOCIN AND BEHAVIOUR, BUT NOT CORTICOSTERONE RESPONSES TO THE 5-HT AGONIST M-CPP AND THE DOPAMINE AGONIST APOMORPHINE ARE DIFFERENTIALLY AFFECTED BY THE LESION OF THE HYPOTHALAMIC PARAVENTRICULAR NUCLEUS.

G. Bagdy, K. Gerber, Laboratory of Experimental Medicine, National Institute of Psychiatry and Neurology, Budapest, Hungary, H-1021

There is evidence that administrations of the dopamine agonist apomorphine or the serotonin-2C (5-HT_{2C}) receptor agonist m-chlorophenylpiperazine (m-CPP) increase plasma concentrations of oxytocin, corticosterone and induce penile erections (PE) in male rats, and lesion of the hypothalamic paraventricular nucleus (PVN) prevents apomorphine-induced penile erections. To test the hypothesis that the PVN mediates m-CPP-induced oxytocin, corticosterone and PE responses, we measured the effects of m-CPP (0.6 mg/kg iv) on these parameters in chronically cannulated, freely moving male rats after surgical PVN lesion or sham operation. In addition, the effects of PVN lesion on apomorphine-induced (0.05 mg/kg iv) oxytocin and corticosterone responses have also been tested. Surgical PVN lesion markedly attenuated corticosterone, but not oxytocin and PE responses to m-CPP. In contrary, apomorphine-induced oxytocin and corticosterone responses were significantly lower in PVN lesioned animals than in controls.

The present studies suggest that the PVN mediates m-CPP-induced corticosterone but not oxytocin and PE responses. Apomorphine-induced oxytocin and corticosterone responses, however, are mediated mainly by the PVN. Thus, the mechanisms of action of these drugs on oxytocin secretion and PE responses differ. 5-HT_{2C} receptor-mediated oxytocin and PE responses are independent of dopaminergic mechanisms.

P3.42

DISTRIBUTION OF NEUROTENSIN BINDING SITES IN THE HUMAN AMYGDALOID COMPLEX

T.A. Lantos*[1], A. Bérod[1], M. Palkovits[2] and W. Rostène[1]
[1] INSERM U. 339 Hôpital St. Antoine, 75571 Paris Cedex 12, France,
[2] Laboratory of Neuromorphology, Semmelweis University Medical School, Budapest, Hungary

Recent studies indicate that the amygdala is involved in various mental functions such as emotional and social behavior, learning and memory. It is well known that neurotensin (NT) is widely distributed throughout the amygdaloid complex. In our present work we investigated the topographical distribution of NT binding sites by quantitative autoradiography using monoiodo ^{125}I-Tyr_3-NT on amygdala sections of adult humans. High concentrations of ^{125}I-NT binding sites were found in the anterior amygdaloid area, the central amygdaloid nucleus and the amygdalo-piriform and amygdalo-hippocampal transition areas. Moderate to low densities were detected in the medial, cortical, accessory basal, basal, and lateral amygdaloid nuclei. The distribution of NT binding sites roughly matches with the findings of NT-immunocytochemistry. These data and the partial overlapping with the dopaminergic terminals suggest that NT may be involved in certain mental disorders including dementia and schizophrenia.

P3.43

GLUCOCORTCOIDS MODULATE D1 AGONIST INDUCED PRODUCTION AND RELEASE OF ATRIAL NATRIURETIC FACTOR (ANF) FROM RAT HYPOTHALAMIC NEURONS IN CULTURE

A.T. Lim*, D. Lee, W. Huang, D. Copolov. Cell Biology Unit, Mental Health Research Institute, Parkville 3052, Victoria, AUSTRALIA.

Although ANF modulates the release of dopamine in the hypothalamus, it remains unclear whether the latter reciprocally affects the function of ANF neurons. Employing long term monolayer cultures of hypothalamic neurons prepared from neonatal rats (Lee et al, ENDOCRINOLOGY 131:911, 1992), treatment with SKF38393, a D1 agonist was found to enhance the release of immunoreactive (ir)ANF in a dose related manner. Furthermore, the changes were accompanied with an increase in the abundance of pro-ANF mRNA in the cultures as determined by colorimetric Northern blot using synthetic antisense oligonucleotide probes (Huang et al, ENDOCRINOLOGY 131:1562 1992). These changes induced by SKF38393 were abolished in the presence of D1 receptor antagonist SCH23390 but not sulpiride, a D2 receptor antagonist. That ANF neurons expressed D1 receptors is supported by findings from studies employing combined in situ hybridization and immunocytochemistry to localise D1 receptor mRNA in greater than 85% of the irANF positive cells. Furthermore, although by itself dexamethasone (DM) was shown to have little effect on the basal release and production of ANF, the glucocorticoid significantly suppressed D1 agonist, SKF38393, induced stimulation in a dose and time dependent manner. This inhibition of DM was abolished by glucocorticoid receptor antagonist, RU38486 but not by mineralocorticoid receptor antagonist, RU28318. We thus conclude that in rats, hypothalamic ANF neurons are directly responsive to D1 agonist stimulation and that this effect is suppressed specifically by glucocorticoids.

P3.44

KINETICS AND AUTORADIOGRAPHIC LOCALIZATION OF BINDING SITES FOR NEUROPEPTIDE Y (NPY) IN THE BRAIN OF THE CHICKEN (GALLUS DOMESTICUS).

J. Merckaert*, F. Vandesande. Labo for Neuroendocrinology and Immunological Biotechnology, Catholic University Leuven, Naamsestraat 59, 3000 Leuven, Belgium.

Broiler and leghorn chickens show an extreme difference in ingestive and reproductive behavior. As NPY influences both of them we studied the distribution of the NPY receptors in both chicken models using receptor autoradiography.

15 µm sections of the brains were made and used for receptor localization. The sections were incubated with ^{3}H-NPY as a tracer and NPY as the displacer.

Receptors for NPY are localized in the striatum griseum, the neostriatum, the hippocampus, the cerebellum, the preoptic region, the hypothalamic region with the nucleus paraventricularis magnocellularis and the nucleus preopticus medialis, the pituitary. There were no receptors found in the ectostriatum and the paleostriatum.

Our results showed no differences in localization of NPY receptors in leghorns and broilers and math very well with the localization of immunoreactive NPY in the chicken brain as described by W.Kuenzel.

Using a NPY antagonist, specific for the mammalian NPY Y_1 receptor, our binding studies showed the presence of two receptor populations in the chicken brain. The localization of both receptors is very similar except for the Y_1 receptor which seems to be predominant in the cerebellum.

Further kinetic studies are in progress to determine the K_D and B_{max} of these receptors in the brain of broilers and leghorns.

P3.45

DOPAMINE AND ESTRADIOL ARE MODULATORS OF IN VITRO PROLIFERATION RATE OF RAT PITUITARY VIP-IMMUNOREACTIVE CELLS. J. Carretero, M. Rubio, F. Sánchez, R.J. Vázquez, J.M. Riesco, E. Blanco, J.A. Juanes y R. Vázquez. Dept. of Human Anatomy and Histology, Faculty of Medicine, University of Salamanca, Spain.

Using double labelling for Proliferating Cell Nuclear Antigen (PCNA) and Vasoactive Intestinal Peptide (VIP) by immunocytochemistry, a dose-time study was conducted to elucidate the repercussions of the addition of 17ß-estradiol or dopamine to rat monolayer pituitary cultures on morphology, size, number and PCNA-labelling index of VIP-immunoreactive cells, comparing the results with those obtained in control cultures. Estradiol led to a dose- and time-related significant increase in the parameters evaluated. Dopamine, however, induces significant decreases. The results obtained suggest that estradiol and dopamine are physiological regulators of activity of rat pituitary VIP-immunoreactive cells and they are in vitro modulators of the proliferation rate of this cells.

Supported by spanish grant DGICYT, PM91-0105.

P3.46

VASOPRESSIN AND CATECHOLAMINE CONTROL OF THE THYROID GLAND RESPONSE UNDER STRESS CONDITIONS IN RATS. IN VIVO AND IN VITRO STUDY. I.A. Krasnovskaya*, A.L. Polenov. Laboratory of Neuroendocrinology, Sechenov Institute of Evolutionary Physiology and Biochemistry RAS, St.Petersburg, Russia, 194223.

The thyroid gland (TG) response was studied in experiments simulated a stress increase of vasopressin (AVP) and adrenaline (A) level in blood. For this aim AVP (50pg/100g) and/or A (0.4pM/100g) was injected intraperitoneally and 20 min later the rats were decapitated. In the rats with intact hypophysis A caused a thyroinhibiting effect: the thyrocyte height decreased (78%, $P<0.05$) but the thyroid hormone blood level was constant. The AVP injection resulted in activation of TG: thyrocytes enlarged (112%, $P<0.05$), and thyroid hormone level increased (T3 - 190%, T4 - 110%, $P<0.05$). The injection of A and AVP simultaneously caused no TG stimulation. In hypophysectomized rats the pattern of the TG reaction was the same. In in vitro study the TG slices were incubated in the medium containing AVP (50pM/l) or A (50pM/l) or noradrenaline (NA, 5pM/l) or their combination. The thyrocyte activity was estimated by uptake and release of 3H-leucine diluted in the medium and by the height of the thyrocytes. A and NA in vitro did not change the thyrocyte activity essentially. AVP per se stimulated the thyroid hormone synthesis and release from the cells. The combination of AVP and A in the incubation medium stopped the release of hormones from the thyrocytes. The combination of AVP and NA stimulated both synthesis and release of the hormones from the thyrocytes.
Thus the pattern of the TG stress reaction depends on combination of AVP and catecholamine neurohormones released into blood.

P3.47

EVIDENCE FOR THE INVOLVEMENT OF ENDOGENOUS OPIOIDS IN THE REGULATION OF OVARIAN DEVELOPMENT IN THE FIDDLER CRAB, UCA PUGILATOR. M. Fingerman*, R. Sarojini, R. Nagabhushanam. Dept. of Ecology, Evolution, and Organismal Biology, Tulane University, New Orleans, Louisiana, U.S.A., 70118.

The potential involvement of an endogenous opioid system in the regulation of ovarian development in the fiddler crab, *Uca pugilator*, was investigated *in vivo*. Injection of synthetic methionine enkephalin into female crabs significantly slowed ovarian maturation. The inhibition was dose-dependent. The mean ovarian index and mean oocyte diameter of the crabs that received the opioid were significantly less than the corresponding values for the saline injected concurrent control specimens. Injection of the opioid antagonist, naloxone, produced dose-related ovarian maturation. These results provide the first evidence that an opioid system is involved in the control of reproduction in a crustacean.

P3.48

RECIPROCAL CONNECTIONS BETWEEN VASOPRESSIN AND β-ENDORPHIN IMMUNOREACTIVE NEURONS OF THE RAT HYPOTHALAMIC PARAVENTRICULAR(PVN) AND ARCUATE NUCLEUS(AN). J.Kiss, T.J.Görcs, V.M.Wiegant and B.Halász. Dept. Neuroendocrinology and Dept. Neurobiology, Joint Research Organization of the Hungarian Acad. and Semmelweis Univ. Med. Budapest, Hungary, H-1094 and Rudolph Magnus Institute Dept. of Med. Pharmacology, Univ. Utrecht, Utrecht, the Netherlands,3508TA

Using single- and double-label immunocytochemical techniques at light and electron microscopic level, arginine-vasopressin-immunoreactive (AVPir) varicose axons coursing towards the median eminence established close topographical contacts with β-endorphin immunoreactive (BEir) neuronal somata and dendrites of the AN. At the electron microscope level AVPir axons were in synaptic contact with BEir dendrites of AN neurons. In the PVN intensely stained varicose BEir fibres formed dense networks and contacted AVPir somata and dendrites. Electron microscopic investigations revealed BEir boutons forming synapse with AVPir perikarya and dendrites of PVN neurons.
The findings provide morphological basis for the view that AVPir axons (presumably coming from the PVN or supraoptic nucleus) may act directly on BE-neurons to release this peptide, and vice versa that BE-containing fibres, presumably arising from the AN may exert their influence directly on the vasopressin synthesizing neurons of the PVN.
Supported by OTKA 2615A and T 6372 grants.

P3.49

COEXISTENCE OF NADPH-DIAPHORASE WITH VASOPRESSIN BUT NOT WITH VASOTOCIN IN THE HYPOTHALAMUS.

C.Viglietti-Panzica, N.Aste, G.C.Panzica, F. Sánchez, R. Arévalo, J.-R. Alonso. Dept. Hum. Anatomy & Physiology, Torino (Italy), Dept. Hum. Anat. Histol. and Dept. Cell Biol., Salamanca (Spain).

At present, the presence of NADPH-diaphorase (ND) in the hypothalamus of the rat (Arévalo et al., 1992) and quail (Panzica et al., 1994) is well-known. In a previous paper, we have described partial coexistence of ND with vasopressin in the hypothalamus of the rat (Sánchez et al., 1994). However no information is available concerning the possible coexistence of ND with vasotocin (VT), the nonapeptide, of the family of vasopressin, produced in the hypothalamo-hypophysial system of non-mammalian vertebrates. Based upon the foregoing, a combined histochemical-immunocytochemical study was carried out to elucidate whether or not there is a coexistence of ND and VT. Additionally, in order to compare the results with the rat, the same analysis was developped for vasopressin. No coexistence was found for ND and VT. Confirming our previous studies coexistence with vasopressin was found. However, the degree of coexistence was never higher than 12%. The present findings obtained in the hypothalamus of mammalian and non-mammalian vertebrates suggest that ND is not related to intracellular regulative mechanisms involving the antidiuretic hormone, especially in birds. The presence of close contacts between ND containing fibers and small clusters of VT positive neurons suggests, yet, potential functional relationships between these two systems.

This work was supported by the University of Salamanca, MURST, and CNR.

P3.50

COEXISTENCE OF NADPH-DIAPHORASE WITH TYROSINE HYDROXYLASE IN MAGNOCELLULAR HYPOTHALAMIC NEURONS OF THE RAT.

E. Blanco*, J.M. Riesco, F. Sánchez, J.A. Juanes, J. Carretero, M. Rubio, R. Vázquez. Dpto. de Anatomía e Histología Humanas. Facultad de Medicina. Universidad de Salamanca. 37007 Salamanca. Spain.

The presence and distribution of NADPH-diaphorase (ND) neurons as well as tyrosine hydroxylase-immunoreactive (TH) neurons in the hypothalamus are well established. Previous studies by our group have shown the coexistence of ND with neuroactive substances such as calbindin, somatostatin, vasopressin and oxytocin in neurons of this region of the brain. Since the topographical patterns of distribution of ND and TH coincide in many cases, the aim of this study was to determine the possible coexistence of both substances in the main hypothalamic magnocellular nuclei of the albino rat. Histochemical-immunocytochemical double labelling was employed on the same sections as well as a morphometric study. NADPH-diaphorase and tyrosine hydroxylase neurons were observed in all the nuclei under study (supraoptic, paraventricular and accessory nuclei), although most neurons showing the coexistence of both substances were mainly located in the supraoptic nucleus, finding isolated neurons with double labelling in the magnocellular parts of the paraventricular nucleus and in some of the accessory nuclei. Although both substances have previously been shown to be modified in hypothalamic neurons after osmotic stimuli, the range of functions of ND in the CNS is only beginning to be understood. Further studies are needed to elucidate the functional role that ND/TH neurons play in the nervous system.

P3.51

EFFECT OF ADRENALECTOMY ON THE NADPH-DIAPHORASE EXPRESSION IN THE PARAVENTRICULAR AND SUPRAOPTIC NUCLEI OF THE RAT.

F. Sánchez*, M. Rubio, V. Hernández, J. Carretero, J.M. Riesco, J.A. Juanes and E. Blanco. Dept. Human Anatomy. Faculty of Medicine. University of Salamanca. 37007. Salamanca. Spain.

A histochemical study of NADPH-diaphorase staining in the supraoptic and paraventricular nuclei of the rat, following adrenalectomy was carried out. In normal and sham operated animals NADPH-diaphorase was present in the magnocellular neurons of both nuclei, and in less degree in the parvicellular neurons of the paraventricular nucleus. Following billateral adrenalectomy (14 days) an increase of the number of stained neurons was detected. When the adrenalectomized animals received a daily dosis of corticosterone no differences were seen when compared to the nomal and sham operated groups. These results suggest that nitric oxide could be related, as a modulator, with the morphology and function of the magnocellular neurons located in both nuclei. In addition, glucocorticoids seems to regulate the NADPH-diaphorase expression negatively.

P3.52

IMMUNOCYTOCHEMICAL STUDY OF THE MONOAMINERGIC INNERVATION OF NEUROPEPTIDERGIC CELLS IN THE CHICKEN HYPOTHALAMUS.

L. Moons*, E. D'Hondt, K. Pijcke and F. Vandesande, Zoological Institute, Naamsestraat 59, 3000 Leuven, Belgium.

Intensive selection for increased muscle growth in meat-type chickens has led to a decrease in the reproductive performance of the parent stocks. For some time, we have been interested in the neuroendocrine background of this negative correlation between body weight and reproductive capacity in the chicken. It is generally known that in the hypothalamus the control of both the reproductive and feeding behavior often happens through identical neurotransmitters (catecholamines and serotonin) and neuropeptides (LHRH-I, CCK, GAL, END, NPY). From our previously performed immunocytochemical (ICC) stainings in the brain of the chicken, it became obvious that the biogenic amines, (L-DOPA, DA, NA and 5-HT) as well as several neuropeptides (LHRH-I, NPY, GAL, CCK and END) are all present in most of the hypothalamic nuclei, involved in the control of reproduction and growth. The poor information concerning functional interactions between monoaminergic neurotransmitters and neuropeptides in the hypothalamus of birds encouraged us to start with some double ICC stainings. Although we could not find any colocalizations between monoamines and peptides at the hypothalamic level, this light microscopical ICC study did reveal very close associations between DA- and 5-HT-containing fibers or terminals and perikarya showing immunoreactivity for the various peptides. The close interactions between the aminergic fibers and the peptidergic neurons occur in several hypothalamic nuclei but are most abundant in the preoptic region and in the periventricular region of the hypothalamus. These results suggest an important role for DA and 5-HT in the control of neurosecretion of peptide hormones from hypothalamic cells in the chicken brain. The ICC data provide an excellent basis for further research on the functional significance of the different peptide-amine interactions in the hypothalamus of the chicken.

P3.53

ULTRASTRUCTURAL ORGANIZATION OF IMMORTALIZED LUTEINIZING HORMONE-RELEASING HORMONE NEURONS IMPLANTED INTO THE THIRD VENTRICLE OF THE RAT BRAIN.

Zs. Liposits#*, W. C. Wetsel@, W. A. Eckert#, J. J. Reid#, I. Merchenthaler#. *Department of Anatomy, Albert Szent-Györgyi Medical University, H-6701 Szeged, Hungary, #Functional Morphology Group, Laboratory of Molecular and Integrative Neuroscience, and @Hormone Action Group, Laboratory of Cellular and Molecular Pharmacology, NIEHS, Research Triangle Park, NC 27709, U. S. A.

Immortalized luteinizing hormone-releasing hormone-synthesizing neurons (GT1-7) were stereotaxically implanted into the basal part of the third ventricle of adult rats and the abilities of these neurons to establish connections with the host and to target the median eminence were evaluated. At the end of 8 weeks, the immortalized GT1-7 neurons had established connections both with neurons in the arcuate nucleus and with the fenestrated capillaries of the median eminence. The grafted GT1-7 cells became anchored at the targeted site and mutual connections developed between the host and graft tissues. Implanted GT1-7 neurons developed contacts with each other and displayed organelles indicative of active protein synthesis. The immortalized neurons appeared to be more differentiated at locations where few cells were present than at sites where dense clusters of GT1-7 neurons appeared. Axons of the host also established contacts with the implanted GT1-7 cells. Processes and perikarya of the immortalized neurons appeared in the arcuate nucleus and median eminence. In the latter region, GT1-7 processes terminated on the limiting membrane where they interdigitated with genuine hypophysiotropic axons of the host. These data indicate that the immortalized LHRH neurons are capable of establishing connections with the host neural tissue and targeting the hypophyseal portal circulation. This neuronal model may be useful in determining the chemical and morphological signals that are important for appropriate cellular targeting.

P3.54

VASOACTIVE INTESTINAL PEPTIDE (VIP)-LIKE IMMUNOREACTIVE CEREBROSPINAL FLUID (CSF)-CONTACTING NEURONS IN THE AVIAN LATERAL SEPTUM.

K. Hirunagi[1*], K. Kiyoshi[1], A. Adachi[2], S. Ebihara[2], K. Maeda[3], H. -W. Korf [4]. Depts. of Veterinary Anatomy[1], Animal Physiology[2] and Animal Reproduction[3], School of Agricultural Sciences, Nagoya Univ., Nagoya, Japan, 464-01, Center of Morphology [4], Section Neurobiology, Johan Wolfgang Goethe Univ. Frankfurt/Main, Germany, D-60590

By means of immunocytochemical demonstration of VIP an accumulation of CSF-contacting neurons was found in a circumscribed region of the lateral septum/nucleus accumbens in the duck and pigeon. VIP-like immunoreactive(ir) CSF-contacting neurons were bipolar cells. Their perikarya accumulated in the subependymal region of the ventromedial wall of both lateral ventricles at the level of the pars medialis of the lateral septal organ (LSO)(Kuenzel and Blähser 1994). The neuron bore a ventricular process and a basal process. The ventricular process penetrated the ependyma and terminated in the lateral ventricle as a knob-like structure. The basal processes could be followed into the deeper neuropil areas. Immunoelectron microscopy revealed more details of fine structures of VIP-like ir neuronal elements. VIP-like ir CSF-contacting neurons had common features of CSF-contacting neurons such as a cilium and an aggregation of mitochondria in ventricular terminals in the duck. Immunolabeled dense vesicles were found in ventricular terminals and processes, perikarya, immunolabeled axon-like processes and axon terminals in the septal area. VIP-like ir terminal fields were examined in the lateral septum of the pigeon. VIP-like ir axon terminals had synaptoid contacts with perikarya of small VIP-immunonegative neurons of the lateral septum, which were characterized by an invaginated nucleus, numerous mitochondria, well-developed Golgi apparatus, endoplasmic reticulum and a small number of dense-core vesicles (about 100nm in diameter). VIP-like ir axons were also seen in contact with immunonegative dendrites in the lateral septum. These findings suggest that VIP-like ir neurons of the lateral septum project to small, presumably peptidergic neurons of the lateral septum. Preliminary examinations of the pigeon revealed that GnRH-like ir fibers and cell bodies accumulated in the pars medialis of the LSO.

P3.55

PUBERTAL INCREASE OF INSULIN-LIKE GROWTH FACTOR-I-LIKE IMMUNOREACTIVITY IN RAT HYPOTHALAMIC ASTROGLIA.

M. Dueñas, S. Luquín, J.A. Chowen, I. Torres-Alemán, F. Naftolin and L.M. Garcia-Segura. Instituto Cajal, C.S.I.C., 28002 Madrid, Spain and Dept. OB/GYN, Yale University School of Medicine, New Haven, CT 06510, USA

The surface density of insulin-like growth factor I-like immunoreactive cells (SvIGF-I) was assessed in the rat arcuate nucleus, a hypothalamic area that regulates pituitary secretion. Immunoreactivity was observed in astroglial cells with the morphological aspect of tanycytes. SvIGF-I increased with puberty in the arcuate of males and females, while decreasing with age in other brain areas. In females, SvIGF-I rose markedly between the morning and the afternoon of the first day of proestrus, remained high in the morning of the first day of estrus and then declined by the morning of the first day of metestrus. Fluctuations in SvIGF-I were regulated by 17β-estradiol and progesterone. *In situ* hybridization histochemistry for IGF-I mRNA resulted in an absence of labeling in astroglial cells, suggesting an extracerebral origin for IGF-I.

P3.56

POMC NEURONS INNERVATE SOMATOSTATIN CELLS IN THE HYPOTHALAMIC PERIVENTRICULAR NUCLEUS.

M. Fodor*, Zs. Csaba, C. Kordon, J. Epelbaum. INSERM U 159., Paris, France, 75014

It has been reported that opioid peptides alters growth hormone secretion via central hypothalamic mechanisms. In the present study we used retrograde transport of wheat germ agglutinin-apohorseradish peroxidase-gold complex (WGA-HRP-gold) and imunohistochemistry to identify the precise origin and possible input of the POMC terminals to the periventricular somatostatin-containing cells. In the first group of animals discrete pressure injection of the WGA-HRP-gold restricted to the periventricular nucleus were carried out. Following the tracer injection and subsequent immunostaining for β-endorphin, a significant proportion (15.1±2.1%) of the immunostained neurons was double labeled. These neurons were evenly distributed among the single labeled immunoreactive cell bodies throughout the entire rostro-caudal extent of the arcuate nucleus. To determine whether the POMC-containing axons are contacted with somatostatinergic perikarya, in a second group of intact animals dual immunostaining procedure was performed. Nickel intensified POMC-containing fibers were observed in apposition to a majority of the somatostatinergic neurons in the anterior periventricular area by means of light microscopy. The present results indicate that POMC peptides originating in the arcuate nucleus may modulate GH release via a direct influence on periventricular somatostatin neurons.

P3.57

AROMATIZATION MEDIATES THE EFFECT OF TESTOSTERONE ON AROMATASE IMMUNOREACTIVE CELLS IN THE QUAIL MEDIAL PREOPTIC NUCLEUS.

N.Aste, P.Aimar, A.Foidart°, J.Balthazart°, C.Viglietti-Panzica, G.C.Panzica. Dept. Hum. Anat. & Physiol., Torino (Italy), °Lab. Biochem., Liège (Belgium).

The conversion of testosterone (T) into 17ß-estradiol (E_2, aromatization) plays a key role in the activation of male sexual behaviour. In quail, T and E_2 mainly act in the medial preoptic nucleus (POM) to activate male copulation. The volume and cytoarchitectonic organization of POM are sensitive to plasma levels of T and this nucleus contains a dense population of aromatase-immunoreactive (ARO-ir) cells. Previous studies have shown that, in castrated quail, T and its metabolites increase the size of the large neurons located in the lateral part of the POM. This area also contains large ARO-ir cells and we hypothesized that the steroids were primarily acting on these cells. To test this idea castrated male quail were gonadectomized (n=27) and treated with Silastic implants filled with T, E_2, 5α-dihydrotestosterone (DHT), E_2 and DHT (E_2+DHT), or left empty as control. Gonadally intact males (n=6) were also included as intact controls. The number and size of ARO-ir cells were measured in the POM of these birds by computer-assisted image analysis. As a mean, the ARO-ir elements were largest size than the other cells in POM. The size and the number of ARO-ir cells decreased after castration and returned to intact level after T treatment in both the lateral and medial part of the nucleus. The ARO-ir cell size was significantly increased by E_2 and E_2+DHT treatments in both parts of POM but did not reach the level of the intact control group. These treatments also increased the number of ARO-ir cells in the lateral part of the nucleus. DHT alone had no effect on ARO-ir cells. These data are similar to those obtained in the study of Nissl-stained material. They suggest that ARO-ir cells are a major target of T and of E_2 in POM. The specificity of the hormonal control of ARO-ir cells and of male copulation are very similar which provides additional evidence for a causal link between these two processes. *This study was supported by grants from MURST, FNRS, and ESF.*

P3.58

TREFOIL FACTOR-LIKE IMMUNOREACTIVITY IN THE HUMAN HYPOTHALAMUS AND PITUITARY.

J. C. Probst, T. Zetzsche, T. Skutella and G. F. Jirikowski,
Max Planck Institute of Psychiatry, Clinical Institute, Dept. of Neuroendocrinology, Munich, Germany D-80804

Trefoil factor peptides represent a new and growing family of cysteine-rich polypeptides which are characterized by their distinctive structure. This subunit or module, also termed p-domain, is found in polypeptides consisting of one, two or four p-domains, being expressed mainly in the gut of mammals but also in the gut and skin of the south african clawed toad *Xenopus laevis*. Recently, molecular cloning of a central nervous system homolog of rat intestinal trefoil factor (rITF) was successful and established a new gut-brain peptide which was termed rP1.B/rat brain trefoil factor (rBTF). The messenger RNA for rBTF was shown to be expressed mainly in the nucleus arcuatus and the supraoptic nucleus of the rat hypothalamus. Additionally, with immunohistochemical studies rBTF could be detected in the posterior and anterior pituitary. rBTF therefore represents a yet not described, novel hypothalamic-hypophysiotropic peptide. Because of the high degree of homology between the intestinal and brain derived peptide of 98-99 % , it was irrevocable to test an antibody directed against human ITF. Paraffin-embeded human hypothalamus sections were immunostained with anti-hITF with the biotin-avidin method. Positively stained cells could be localized in the periventricular and paraventricular nucleus and in the posterior and anterior lobe of the pituitary. This result strongly suggests that, as in rat, a brain homolog of hITF is existing. In order to verify the hormone and growth factor-like properties which are discussed, expression systems have to be designed for the production of sufficient amounts of trefoil peptides for physiological and biochemical studies of the peptides.

P3.59

MELANIN CONCENTRATING HORMONE IN HUMAN AND RAT

K Takahashi*, H Suzuki, K Totsune#, F Satoh#, O Murakami#, H Sasano##, T Mouri##, S Shibahara. Dept of Applied Physiol & Mol Biol,#the 2nd Dept of Int Med and ##the 2nd Dept of Pathol, Tohoku Univ Sch of Med, Sendai, Japan 980

Melanin concentrating hormone (MCH), originally isolated from salmon pituitary, acts as a circulating hormone in the pigment regulation in the salmon. MCH is present in human and rat brain, but its physiological significance has not been clarified. We have previously reported the presence of high concentrations of MCH in the human brain and numerous MCH immunoreactive neurons in the human hypothalamus. In the present study, to clarify whether MCH is a circulating hormone, a neurotransmitter or a neuromodulator in mammals, 1) the presence of MCH mRNA in human brain and rat tissues was studied by Northern blot hybridization, and 2) the presence of MCH in human plasma, adrenal glands and adrenal tumors by radioimmunoassay. The probe for the Northern blot analysis was prepared by PCR from rat brain cDNA. Human/rat MCH was used as standard and the antiserum to salmon MCH with 100% cross reaction with human/rat MCH was used in radioimmunoassay. Northern blot hybridization showed a band of approximately 1 kb in rat and human hypothalamus. MCH mRNA was not detectable from any other regions of brain, pituitary and rat peripheral tissues. Immunoreactive MCH was not detected in human plasma (<1.5 pmol/l, n=4), human adrenal glands (<1 pmol/g wet weight, n=9), adrenocortical tumors (n=9), and pheochromocytomas (n=13). These findings indicate that MCH is mainly produced in the hypothalamus and may be a neurotransmitter or a neuromodulator rather than a circulating hormone in human and rat.

P3.60

GAMMA KNIFE AND HYPOTHALAMO-PITUITARY FUNCTION IN CUSHING'S DISEASE

O Murakami*, F Satoh, H Ikeda#, H Jyokura##, K Takahashi, K Itoi, K Totsune, M Sone, A Sugawara, M Ohneda, K Hanew, T Mouri###, T Yoshimoto#, K Abe. The 2nd Dept of Int Med, #the Dept of Neurosurgery and ###the 2nd Dept of Pathol, Tohoku University School of Medicine, Sendai and ## the Gamma House, Jiro Suzuki Memorial Clinic, Furukawa, Japan

Irradiation therapy of the intracranial mass lesion with gamma knife is lesion-specific and appropriate for the relatively small mass lesions. The effects of the gamma knife therapy was studied in 4 patients with Cushing's disease, in whom the prior therapy of Hardy's operation had been ineffective. These patients were treated with the gamma knife (the marginal dose: 28.7-35.0 Gy). Plasma cortisol concentrations in all patients were decreased within 1 - 3 months and reached the nadir 3 - 6 months after the therapy. One patient was supplemented with glucocorticoid due to the low plasma cortisol concentrations 4 months after the therapy. Plasma ACTH concentrations were also decreased in all patients. Plasma ACTH concentrations in 2 cases were less than 50% of the values before the therapy in 3 - 6 months. CRH test was performed before and after the gamma knife therapy in 3 patients. During the periods of well controlled plasma cortisol, the maximal response of ACTH in CRH test was less than 50% compared to the response before the therapy in 2 of 3 patients. No remarkable decrease in other pituitary hormones was noted in hypothalamic hormone (TRH, LH-RH, GRH) tests after the therapy. Secondary hypofunction of thyroid and gonad did not occur. The gamma knife therapy in Cushing's disease was effective in lowering plasma ACTH and cortisol concentrations. These effects were observed earlier than those in the conventional irradiation therapy. No adverse effects in hypothalamo-pituitary function or in CNS were observed.

P3.61

ABSENCE OF INTERLEUKIN-6 RELEASE AFTER CRH-41 STIMULATION DURING BILATERAL INFERIOR PETROSAL SAMPLING IN PATIENTS WITH CUSHING'S DISEASE.

S. Tsagarakis, E. Vasilatou, J. Kaskarelis*, P. Giannou^, G. Kontogeorgos^, E. Botoula, N. Thalassinos.
Department of Endocrinology and *Radiology "Evangelismos" Hospital, ^Department of Pathology General Athens Hospital, Athens, Greece.

We have previously demonstrated the presence of immunohistochemically detectable interleukin-6 (IL-6) in pituitary adenoma cells, in the majority of patients with pituitary tumours. Although IL-6 release from pituitary adenomas has already been shown in cultures, in vivo IL-6 secretion has never been investigated. In the present study therefore, IL-6 secretion in inferior petrosal sinuses (IPS), a venous district close to the pituitary drainage, was investigated in 5 patients with Cushing's disease subjected to bilateral IPS sampling for diagnostic purposes. Plasma ACTH and IL-6 concentrations from IPS and peripheral samples were measured before and after a bolus iv dose of 100μg human CRH-41. Central:Peripheral (C:P) ratios for ACTH after CRH-41 stimulation were consistent with pituitary ACTH hypersecretion in all 5 patients. Peak C:P ACTH ratios at the dominant ACTH-secreting site ranged from 3 to 14.8 (mean±SD: 8±4.8). However no significant gradient for IL-6 was found on either basal or post-CRH stimulation samples (Basal C:P ratio: 1±0.07, post-CRH C:P ratio dominant site:1.02±0.09). All 5 patients proceeded to transsphenoidal surgery and 4 of them were cured (undetectable cortisol levels postoperatively). In 2 of those cured patients a corticotroph adenoma was demonstrated on pathology, and both adenomas were IL-6 positive by immunohistohemistry. In the remaining 2 cured patients adenoma tissue was not available for immunohistochemistry. It is concluded that IL-6 produced in tumorous pituitary corticotroph cells is not released in the systemic pituitary drainage, and therefore a local paracrine/autocrine effect is most likely and requires further investigation.

P3.62

TRANSFORMATION OF A HUMAN PITUITARY TUMOUR CELL POPULATION IN RESPONSE TO THERAPY: AN EM IMMUNOCYTOCHEMICAL STUDY. E. Bácsy, I. Fazekas, F. Slowik, E. Pásztor, S. Czirják. Institute of Experimental Medicine and National Institute of Neurosurgery, Budapest, Hungary

A growth hormone (GH) and prolactin (PRL) secreting pituitary adenoma was removed from a 4.5 years old girl. The child was reoperated on twice (at ages 5 and 10) because of recidives of the tumour. In the meantime, she was regularly treated with bromocriptine. The characteristics of the tumour cell population collected after the first and the third operations were examined by electron microscopy, immunocytochemistry, and in tissue culture. After the first intervention the tissue consisted of two morphologically distinct cell types: the GH-type and the PRL-type cells; in many cells of both populations the two hormones were co-localized. In the tissue removed 5 years later the GH-type cells showed no alteration. On the other hand, there was a number of pleomorphous cells with sparse, smaller secretory granules with weak PRL or both PRL and GH immunoreactivity, and lysosome-like structures. Both characteristic cell types could be identified in cultures. The structural difference between the PRL-type cells of the two tissue samples was preserved in vitro. We conclude that PRL-type cells are altered by chronic bromocriptine treatment; this alteration persists during in vitro culture but does not prevent survival or growth.

P3.63

EFFECT OF VASOACTIVE INTESTINAL POLYPEPTIDE (VIP) ON GROWTH HORMONE- AND PROLACTIN-PRODUCING HUMAN PITUITARY ADENOMA CELL CULTURES. I. Fazekas, I. Varga, F. Slowik, K. Bálint, K. Rácz, K. Mohari, E. Pásztor, E. Gláz. Nat. Inst. Neurosurgery; F.J.C.Nat.Res.Inst.Radiobiol.; 2nd Dept. Medicine, Semmelweis Univ., Budapest, Hungary.

Adenomas of five acromegalic patients and three prolactinomas were investigated by morphological methods and the effect of VIP on growth hormone (GH) and prolactin (PRL) secretion was tested in vitro. The preoperative serum level of GH and PRL were elevated. Immunocytochemical examinations revealed the presence of immunoreactive GH and PRL cells in the tumors. By electron microscopy the tumors were classified as two densely granulated GH cell adenomas, two sparsely granulated GH cell adenomas, one mixed GH/PRL cell adenoma and three sparsely granulated PRL adenomas. The dissociated cells were explanted into micro test plates. The cultures were treated with VIP (10^{-6}-10^{-12} M). GH and PRL contents in the culture media were measured by radioimmunoassay. GH release was significantly stimulated by VIP in a dose-dependent manner while only 10^{-6}-10^{-7} M VIP was effective on the PRL release. Since the cells showed strong immunostaining for VIP in all our adenomas it may be supposed that VIP acts in an autocrine or paracrine fashion within the pituitary.

P3.64

A REEVALUATION OF THE PROLACTIN-RELEASING ACTIVITY OF GROWTH HORMONE-RELEASING HORMONE IN ACROMEGALY IN VIVO

K. Kageyama*, H. Watanobe, T. Tamura, K. Takebe.
Third Department of Internal Medicine, Hirosaki University School of Medicine (KK, HW, KT), Hirosaki, Japan, 036; and Department of Neurosurgery, Brain Research Institute, Niigata University(TT), Niigata, Japan, 951

We examined a large number (51 patients) of active acromegalics in order to obtain reliable data on the incidence of the paradoxical PRL response to GHRH in this disorder. Each patient underwent iv bolus injections of GHRH(100 μg) and TRH(500 μg) on separate days, and plasma levels of GH and PRL were measured. The plasma PRL response to GHRH was considered positive (a paradoxical increase) when an increase over baseline of at least 50% occurred. We found that only 6 patients (12%) showed a positive PRL response to GHRH. These PRL-responders to GHRH had higher GH responses to this peptide than PRL-nonresponders to GHRH. Although PRL-responders and nonresponders to GHRH had a similar PRL responsiveness to TRH, the GH response to TRH was lower in PRL-responders to GHRH than in PRL-nonresponders to this peptide. In addition, PRL-nonresponders to GHRH had lower basal GH and higher basal PRL levels than PRL-responers to GHRH. These results suggest that (1) the alleged PRL-releasing activity of GHRH in acromegaly may be much weaker than was originally reported by Losa et al.(1985), and (2) the positive PRL response to GHRH may be associated with a relatively high GH response to this peptide, and also with a relatively low GH response to TRH.

P3.65

INSULIN SECRETION, INSULIN-LIKE GROWTH FACTOR-I LEVELS, AND GROWTH HORMONE CONCENTRATIONS IN ACROMEGALY. M.I. Goth*, I. Szabolcs, O. Dohan, L. Kovacs, G. Szilagyi. Div. of Endocrinology, First Dept. of Medicine, Imre Haynal Univ. of Health Sciences, Budapest, Hungary, 1389.

Acromegaly is associated with altered GH, IGF-I and insulin secretion. Their interrelationships were investigated in active and inactive (minimum serum GH after oral glucose load, OGTT >2µg/l, n=15; or <2µg/l, n=19) disease. A significant positive correlation ($p<0.05$) was found between IGF-I and fasting GH concentration only in those with inactive disease. IGF-I did not correlate with the minimum serum GH and the area under the GH curve (AUC-GH during OGTT) in either groups. When GH secretion was stimulated by TRH, the relation between IGF-I and AUC-GH during TRH was significant ($p<0.05$) only in the active group. No relationship between IGF-I, GH, insulin concentrations and various parameters of serum glucose levels was found. A significant positive correlation was shown to exist between the fasting serum GH concentration ($P<0.05$), the minimum GH ($p<0.01$), the AUC-GH ($p<0.01$) during OGTT and the fasting serum insulin level in patients with active, but not in patients with controlled disease. In contrast to the active group, the body mass index of controlled patients correlated with the fasting blood glucose levels ($p<0.05$). Our data show different relations of IGF-I, GH and insulin levels in active and controlled acromegaly. The most striking observations are the significant positive correlations between plasma IGF-I levels, various parameters of serum GH values and fasting insulin concentration and the lack of these relations in patients with inactive disease.

P3.66

GROWTH HORMONE RESPONSE AFTER GHRP-6 IN PATIENTS WITH ACROMEGALY. Popović V., Damjanović S., Micić D., Petakov M., Djurović M., Doknić M., Dieguez C. and Casanueva F., Institute of Endocrinology, University Belgrade, YU and Endocrine Section, University Santiago de Compostela, Spain

Hexapeptide GHRP-6 is a synthetic compound that releases growth hormone in dose related and specific manner. The exact site of its action is a matter of debate. We studied the effect of so called GHRP-6 on growth hormone secretion in patients with somatotroph adenomas (acromegaly). Thirteen newly diagnosed acromegalics were studied, 9 males and 4 females aged from 25-70 years (mean 45 yrs). GHRP-6 (Peninsula, UK) 100 mcg i.v. bolus was administered at 0 min. Another day they received 100 mcg i.v. bolus GHRH (GHRH 1-29 Serono, Spain) at 0 min. Plasma growth hormone levels (GH, mU/L) were measured by Pharmacia-Delfia, every 15 min for 2h. The data are presented as mean peak value during the tests and as area under the secretory curve (AUC) calculated by trapezoidal method. T test for paired data was then used. Mean basal GH was 82 +/- 27 mU/L while mean peak GH level after GHRP-6 was 222 +/- 39 mU/L ($p<0.05$). Mean GH peak level after GHRH was 146 +/- 31 mU/L ($p<0.05$). AUC after GHRP-6 was 17101 mU/L/ml/min while AUC after GHRH was 13651 mU/ml/min the difference being statistically significant ($p<0.01$). GHRP-6 is more potent than GHRH in GH release from adenomatous somatotrophs. Three acromegalics who did not respond after GHRH responded by further GH discharge after GHRP-6 ($p<0.05$) suggesting synergistic action upon maximally stimulated andenylate cyclase in the adenomas of these patients.

P3.67

SUMATRIPTAN DOES NOT MODULATE GHRH-INDUCED GH SECRETION IN MIDDLE-AGED NORMAL VOLUNTEERS AND ACROMEGALICS. C.M. Cuttica*, M. Giusti, L. Foppiani, S. Valenti, P. Sessarego and G. Giordano. DISEM, Cattedra di Endocrinologia, University of Genova, Genoa, Italy. Sumatriptan (SU), a 5-HT_{1D} receptor agonist has been reported as stimulating GH release in normal young adults (Rolandi et al, Lancet 339:1335, 1992). Recently we further showed that SU is a weak GH secretagogue in normal volunteers (NORM) but not in acromegalics (ACRO) (Cuttica et al, J Endocrinol Invest 16(1):160, 1993). This study was designed to asses the effect of SU on GHRH-induced GH secretion in middle-aged NORM (2 males, 4 females; 38±6 years) and ACRO (2 males, 4 females; 50±6 years). The following tests were performed: GHRH (1µg/kg bw iv), SU (6 mg sc) and SU (given 30 min before, sc) plus GHRH. GH and PRL were evaluated by IRMA. SU did not induce changes in GH release both in NORM and ACRO. In NORM GH response to GHRH was not modified by SU priming (peak: GHRH 16.3±7.3 ng/ml; SU+GHRH 15.1±4.5 ng/ml). Maximal GH increase from basal was similar in ACRO after GHRH (514±305%) and SU plus GHRH (507±319%). No increases in PRL levels after SU, GHRH or SU plus GHRH were observed in both groups. Our data show that SU does not potentiate spontaneous or GHRH-induced GH release in both groups. To explain this evidence, an autonomous GH secretion, partially independent by the hypothalamic control, could be suggested in ACRO. Moreover, age-related changes in GH responsiveness to SU seem to exist in normal volunteers.

P3.68

THREE INTRAGRANIAL TUMORS IN ONE PATIENT
Z.Penezić*,M.Drezgić,S.Ivanović,S.Vujović,D.Slijepčević. Institute of Endocrinology,KCS,Belgrade,Yugoslavia

A 57-y old woman with 5-y history of enlarging hands and feet,change in facial apperance,headache,arthalgias and hypertension,by wich time she had gained 20kg in weight. Glucose tolerance was impared for 6-m.The clinical impression of acromegaly was comfirmed by high plasma GH level 142-153 (RIA CIS n.v.0-14 nmol/L),with no supression on OGTT,137 to 122.Neuroimaging by MR revealed a pituitary macroadenoma with supraselar extension,second tumor along falx cerebri,and third in the region of crista galli.
Histological evaluation showed a mixed chromophob and eosinophil adenoma, meningothelial meningioma and as third tissue of osteoma. Transcranial adenectomiam were performed with simulaneous removal of meningioma and reduction of osteoma.Normal GH level and reaction to glucose load were found.Irradiation of the sellar region was subsequentlu undertaken.LTH,TSH,FSH,LH and ACTH were normal before the operation as well as after.
The association of meningiomas and acromegaly is rare,only 9 cases were published (Irsy,1985).The role of irradiation on the development of meningiomas is known (AlMefty,1990), but in some cases there were no previous irradiation,and acromegaly preceaded meningioma.In acromegaly the overall rate of both benign and malignant growths is increased and certan types are more commonly seen (Barzilay,1991).This increased rate could be attributet to stimulatory effect of GH,or more likely IGF-I as its principal mediator.Patients with untreated acromegaly also have increased rate of frontal sinus osteoma (Spencer,1987).According to aveilable published data,we haven't found association of pituitary adenoma,meningioma and osteoma at the same patient.

P3.69

LONGTERM FOLLOW UP OF PATIENTS WITH MAKROPROLACTINOMAS.

J. Schopohl*, B. Reichardt, B. Kohler[1] C.J. Strasburger, K.v. Werder[1]. Med. Klinik, Klinikum Innenstadt, 80336 München. [1]Schlossparkklinik, 14059 Berlin. Germany.

We report on our experience of longterm follow up (10.5 years {median}; 6.25 - 18.5 {range}) of 27 patients (pat) with macroprolactinomas (>10 mm diameter; 13 female, 10 male, median age at diagnosis 40 years; range 18 - 65). Operation lowered PRL levels by 75 % in 13 pat, however only two pat had normalized PRL levels, which increased again after 1 year to pathological levels. In all pat dopaminergic therapy (DT) with bromocriptine (BC) was started. PRL levels fell from 21100 mU/L (median) (200 - 250000 mU/L {range}) to 40 mU/L (23 - 2700 mU/L). Only in 5 pat PRL levels remained above 400 mU/L. Maximal BC dosis used during the first months of therapy was 7.5 mg/day (2.5-40 mg/day). PRL levels dropped to a minimum after 5 months (0.25 - 84 months) of BC the-rapy and the dosis could be sucessively reduced to 2.5 mg/day (1.25-30 mg/day). In 19 patients BC therapy was withdrawn after 2,5 years (0.25-7 years) and PRL levels increased to 3600 mU/L (233 - 100000 mU/L). Only 1 pat showed normal PRL levels during the last 4 years. A small PRL increase to 1600 mU/L was observed in 3 pat without change during the last 5 to 9 years. In the others DT had to be continued. After 6.5 years (0.75-10 years) in 8 pa-tients the therapy was again stopped. In 1 pat PRL levels stayed normal since 4.5 years, in another pat there was only a slight PRL increase to 800 mU/L without change during the last 6 years. In these 6 pat DT could be omitted completly after a treatment period of 4.25 years (0.5-8 years). In 16 pat NMR or CT scan showed complete disappearance of the macroadenoma during DT and in 5 pat tumor reduction between 60 and 80% was seen. In two pat no tumor reduction was obtained due to short duration of treatment because of untolarable side effects. 14 pat had no or only minor side effects and 9 pat had severe or untolarable side effects. Conclusion:Dopaminergic therapy normalized PRL levels in 74 % of the pat and reduced PRL levels effectively in over 90 %. In few pat DT can be stopped without relapse, and this has to be tested individually.

P3.70

CLINICAL,NEUROENDOCRINOLOGICAL FEATURES AND IMAGING TECHNIQUES OF INFUNDIBULOMA

J. Bérczy, Gy. Gyetvai, K. Karlinger[x] IIIth Department of Internal Medicine County Hospital Eger[x] Semmelweis University of Medicine
Eger, Hungary, H-3300 Pf.15.

Infundibuloma may present with endocrinologic disorders such as diabetes insipidus, hyperprolactinemia. Subject and methods: Infundibuloma were established on CT or MRI scan in three cases. Dynamic tests of hypothalamic-pituitary functions were performed /TRH,LHRH, CRF,Metoclopramid/, and hormon levels were measured by radioimmunoassay. The main clinical signs were polyuria and polydipsia. Central diabetes insipidus was diagnosed all cases. First case: hyperprolactinemia, second case: tertier hypadrenia were also established. In the first case, for years later the infundibuloma was growing and multiple cerebral lesions developed. Other two cases the infundibuloma has been unchanged for five years. Conclusions: 1. hypothalamic-pituitary functions have to evaluate because one or more hormonal deficiences often accompany infundibuloma. 2. there is evidence the regular CT or MRI scan and neuroendocrinological control of patients having infundibuloma.

P3.71

STUDY OF PRL RECEPTORS IN HUMAN ADENOMAS.

E. Ciccarelli*, S. Grottoli, P. Razzore, A. Bertagna, A. Longo°, G.C. Abbona+, C.Ghè§, G. Muccioli§
Department di Clinical Physiopathology, Division of Endocrinology, § Institut of Pharmacology and Experimental Therapy and Department of Biomedical Science ed Human Oncology, University of Turin; °Division of Neurosurgery, CTO Hospital, C.so Dogliotti 14, 10126, Turin, Italy.

Prolactin receptors (PRL-R) were previously identified either in anterior pituitary tumour induced by estradiol or in normal cells of rat origin in culture. These studies suggested the possibility that all PRL-secreting and non-PRL secreting cells could carry specific binding sites; no clear differentiation was made between PRL-secreting (PS) and non-PRL secreting (NPS) cells. We studied the presence of free and total PRL-R in pituitary tumour membranes from 19 pts (aged 20-72 yrs, 8 F and 11 M).
Immunostaining was positive for PRL in 3 pts, mixed GH and PRL in 3 pts, GH in 3 pts, glicoproteic hormones (FSH, LH and TSH) and subunit in 8 pts; the remaining 2 pts had null cell adenoma. Mean PRL levels before surgery were 295.7 ng/ml (37-562 ng/ml) in PS tumours, 34.8 ng/ml (range 24.7-51.6 ng/ml) in mixed PRL and GH secreting tumours and 17.1± 5.25 (range 2.2-71.0 ng/ml) in NPS tumours.Six cadaveric pituitary from subjects whose death was unrelated with brain and endocrine diseases were also studied as control group. In all pituitary tumours, specific PRL binding (mean SEM, free PRL-R) was 0.41 0.11% (range 0-1.96%); superimposable results were shown in controls (0.41 0.10 %, range 0.10-0.78%). In NPS tumours and in mixed tumours the free PRL-R were 0.25±0,11% and 0.28 0.16%, respectively. An increased specific binding (1.25 and 1.96%, respectively) was shown in 2/3 prolactinomas in whom PRL levels were markedly elevated (288 and 562 ng/ml); the remaining patients with prolactinoma had lower PRL-R (0.45%) and only mildly elevated PRL levels (37 ng/ml). Treatment of all tumour membranes with 4 M $MgCl_2$, increased the specific binding (total PRL-R; 0.54±0.11%). Also with this procedure only the 2 prolactinomas were conferemed PRL-R + (1.84% and 2.58%). A positive correlation was shown between free or total PRL-R and PRL levels (r=0.7409 and 0,7903; p<0.001). We conclude that no significant amount of PRL receptor was shown in NPS human pituitary tumours. In PS tumours, PRL receptors were increased only in presence of very high serum PRL levels suggesting only in these conditions the possibility of a positive feed-back between serum PRL and its receptor.

P3.72

OE_2 BAND: A PROTEIN PRODUCED BY EXPERIMENTAL PITUITARY TUMORS.

L. Bokser, R. Vidal, J.L. Zugaza, M. Lage, F. Perez, J. Perez, F.F. Casanueva. Molecular & Cellular Endocrine Laboratory. Department of Medicine, Universidad de Santiago, 15780 Santiago de Compostela, Spain.

Chronic estrogen treatment induces prolactin secreting pituitary tumors in rats. Recently, we have described using SDS-PAGE that these tumors produce a novel protein (OE_2 band) with a Mr of 38 kDa(1). This protein isolated from culture medium was never detected in tissue extracts. In an attempt to further characterize the OE_2 band, possible mechanisms for OE_2 protein degradation were studied. Sprague-Dawley rats were injected s.c. with 2 mg of estradiol depot every 30 days for 3 months. Pituitary tumor tissue samples were incubated at 37°C for 6 h in DMEN methionine free, supplemented with ^{35}S-methionine (150 µCi/ml). Proteins in the incubation medium and cell extracts were analyzed by SDS-PAGE. In some experiments labelled incubation medium was mixed with non-radioactive tissue extracts. The culture medium was also submitted to different conditions of pH and temperatures. The OE_2 protein was consistently present in the incubation media. However when it was combined with tissue extracts this protein was completely degraded. This effect was attenuated by the addition of a cocktail of protease inhibitors. With exception of the incubation at 65°C, most of the different conditions of pH and temperature did not affect the OE_2 band. These results suggest that the OE_2 band is not detected in tissue extracts because tissue proteolitic factors could be destroying it. The OE_2 protein is highly resistant to degradation in a wide spectrum of manipulation conditions. Although further studies are necessary, the OE_2 protein could be useful in the future as a pituitary tumor marker.

(1) *Casabiell et al, J. Mol. Endocrinol. 10:345-357, 1993*

P3.73

THE INFLUENCE OF ANGIOGENESIS INHIBITORS FUMAGILIN AND ITS SYNTHETIC ANALOG AGM-1470 ON GROWTH AND ANGIOGENESIS OF PITUITARY PROLACTINOMAS INDUCES IN FISCHER F344 RATS.

Grochal M.,Zielinski K., Kulig A., Pawlikowski M., Kunert-Radek J., Radek A., Stepien H. Dept.of Neurosurgery (1) and Patomorphology (2) Military Medical Academy and Institut of Endocrynology University Medical School, Lodz, Poland.

Angiogenesis, the process a new blood vassels formation, is essential to solid tumors growth and metastasis development. The purpose of present study was evaluation of two selective angiogenesis inhibitors (Fumagilin and its analog AGM-1470; gift from Dr Katsuichi Sudo,Takeda Chemical industries, Osaka, Japan) on growth and microvassels formation in the prolactin-secreting pituitary tumors in male Fischer F344 rats. The pituitary tumors were induced by subcutabeous implantation of the silastic tubes containing 10 mg of diethylstilboestrol for seven weeks. The tumor growth and density of microvassels (a meaesure of angiogenesis) was evaluated on the basis of the tumor weight and light-microscopic pituitary sections morphometric analysis using IBAS 2000 version 4.4 computer programm. Microangiography with 10% $BaSo_4$ was used to show new microvassels formation in normal and adenomatous pituitary gland. It has been shown, that fumagilin and its potent, synthetic analog AGM-1470 injected in the s.c.doses of 10 mg per kg body weight during the last 21 days of the experiment significantly decreased pituitary tumor weight and new vassels formation in DES-traeted animals. Our results show that both angiogenesis inhibitors have the significant suppressive effect on the development of DES-induced pituitary prolactinomas in rats. Such agents may prove to be valuable chemotherapeutic agents in the pharmacological treatment of prolactin-secreting adenomas.

Suppored by the Comittee of Scintific Research of Poland, Grant No 6P20708904

P3.74

GH BINDING PROTEINS (GHBPs) IN TURNER'S SYNDROME (TS) AND IN SLOW GROWING CHILDREN (SGC)._

E. Rossi*, B. Merola,, V. Esposito, G. D'Amore, Ph Jaquet°, S. Longobardi, A. Colao, F. Orio Jr, M. Cataldi, G. Lombardi, Dept. of Endocrinology and Clinical and Molecular Oncology, "Federico II" University, Naples, Italy. ° Service of Endocrinology, C.H.U Nord, Marseille, France.

Aim of this study was to assess the GHBPs in SGC and in TS in order to define whether binding abnormalities are involved in the pathogenesis of growth defect in these patients. The GHBPs was assayed by elution of serum + I-125-GH* (20000 cpm) pre-incubated with or without 10 mcg of unlabelled GH, on a column of Ultragel AcA 44 (50x0.5 cm). Both in TS and in SGC the GHBPs was low vs two sex- and age- matched control groups, with a mean value of 10% in TS and 12% in SGC ($p< 0.05$). Many studies have suggested that GH is able to up-regulate the high affinity GHBP. Our results are in agreement with previous reports because we demonstrate low serum GHBPs in SGC, with growth defect and impaired GH secretion during 24 hours. Taking into account the GH regulation on GHBPs, the reduced GHBPs in SGC confirms an impaired GH action in these patients. Furthermore, since the high affinity GHBP represents an estimation of the expression of tissue GH receptors, the low GHBP suggests a low concentration of tissue GH receptor, which could contribute to the short stature in TS and in SGC.

P3.75

α-MELANOCYTE-STIMULATING HORMONE (αMSH) INCREASES AFTER CRH ADMINISTRATION IN THE INFERIOR PETROSAL SINUS IPSILATERAL TO THE ACTH-SECRETING ADENOMA IN CUSHING'S DISEASE.

A.Colao*, B. Merola, F. Tripodi, A. Di Sarno, D. Ferone, S. Longobardi, C. Di Somma, E. Rossi, G. Lombardi. Dept. of Clinical & Molecular Endocrinology and Oncology, "Federico II" University of Naples, Italy 80131.

An increase of αMSH was found in the inferior petrosal sinuses (IPS's) in Cushing's disease (Colao A., et al. *Neuroendocrinology* 1993;58:227-33). In order to evaluate if CRH can stimulate the release of αMSH we assayed ACTH, β-Endorphin (βEPH) and αMSH concentrations before and 5, 10 and 15 min after CRH test in 30 patients subjected to simultaneous and bilateral IPS sampling for diagnostic purposes. ACTH and βEPH increased significantly after CRH both in periphery and in the IPS's, overall in the IPS ipsilateral to the adenoma ($p<0.001$). Conversely, no significant change of αMSH was found in all the 3 venous districts examined. Only in 7/30 patients, however, a significant increase of αMSH after CRH was found in the IPS ipsilateral to the ACTH-secreting adenoma (50-115.5% of baseline). In conclusion, the results of the present study suggest that only in a subset of patients with ACTH-secreting adenoma αMSH can be released together with ACTH and βEPH by adenomatous corticotrophs.

P3.76

ADULTS WITH CHILDHOOD-ONSET GH DEFICIENCY HAVE A REDUCTION OF LUNG VOLUMES.

B. Merola[1]*, S. Longobardi[1], A. Colao[1], M. Sofia[2], C. Di Somma[1], A. Micco[2], F. Di Rella[1], F. De Simone[2], G. Lombardi [1]. [1]Dept. of Clinical & Molecular Endocrinology and Oncology and [2]Institute of Respiratory diseases,"Federico II" University, Naples, Italy, 80131.

Aim of this study was to evaluate lung volumes, by spirometry in 10 patients diagnosed as GHD during childhood (**GHDc**), 10 patients as GHD during adult age (**GHDa**) and 10 healthy subjects (**HS**). The respiratory muscles strength was assessed under static condition measuring Maximal Inspiratory (PImax) and Espiratory (PEmax) pressures. Both PImax, PEmax and lung volumes were significantly lower in GHDc than HS [91.2±30.1 vs. 114.1±13.4 and 94.4±43.1 vs. 160±42 cmH_2O, Forced Vital Capacity (FVC): 3.4±0.8 vs. 4.4±1.2 L; Forced Expiratory Volume at 1 sec (FEV1): 2.7±0.7 vs. 3.7±0.9 L; Total Lung Capacity (TLC): 4.8±1.4 vs. 6±1.2 L]. Conversely, no change was found between GHDa and HS, except for a PEMax significantly reduced (106±38.9 vs.160±42). In conclusion, GHDc patients show a reduction of TLC, FVC and FEV1, therefore having an impairment of ventilatory function, despite of a relatively preserved residual volume. By contrast, GHDa patients show only a significant reduction of PEmax probably due to an impairment of respiratory muscles strength and mass.

P3.77

TUMOR NECROSIS FACTOR ALPHA INCREASES AFTER CORTICOTROPIN-RELEASING HORMONE STIMULATION IN CUSHING'S DISEASE: *in vivo* AND *in vitro* STUDIES.
S. Longobardi*, A. Colao, B. Merola, C. Di Somma, D. Ferone, R. Pivonello, V. Covelli[1], G. Lombardi. Dept. of Clinical & Molecular Endocrinology and Oncology, and [1]Neurology, "Federico II" University of Naples, Italy 80131.

Aim of this study was to evaluate the effect of CRH on αTNF in 5 patients with Cushing's disease subjected to inferior petrosal sinus (IPS) sampling for diagnostic purposes. All the 5 patients underwent surgery and a pituitary microadenoma was found. Pituitary tumor tissue available from 2 patients was used for *in vitro* study. ACTH and ß-EPH levels were significantly higher, whereas αTNF were sligtly decreased in the IPS ipsilateral to the ACTH-secreting adenoma than in the contralateral one and in the periphery. CRH caused a significant increase of ACTH and ß-EPH in both IPS's and in the periphery, overall in the ipsilateral IPS. Similarly, a significant increase of αTNF levels occurred in the IPS ipsilateral to the adenoma and in the periphery but not in the contralateral one. Moreover, CRH increased ACTH, ß-EPH and αTNF levels in culture medium from the two ACTH-secreting tumors (over 300%, 250% and 110% of baseline levels, respectively). These data demonstrate that αTNF is detectable in blood collected in the IPS's, and that pituitary adenomatous corticotrophs may release αTNF when stimulated by CRH.

P4.1

SUPRACHIASMATIC CONTROL OF CORTICOSTERONE AND MELATONIN RELEASE VIA ITS PEPTIDERGIC TRANSMITTERS.
A. Kalsbeek and R.M. Buijs. Netherlands Institute for Brain Research, Amsterdam, The Netherlands.

The PVN/DMH area harbours a major population of hypophysiotrophic neurons and provides axonal pathways to all autonomic preganglionic cellgroups. By infusing SCN-peptides via permanent microdialysis probes in these SCN target areas, it was possible to mimick SCN output selectively. At the same time bloodsamples were taken for measuring hormonal release. Initial results showed that infusion of VP, but not VIP, in the PVN/DMH area inhibits the release of corticosterone. The physiological significance of this inhibitory effect of VP was certified by infusing a VP-antagonist at the same brain site in intact animals. The immediate increase of plasma corticosterone (and ACTH) levels evoked by the VP-antagonist indicates that the high release of VP by SCN terminals during the daytime may be responsible for the basal corticosterone levels observed during daytime.
Comparable experiments showed that both AVP and VIP, but not oxytocin, infused at the level of the PVN/DMH area are able to enhance plasma melatonin levels in the middle of the dark period.
Currently we are investigating the chemical identity of the specific populations of hypothalamic neurons activated by the peptide transmitter(s) infused through the microdialysis probe by using c-fos immunocytochemistry.

Kalsbeek et al. Brain Res. 580(1992)62-67
Kalsbeek et al. J.Comp.Neurol. 332(1993)293-314
Kalsbeek & Buijs Prog.Brain Res. 92(1992)321-333
Kalsbeek et al. J.Pineal Res. 15(1993)46-52
Buijs et al. Am.J.Physiol. 264(1993)R1186-R1192
Buijs et al. J.Comp.Neurol. 335(1993)42-54

P4.2

THE INFLUENCE OF HREC TNF ALPHA THERAPY ON THE CIRCADIAN RHYTHM OF CORTISOL SECRETION IN PATIENTS WITH NEOPLASMS.
B.Zubelewicz, R.Brączkowski
5th Dep. of Internal Medicine Silesian University School of Medicine Bytom Poland

There is a lot of reports about connections betwe en cytokines and endocrine system. It is generally know that such cytokines like interleukin 1,2, interferon influence the cortisol secretion. But the opinions about the influence of egzogenous THF alpha on it are not univocal. The majority of works show that TNF alpha increases the level of cortisol in blood / regarding the animal model of experiment /. In our work we want to check how do therapeutic doses of hrec TNF alpha influence the adrenal cortex function. We examed patients with neoplasmatic diseases. The hrec TNF alpha was given intravenously in three 5 days cycles in dosage raises from 50ug/m^2 in 1st cycle to 150ug/m^2 in the last cycle. The blood was taken in the circadian rhythm and the level of cortisol was estimated using RIA method. The level of 17 OHCS and 17 CS was estimated using colorimetric method. Conclusions: The egzogenous hrec TNF alpha in therapeutic doses inhibits the adrenal cortex function. The level of cortisol is decreased and the circadian rhythm is saved.

P4.3

EVIDENCE OF THE EXISTENCE OF A VIP IMMUNOREACTIVE HYPOTHALAMO-RETINAL CONNECTION IN RAT.
Köves, K.*, Fogel, K., Kausz, M., [1]Görcs, T. 2nd Dept. of Anatomy, Semmelweis University Medical School, Budapest, Hungary, H-1450 and [1]1st Dept. of Anatomy, United Research Organization of Hungarian Academy of Sciences and Semmelweis University, Budapest, Hungary, H-1450

Presence of retino-hypothalamic connection is well established. However, the data concerning the existence of a hypothalamo-retinal pathway is very contradictory. In the sagittal sections of the hypothalamus of Sprague-Dawley rats we have observed vasoactive intestinal polypeptide (VIP) immunoreactive (ir) fibers, forming a dorso-medial bundle in the optic chiasm and optic nerve, coming from the suprachiasmatic nucleus (SCH) and the above lying region. The fiber bundle became more prominent two months after enucleation and VIP ir cell bodies appeared in the supraoptic and paraventricular nuclei beside the characteristic localization in the SCH. We have concluded that the ir material accumulated in those neurones which send their axons to the eye, that is in the neurones of the supraoptic and the paraventricular nuclei. Four days after the injection of a retrograde tracer, wheat germ agglutinin (WGA), into the vitreus body, labeled perikarya were also observed in the same nuclei. These observations support the hypothesis of a hypothalamo-retinal projection. Our data also suggest that the hypothalamo-retinal projection in rats contains neuropeptide VIP. This retinal input may play a role in modifying the circadian endocrine rhythms (These studies were supported by OTKA T5443 to K.K. and by OTKA 2615 to B.H.)

P4.4

VARIATIONS IN PLASMA RENIN ACTIVITY (PRA) AND BLOOD PRESSURE DURING SLEEP IN RATS. L. Beranek (1)*, F. Obál Jr. (1), G. Brandenberger (2), Dept. Physiology, A. Szent-Györgyi Medical University, Szeged, Hungary 6720 (1), Laboratoire de Physiologie and Psychologie Environnementales (CNR/INRS), Strasbourg, France, 67087

Increasing PRA coincides with non-rapid eye movement sleep (NREMS) whereas REMS is associated with declining PRA in human subjects (Brandenberger et al., 1988). The aim of our experiments was to determine whether PRA also varies with the sleep states in the rat. The rats were chronically implanted with EEG electrodes and a cardiac catheter. Blood samples were withdrawn in four consecutive NREMS and REMS episodes (approx. at 6 min intervals); occasionally samples were obtained during wakefulness. Sampling started with NREMS in one group (n=14) and with REMS in an other group (n=13) of rats. PRA was determined by RIA of angiotensin I generated after incubation of the plasma. PRA was significantly higher during NREMS than during REMS in both groups of rats. PRA during wakefulness was close to that observed during NREMS. Blood pressure was recorded in rats implanted with a chronic catheter in the aorta. Blood pressure increased significantly during REMS. In conclusion, PRA varies with the sleep states in the rat. The REMS associated low PRA is accompanied by high blood pressure. The mechanisms of the changes in REMS and blood pressure during REMS remain to be determined.

P4.5

MONOAMINE OXIDASE AND ANTIOXIDATIVE ENZYMES IN THE BRAIN OF GROUND SQUIRREL (Citellus citellus) IN RELATION TO THE ANNUAL CYCLE. V.Janić-Šibalić, D.Blagojević*, B.Buzadžić, B.Korać, Z.S.Saičić, M.B.Spasić, V.M.Petrović. Dept. of Physiology, Institute for Biological Research, 29. November 142, 11060 Belgrade, SR Yugoslavia.

The hibernator-ground squirrel was analyzed in different period of the year and different physiological states: prior to the hibernation, after arousal and in normothermic state, during the summer and winter. In the period prior to the hibernation, activities of monoamine oxidase (MAO), catalase (CAT), glutathione-S-transferase (GST) and glutathione reductase (GR) were about at the same level, but superoxide dismutase (SOD) and glutathione peroxidase (GSH-Px) were lower as compared with aroused ones. In experiments undertaken in summer as well as a few data obtained in the winter significantly lower MAO activity than in previous groups was found; the activities of CAT, GSH-Px and GST were also lower, but SOD was at the same level as in corresponding controls. Results suggest the existence of a good correlation between catecholamines degradation and the activity of the antioxidative enzymes studied.

P4.6

THE CIRCADIAN RHYTHM OF MELATONIN SECRETION IN NEOPLASMATIC PATIENTS AFTER HREC TNF ALPHA THERAPY.

R.Braczkowski, B.Zubelewicz, W.Romanowski
5th Dep. of Internal Medicine Silesian University School of Medicine Bytom Poland

There are some reports about connections between the pineal gland and neoplasms. There are a lot of data showing that disturbances in secretion of the main pineal hormone melatonin are connected with the changes in cytokines production. To have a possibility of using hrec TNF alpha in the immunotherapy of cancer, we want to check its influence on the melatonin secretion in those patients. We examed 8 patients. The blood was taken at 8a.m. 2p.m. 8p.m. 2a.m. 4a.m. and 8a.m. next day. The blood was centrifugated and melatonin level was estimated using RIA method. Results were checked statistically using simple t test. The results we obtain to discussion.

P4.7

CHANGES IN PEPTIDYL GLYCINE α-AMIDATING (PAM) ACTIVITY IN THE RAT ANTERIOR PITUITARY (AP) AFTER BILATERAL ADRENALECTOMY (ADX) AND ADRENAL ENUCLEATION (ENUC). M.J. Perone, F.E. Estivariz, A. Chisari, M. Carino, A. Giobambatista, E. Spinedi. IMBICE, 1900 La Plata, Argentina.

To elucidate whether exsists a differential processing in AP POMC peptides due to changes in post-translational PAM activity after adrenal manipulations, AP PAM activity and α-MSH were measured in the adult female rat at different days (2, 7, 14 and 21) after Sham, Enuc and Adx surgeries. The results were expressed in ng α-MSH/AP and for PAM activity in pmol/mg protein/h (mean±SEM). At 2 days, AP α-MSH decreased ($p<0.05$) in Enuc (13±2.3) and Adx (56.6±26) vs. Sham (125±17); at 7 days, Enuc (171±30) restored and Adx (260±57) increased ($p<0.05$) AP α-MSH vs. Sham (134±32); at 14 days, Enuc (200±54) and Adx (208±38) were significantly ($p<0.05$) higher vs. Sham (70±19); finally, at 21 days Enuc (230±40) remained higher, while Adx (90±12) was similar to Sham (91±19). PAM activities were similar at day 2: Sham (1.2±0.4), Enuc (0.7±0.2) and Adx (1.2±0.3); at 7 days, Sham (5.1±0.4), Enuc (6.7±0.5) and Adx (6.5±0.5) although were similar, they increased ($P<0.05$) vs. day-2 values; then remained unchanged, Sham (5.1±0.4), Enuc (6.1±0.6) and Adx (6.5±0.6) at 14 days; while Enuc (7.9±0.6) was similar to Sham (8.2±0.6) at 21 days, Adx (6.4±0.03) was significantly ($p<0.05$) lower than Sham (8.3±0.6). The changes observed in AP α-MSH after Enuc and Adx seem to be related to those found in PAM activity. Differences in proteolytic and PAM activities between Enuc and Adx might be due to particular steroid production during adrenal regeneration.

P4.8

GLUCOCORTICOIDS INCREASE NEUROTENSIN CONTENT AND mRNA IN HYPOTHALAMIC NEURONS IN CULTURE : MODULATION BY FORSKOLIN.
V. Scarcériaux, D. Pélaprat, P. Forgez, A. M. Lhiaubet, W. Rostène*. INSERM U339, 184 rue du Fbg St Antoine, 75571 PARIS Cedex 12, France.

Neurotensin (NT) is a tridecapeptide present in high concentrations in the hypothalamus. Sequences homologous to cAMP- and glucocorticoid-responsive elements have been localized on the NT gene, suggesting that it could be regulated by glucocorticoids and adenylate cyclase activators. However, little is known on the influence of these factors on NT levels in the brain. In order to investigate such regulations, primary cultures of rat fetal hypothalamic neurons were developed. The amount of NT was detected by radioimmunoassay, the number of NTergic cells was counted after immunocytochemistry, and NT mRNA was studied by Northern blot. After ten days in culture, a 48-hour treatment with 1 μM Dex induced a 90% increase of intracellular NT content associated to a doubling of NTergic cell number. This increase was inhibited by the glucocorticoid antagonist RU38486 and mimicked by the glucocorticoid agonist RU 48362, suggesting that the Dex effect was mediated by glucocorticoid receptors. Under the same conditions, no effect of forskolin (Fsk) was noted. However, Fsk potentiated the action of Dex, since a 300% increase in both NT content and number of NTergic cells was observed when both factors were added simultaneausly. Moreover, under those conditions, an increase in NT mRNA levels was also observed by Northern blot, which might reflect a regulation at the transcriptional level. These results demonstrate that NT levels in hypothalamic neurons can be regulated by glucocorticoids, and this effect can be modulated by Fsk.

P4.9

PHORBOL ESTER-INDUCED EXPRESSION OF C-FOS AND NEUROPEPTIDE Y GENES IN SH-SY5Y NEUROBLASTOMA CELLS. P. Magni*, R. Maggi, F. Pimpinelli, M. Motta. Res. Ctr. of Oncological Endocrinology, Dept. of Endocrinology, University of Milano, Milano, Italy, 20133

Neuropeptide Y (NPY) is a widely distributed regulator of mammalian nervous system functions. Its biosynthesis and secretion appear to be regulated by different agents, such as dopamine, insulin and the IGFs; however, little information is available on the molecular mechanisms modulating the expression of the NPY gene, particularly in humans. Several lines of evidence indicate that protein kinase C (PKC)-dependent mechanisms participate in the modulation of NPY gene expression in rats and mice. Furthermore, the regulatory region of the human NPY gene contains a putative consensus sequence for the AP1 transcription complex. The present experiments have been performed in order to elucidate: 1) the expression of the NPY gene in the human neuroblastoma cell line SH-SY5Y in basal conditions and following activation of PKC; 2) the possible role of the activation of immediate early genes (e.g. c-fos) in the stimulation of the expression of NPY gene. C-fos and NPY mRNA levels were evaluated by Northern blot analysis either in the absence or in the presence of 20 nM TPA (12-O-tetradecanoyl-phorbol 13-acetate) in the culture medium. In control experiments, phorbol 12,13-didecanoate (Pdd), an inactive phorbol ester, was used. The results show that SH-SY5Y cells express detectable basal levels of NPY mRNA. TPA treatment induces both c-fos and NPY gene expression. C-fos mRNA levels are transiently increased 30-60 min after treatment, while NPY mRNA levels display a progressive but slower increase; this is already detectable at 1 h, is higher at 3 h, and peaks after 6 h of exposure to TPA. Pdd fails to produce any of these effects. These findings indicate that TPA induces, via a PKC-dependent mechanism, a temporally coordinated expression of c-fos, an early response gene, and of NPY, a slow responding gene, in SH-SY5Y human neuroblastoma cells. The role of early gene expression (c-fos, c-jun and others) and of their products as possible mediators of the TPA induction of the expression of the human NPY gene needs to be further investigated. (Supported by AIRC and by CNR -BTBS #93.01103.PF70, FATMA #93.00700.PF41, Aging #93.00438.PF40, ACRO #93.02197.PF39-, and by MURST)

P4.10

STEROID METABOLITES IN CULTURED OLIGODENDROCYTES AND THEIR EFFECTS ON MYELIN BASIC PROTEIN.

R.C. Melcangi*, A. Poletti, L. Martini.
Department of Endocrinology, University of Milano, Italy

In the brain, testosterone, progesterone and corticosterone are converted, by the action of the enzyme 5α-reductase, into 5α-reduced metabolites. Up to now it is not clear if a single or multiple enzymes are involved in the process of 5α-reduction of different substrates. Recent data obtained in the authors' laboratory have shown that glial cells possess a considerable 5α-reductase activity. In line with these observations, the present work indicates that, purified cultures of oligodendrocytes are able to actively convert testosterone into dihydrotestosterone (DHT), and progesterone into dihydroprogesterone (DHP). Since, oligodendrocytes are actively involved in the production of myelin (a structure that is very rich in 5α-reductase activity), we have now analyzed if the exposure of oligodendrocytes in culture to corticoids, progestagens or androgens might alter the production of a characteristic marker of myelin, the myelin basic protein (MBP). To this purpose the variation of MBP contents in oligodendrocyte cultures using Western and immonodot blot analysis was determined. The results so far obtained have shown that corticosterone, dihydrocorticosterone and deoxycorticosterone are able to increase MBP contents in the oligodendrocytes. More recent data have shown that also progesterone and its 5α-reduced metabolites may alter the MBP contents in the oligodendrocytes, although in a way different from the corticoids. (Grants: BTBS 93.01103 PF70; FATMA 93.00700 PF41; AGING 93.00438 PF40)

P4.11

PYROGLUTAMYL PEPTIDASE II ACTIVITY IS REGULATED BY MULTIPLE SECOND MESSENGERS IN ADENOHYPOPHYSIS. M. A. Vargas, P. Joseph-Bravo, J.-L. Charli*. Inst. Biotecnología, Universidad Nacional Autonoma de Mexico, Cuernavaca, Mor., Mexico, 62271.

Pyroglutamyl peptidase II (PPII, EC 3.4.19.6), an ectoenzyme present in neural cells and lactotrophs, specifically degrades thyrotropin releasing hormone (TRH) in vitro. We have recently observed that in primary cultures of adenohypophysis the enzyme activity is regulated by TRH and somatostatin. We have shown that TRH-induced down regulation may be mediated through TRH receptor induction of a calcium-independent protein kinase C. Because somatostatin receptor couples negatively to adenyl cyclase in lactotrophs, somatostatin induction of PPII activity may be due to inhibition of protein kinase A (PKA). In order to determine whether PPII activity is regulated by additional second messengers and kinases, we have incubated adenohypophyseal cells, grown in primary culture for 5 days, in the presence of agents enhancing PKA activity or intracellular calcium levels. PPII activity was determined with a radiometric assay 16 hrs after initiation of drug treatment; at this time point, TRH effect is maximal. Incubation of cells with 10^{-4} M 8-bromo-cAMP had a small non significant inhibitory effect. 10^{-4} M IBMX, an inhibitor of phosphodiesterases, alone or in combination with 8-bromo-cAMP inhibited PPII activity by 38%. Activation of PKA with forskolin decreased PPII activity in a dose-dependent fashion. Maximum effect (40 %) was attained at $4x10^{-6}$ M; ED50 was 10^{-7} M . Incubation with 10^{-6} M 1,9-dideoxyforskolin, an inactive analogue, had no effect. On the other hand, addition of BAY K 8644, a L type Ca^{++} channel agonist, decreased activity in a dose-related fashion. A 40 % effect was obtained at $3x10^{-6}$ M. 10^{-6} M A23187 also induced PPII inhibition (55%). Our data demonstrate that PPII activity is down regulated by activation of PKA or enhancement of intracellular calcium levels. This suggests that PPII activity may be controlled by multiple intracellular effectors. (supported in part by grants # 00776-N9110 from CONACYT and # IN204791 from DGAPA-UNAM).

P4.12

TRH AND ITS DEGRADING ENZYME, PYROGLUTAMATE PEPTIDASE II REGULATION DURING DEVELOPMENT OF KINDLING. *P. de Gortari[*+], A. Fernández-Guardiola[#], A. Martínez[#], M. Cisneros[*], and P. Joseph-Bravo[*]. *Inst. Biotecnología, UNAM, AP 510-3, Cuernavaca Mor., Mexico 62271;#Inst. Mexicano Psiquiatría,+Dept. Nutrición, U. Iberoamericana.

Pyroglutamate aminopeptidase II (PPII, E.C. 3.4.19.6) is an ectoenzyme present in brain and adenohypophysis, responsible for degradation of released TRH. PPII is modulated under different endocrine conditions where TRH regulates prolactin or thyrotropin secretion (estrous cycle or hyperthyroidism) but only at the adenohypophyseal level. In cultured adenohypophyseal cells TRH downregulates PPII activity. To study whether brain PPII could be regulated when TRHergic neurons are stimulated, we measured TRH and PPII activity during the development of kindling since levels of this peptide increase in amygdala, hyppocampus and cortex. Male Wistar rats were placed with indwelling bipolar electrodes in left temporal lobe amygdala and frontal cortex. After 7 days recovery, threshold stimulation for amygdaline after discharge was established (average 300 uAmp) and kindling (1 sec, 60Hz, 1msec pulses) induced by daily electrical stimulation. Animals were sacrificed in behavioural kindling stages II, IV and V. Regions under study (amygdala, hyppocampus, n. accumbens, frontal cortex, medula oblongata and hypothalamus) were dissected and assayed for TRH immunoreactivity and for PPII activity. TRH levels increased from stage II to V in amygdala, hyppocampus and frontal cortex. In n.accumbens a significant decrease was observed at stage II, but levels increased progressively through stage V. In contrast, PPII activity was at least 2 fold higher than sham animals at stage II in all these regions, decreasing in stage IV and attaining lower levels than sham animals in stage V (30%), as reported for TRH receptors. These results suggest that PPII activity in the central nervous system can be regulated in conditions known to affect TRHergic neurons.
Financed by DGAPA-UNAM.

P4.13

EXPRESSION OF TRH AND TRH PRECURSOR IN THE ANTERIOR PITUITARY: EVIDENCE FOR ITS INVOLVEMENT IN LACTOTROPH AND THYROTROPH FUNCTIONS.

G. Croissandeau, M. Le Dafniet, D. Grouselle[a], P. Pagesy, A.M. Brandi, F. Peillon, J.Y. Li*. Unité INSERM 223, CHU Pitié-Salpêtrière, 75013 Paris and [a]Groupe de Biologie Cellulaire et Moléculaire, Collège de France, 75005 Paris, France.

A growing body of evidence has been gathered by our group to demonstrate that the anterior pituitary is the unforeseen site of TRH synthesis. Human normal and adenomatous anterior pituitaries transcribe the TRH gene, synthesize the TRH precursor. Anterior pituitary TRH tissue contents are much lower than the amounts of TRH secreted in vitro. TRH release by anterior pituitary cells is modulated by exogenous dopamine and SRIH. Anterior pituitary cells synthesizing TRH are distinct from anterior pituitary hormone producing cells, implying that TRH might be involved in paracrine regulatory mechanisms. For instance, TRH expression in prolactinomas might take part in the hypersecretion and proliferation of adenomatous lactotrophs since we have shown that TRH action is not counterbalanced by a local production of dopamine. In the rat anterior pituitary, we have focused our attention on the modulation of TRH expression in antithyroid-induced hypothyroidism. Hypothyroidism after 21 or 48 days of propylthiouracyl treatment significantly increases TRH and TRH precursor contents in the rat anterior pituitary as it does in the hypothalamus. The effect of hypothyroidism is partially reversed by administration of T4 for the last week of antithyroid treatment. These results showing a relation between the thyroid status and the levels of anterior pituitary TRH expression also favor a paracrine role of TRH in this tissue.

Our results fit in the hypothesis that anterior pituitary functions are not only under the well established hypothalamic central control but are also locally regulated by endogenously synthesized neuropeptides.

P4.14

VASOACTIVE INTESTINAL PEPTIDE IS DECREASED IN THE ANTERIOR PITUITARY GLAND OF hGHRH TRANSGENIC MICE.

J.F. Hyde*, D.G. Morrison, J.P. Moore, Jr. Department of Anatomy and Neurobiology, University of Kentucky College of Medicine, Lexington, Kentucky, U.S.A., 40536.

Galanin gene expression is dramatically increased in the anterior pituitary of hGHRH transgenic mice. The increased galanin mRNA and peptide levels are correlated to the development of pituitary hyperplasia/adenomas. To determine if other pituitary peptide hormones are similarly affected, vasoactive intestinal peptide (VIP) concentrations in the hypothalamo-pituitary axis were examined. Six-month old male hGHRH transgenic mice (n=10) were identified by PCR. Non-transgenic siblings (n=12) were used as controls. All mice were derived from a single founder transgenic mouse provided by Dr. L. Frohman. VIP concentrations in the anterior pituitary, neurointermediate lobe (NIL) and hypothalamus were quantified by RIA using a specific VIP antiserum provided by Dr. A. Carrillo. Both the wet weight (5.6±0.4 mg vs. 1.8±0.1 mg) and total protein content (792.7±105.6 μg vs. 210.0±11.9 μg) of the anterior pituitary were significantly ($p<0.001$) greater in hGHRH transgenic mice as compared to non-transgenics. To normalize this difference, pituitary concentrations of VIP were expressed per mg protein. Immunoreactive VIP concentrations in the anterior pituitary of transgenic mice (0.55±0.08 ng/mg protein) were significantly ($p<0.001$) *lower* than the VIP concentrations in non-transgenic siblings (1.30±0.09 ng/mg protein). VIP concentrations in the NIL were also significantly ($p<0.002$) lower in hGHRH mice. In contrast, immunoreactive VIP concentrations in the hypothalamus were similar in transgenic and non-transgenic mice. We hypothesize that VIP levels are decreased in the anterior pituitary as a result of a hyperplasia of cells that do not synthesize VIP. Alternatively, the lower amount of VIP in the anterior pituitary (and NIL) may be the result of increased peptide secretion. (Supported by USPHS DK-45981)

P4.15

TEMPORAL AND CELLULAR CHARACTERIZATION OF ESTROGEN'S ELEVATION OF PREPROENKEPHALIN AND PREPROTACHYKININ mRNA IN THE VENTROMEDIAL NUCLEUS.

C.A. Priest, C. Eckersell, K. Vink, *P.E Micevych. Dept. of Anatomy and Cell Biology, UCLA School of Medicine, Los Angeles, U.S.A., 90024

The ventromedial nucleus of the hypothalamus (VMH) is the primary locus of control estrogen-induced lordosis behavior in female rats.This behavior involves the activity of endogenous opioid and tachykinin circuits.Temporal effects of 50 μg estradiol benzoate on preproenkephalin-A (PPE-A) and β-preprotachykinin (β-PPT) mRNA levels in the VMH were examined using in situ hybridization histochemistry.Estrogen treatment caused a biphasic increase of PPE-A mRNA cells (but not levels) and levels of β-PPT mRNA (but not the number of cells):the number of PPE-A mRNA cells was increased at 1hr,β-PPT mRNA levels were increased at 2hrs both the number of PPE-A mRNA cells and levels of β-PPT mRNA were elevated at 48hrs.These results indicate that estrogen produces differential activation of gene expression in the VMH.The rapid effects may be due to estrogen's direct activation of gene expression but the 48hr effects suggest a more complex mechanism through which estrogen induces the expression of PPE-A and β-PPT mRNA.

P4.16

SEX-RELATED ALTERATIONS IN HYPOTHALAMIC GHRH mRNA- BUT NOT SRIH mRNA-CONTAINING CELLS IN GENETICALLY OBESE ZUCKER RATS.

C. Videau, J. Epelbaum*, J.M. Dubuis, G. Van Vliet, G.S. Tannenbaum. U.159 INSERM, Paris, France 75014, Université de Montréal and McGill University, Montreal, Quebec, Canada H3H 1P3.

The possibility that the GH suppression associated with obesity is due to alterations in hypothalamic GHRH and/or SRIH has been considered, but the data are not consistent. In the present study, we used *in situ* hybridization to localize and quantify the level of expression of GHRH mRNA- and SRIH mRNA-containing neurons in the hypothalamus of male and female lean and obese Zucker rats (12 weeks of age; n=6 per group). In lean littermates, the number of GHRH mRNA-containing cells in the arcuate nucleus and SRIH mRNA-containing neurons in the periventricular nucleus was 2- to 3-fold higher in males compared to females. The obese phenotype in the male was associated with a significant reduction in arcuate GHRH mRNA expression, both in terms of number of cells (-71%) and grains/cell (-45%). In contrast, the number of GHRH mRNA-containing cells in obese females was significantly augmented (+179%) compared to their lean littermates. The small population of GHRH mRNA-containing neurons of the VMN was not modified in male obese rats while it was considerably increased in obese females. SRIH mRNA-containing neurons in periventricular and arcuate nuclei of obese rats of either sex were unchanged when compared to their lean counterparts. These results demonstrate that: 1) the obese male Zucker rat exhibits a marked diminution in GHRH mRNA expression while a reverse pattern is observed in the female; 2) hypothalamic SRIH mRNA-containing neurons are not significantly altered in obese rats of both sexes. Our findings suggest that the impaired GH secretion of the obese Zucker rat is due, at least in part, to alterations in hypothalamic GHRH gene expression and that SRIH does not play a major role.

P4.17

CLONING AND EXPRESSION OF THE MELANIN CONCENTRATING HORMONE GENE IN THE TROUT BRAIN. A. Levy*, B.I. Baker†, L. Hall** and S.L. Lightman* Department of Medicine, Bristol Royal Infirmary, Bristol BS2 8HW. †School of Biology and Biochemistry, Bath University, Bath BA2 7AY. **Department of Biochemistry, Bristol University, Bristol BS2

Melanin-concentrating hormone (MCH) is a hypothalamic neuropeptide present in all vertebrates. In mammals it is a neuromodulator-neurotransmitter responsive to stress and osmotic challenge. In fish, uniquely, it is also a neurohypophyseal hormone that plays a striking role in the regulation of skin colour. In order to follow the expression of MCH under different physiological conditions, we have cloned and sequenced both MCH genes in the tetraploid salmonid *Oncorhynchus mykiss* (the rainbow trout), and have used specific nucleotide probes and antibodies to map MCH neurons in the brain.
Both nucleotide and aminoacid sequences of *O. mykiss* MCH I and II show high homology with the preprohormones of other oncorhynchids, such as the Chum and Chinook salmon. The MCH II gene is expressed in two groups of neurones:- A previously identified group of magnocellular neurones located in the ventral hypothalamus (nucleus lateralis tuberis, NLT) has axons that project mainly to the posterior lobe of the pituitary gland, with fewer axons radiating along the optic tracts and up into the brain. Transcription, translation and release of MCH from these neurons is markedly enhanced by exposure to a pale-coloured environment, and is in part responsible for adaptive skin colour-change used for camouflage (reviewed in[1]). Synthesis and release of MCH in the NLT are also influenced by stress, such as handling[2]. We have now identified a second group of smaller MCH neurones, dorsal and caudal to the NLT, whose axons project, apparently exclusively, into the brain. At the time of writing, nothing is known about the regulation of MCH in these cells. As more MCH-immunoreactive perikarya are visible after handling, however, we anticipate that they will be stress responsive but not necessarily responsive to background colour.

1. Baker, B.I. *Ann NY Acad Sci* **680**, 279-289 (1993).
2. Baker, B.I. *Int Rev Cytol* **126**, 1-47 (1991).

P4.18

DIFFERENT TIME COURSE ACTIVATION OF HYPOTHALAMUS AND BRAIN STEM MAO ACTIVITY AND BLOOD ACTH CONCENTRATION FOLLOWING ADRENALECTOMY

G. Cvijić, Ž. Matijašević and V. Davidović. Institute of Physiology and Biochemistry, Faculty of Biology, Belgrade, Yugoslavia, Akademski Trg 16, Fax: 638-500.

Monoamine oxidase (MAO) activity in the hypothalamus and brain stem, as well as blood ACTH concentration in the adrenalectomized and sham operated rats were determined. Short time after adrenalectomy (5-15 minutes) MAO activity both in the hypothalamus and the brain stem was decreased in respect to sham-operated animals. However, changes in the enzyme activity, arising long time after adrenalectomy (11 days) in these two brain regions, was different. In the hypothalamus MAO activity remained at the level of controls whereas in the brain stem it was much higher. Immediately after adrenalectomy (5 minutes) blood ACTH concentration was decreased and 11 days later elevated, as compared to sham operated rats. On the basis of our results it may be concluded that changes in brain MAO activity depend on adrenalectomy postoperative time, the site of its action and the lack of glucocorticoids rather than changed ACTH secretion.

P4.19

EFFECT OF NALOXONE ADMINISTRATION ON THE SECRETION OF CRH, AVP AND ACTH IN THE HORSE. S.L. Alexander*, C.H.G. Irvine. Endolab, Christchurch Public Hospital, Christchurch, New Zealand.

To study the role of endogenous opioids in regulating ACTH secretion under resting conditions, we used our nonsurgical method to collect pituitary venous (PV) blood from 9 horses every 0.5-1 min for 30 min before and 80 min after giving the opioid receptor blocker, naloxone (NAL) at several dose rates (0.5-2 mg/kg, N=5, or 0.1-0.2 mg/kg, N=4).

All NAL doses increased ACTH secretion (P=0.004, two-way ANOVA of mean secretion rates over 30-min periods). Peak ACTH secretion was accompanied by a rise (P<0.05) in CRH only in horses given NAL at 0.5-2 mg/kg. Although AVP secretion clearly increased after NAL in 7 of 9 horses, the timing and size of responses varied so that no significant change could be shown. In all horses, the magnitude of peak ACTH increases exceeded (P<0.05) those in CRH, leading to an elevation (P=0.036) in the ratio, PV ACTH:CRH, 30-80 min after NAL. The ratio, PV ACTH:AVP, was raised (P=0.038) 0-60 min after NAL at 0.5-2 mg/kg. Multiple linear regression showed that CRH and AVP explained some of the variance in ACTH (P=0.0002), with an overall adjusted r^2 value of 0.40. However, CRH alone accounted for most of this correlation, since addition of AVP data did not improve the fit to the model (r^2,CRH only = 0.37, F=1.07).

We conclude that blockade of opioid action in unperturbed horses increases ACTH primarily by raising CRH secretion. However, because CRH, AVP and ACTH secretion rates were only modestly correlated and the ACTH:CRH and ACTH:AVP ratios increased, we suggest that opioids may also block secretion of a third ACTH secretagogue or stimulate production of an ACTH inhibitor.

P4.20

MULTIPLE HORMONAL RESPONSE TO EXERCISE IN RELATION TO PHYSICAL TRAINING: PROLACTINE ADAPTIONS TO ENDURANCE EXERCISE.

Gómez-Balaguer M, Tornero C, Saurina J, Piñón F. Department of Endocrinology and Internal Medicine Dr.Peset Hospital. Valencia. Spain

In an attempt to determine the hormonal and metabolic response during maximun exercise we studied 31 healthy puberals boys (14±2 years) with the Bruce protocol and the Ruffier test. The endocrinological and metabolic parameters was measured at different moments during de test and training (FSH, LH, testosterone, T3, T4, TSH, GH, PRL, ACTH, cortisol, cathecholamines, IRI, peptid-C, FFA, ADH, ARP-Aldosterone). Individuals in training exerted more effort and achieved improved aerobiosis capacity with lower lactic acidosis, higher cortisol, ACTH GH, PRL and LH, lower rise in blood pressure, higher insulin levels and lower peptide-C/insulin ratio. Increased ARP-Aldosterone and cathecholamines found increased during excercise in both groups. Plasma testosterone levels, ADH, T3, T4, FSH and TSH did not appear with significant diferences. Lower levels of FFA is present in training exerted more effort. The Bruce and Ruttier test did not appear very useful for determination of the aerobiosis threshold. Only PRL plasmatic level apper with a significant correlation with the aerobiosis threshold.

P4.21

DO OPIOIDS PLAY A MAJOR ROLE IN SEASONAL BREEDING IN THE MARE? C.H.G. Irvine*, J.E. Turner, S L. Alexander. Lincoln University, New Zealand.

We investigated the role of endogenous opioid peptides (EOP) in regulating the seasonal cycle of FSH and LH secretion in mares by measuring LH and FSH responses to graded doses of naloxone (NAL; 0.02-1 mg/kg) given in random order to each of 6 mares in deep anestrus and again, when the mares were cyclic, in the luteal (LP) and follicular (FP) phases. At each state, GnRH dose-FSH or LH response curves were also determined.

In anestrus and LP, but not FP, NAL significantly (ANOVA) increased plasma FSH and LH concentrations. In anestrus, responses to 0.1 mg/kg NAL were greater ($P<0.05$) than those to bigger or smaller doses, whereas in LP, responses to all NAL doses were similar. Neither absolute nor fractional responses to 0.04 mg/kg NAL differed between anestrus and LP. However, responses to 0.1 mg/kg NAL were greater ($P<0.02$) in anestrus than LP. Pituitary responsiveness to GnRH was also greater in anestrus. As estimated from GnRH dose-response curves, the GnRH doses required to replicate anestrous and LP gonadotropin responses (respectively) to 0.04 mg/kg NAL were 1.9 and 6.1 µg, and to 0.1 mg/kg NAL were 11.9 and 5.8 µg.

We conclude that EOP inhibit the mare's reproductive axis in both anestrus and LP, but that larger NAL doses are needed to counteract completely the effect of EOP in anestrus. This indicates that opioid tone is enhanced during anestrus and implies therefore that EOP play a major role in controlling seasonal breeding in the mare. Preliminary results suggest that larger NAL doses induce decreasing gonadotropin responses in anestrous mares because they stimulate corticotropin-releasing hormone release which then inhibits GnRH secretion.

P4.22

CENTRAL EFFECTS OF MORPHINE, SEROTONIN AND ACETYLCHOLINE UPON MILK EJECTION IN RATS. Morales, M.T.* Shapiro, E. and Mena, F. Center of Neurobiology, National University of México, México, D.F. México 04510.

We showed previously that central adrenergic and peptidergic mechanisms may regulate milk ejection in rats through the direct innervation, i.e., sympathetic, of the mammary glands. In the present study we analyzed whether serotonin (5-HT), acetylcholine (Ach) and morphine may influence milk ejection through a similar mechanism. <u>Methods:</u> Wistar lactating rats were chronically implanted with stainless steel cannulae into each lateral ventricle (ICV) or with a polyethylene catheter intrathecally (IT, T10-T11 level). Intramammary pressure (IMP) responses to intravenous oxytocin (OT) were isometrically recorded from an abdominal gland in urethane anesthetized rats. In other rats, to determine the rate of milk ejection the litter was first isolated from their mother for 6h. Following this, the mothers were given two consecutive 15 min suckling periods. OT was injected to the mothers before the second period of suckling. Milk yield was expressed as percentage of the total yield, in both periods combined. <u>Results and discussion:</u> In anesthetized rats, amplitude of IMP responses to OT doses was increased following ICV or IT morphine (1-100ng) or Ach (0.25-1μg), while 5-HT (0.25-5μg) had no effect. In conscious rats, milk ejection was inhibited in variable degree following the ICV or IT administration of 10μg of each of the drugs. These results suggest that each of these substances may participate in a central inhibitory regulation of milk ejection. On the other hand, the fact that morphine and Ach provoked opposite effects in conscious than in anesthetized animals, suggests that functional changes may occur in the neural elements of the spinal cord during anesthesia which may determine a different action of the drugs.

P4.23

GLUCOSE UTILIZATION AND EXPRESSION OF FOS IN THE MAGNOCELLULAR NEUROENDOCRINE SYSTEM ARE ATTENUATED DURING OSMOTIC STIMULATION IN LACTATING RATS. J.Y.Summy-Long*, S.Gestl, M.L.Terrell[1], G.Wolz[2], J.Weisz[2], M.Kadekaro[1]. Dept. Pharmacol. or Dept. OBGYN[2], M.S. Hershey Med. Ctr., Hershey, PA 17033 and Div. Neurosurgery[1], UTMB, Galveston, TX, 77555, USA.

During lactation, responsiveness of the hypothalamo-neurohypophysial system (HNS) to hypertonic saline (HS) is reduced, such that sensitivity decreases without change in osmotic threshold for oxytocin and vasopressin release (Koehler et al., Am.J.Physiol.264:R555,1993). To examine if this change results from an attenuated activation of magnocellular neurons during lactation, we quantified glucose utilization (GU) in the HNS and, in alternating tissue sections, the number of cells expressing immunoreactive FOS protein in the supraoptic nucleus (SON). Conscious virgin (V) or lactating (L; 8-13D) rats were given [^{14}C]deoxyglucose iv 30 min after normal saline(NS) or HS(sc; 0.85M or 1.5M NaCl; 15 ml/kg) and 45 min before death. Data were analyzed by 2-way AOV and Newman Keuls- or Student- t tests (changes significant at $p<0.05$). Osmotic stimulation increased the number of FOS positive cells in the SON of V (NS<0.85M & 1.5M HS;n=6,7) and L (NS<0.85M HS<1.5M HS;n=7) rats. Lactating rats given NS had more Fos positive cells (average #/section ± SEM) in the SON (V 0.8±0.1<L 1.3±0.2) whereas after 0.85M HS, fewer were present (16.8±3.5) compared with V (31.4±4.4) rats. GU (uM/100g/min; x±SEM;n=6-13) in L rats was attenuated in the SON after 1.5M HS (V 101±7>L 59±6) and in the neural lobe following 0.85M HS (V 55±3>L 36±3) and 1.5M HS (V 100±7>L 51±4). Utilization of ketone bodies or fatty acids is unlikely as plasma levels in another group of L rats were negligible or lower than in V, respectively. Thus, during lactation, fewer cells in the SON respond to osmotic stimulation. **(Funding: 5RO1 HD25498,JS-L and 2RO1 NS23055 MK).**

P4.24

SEX DEPENDENCE OF THE HYPOTHALAMIC PARAVENTRICULO-VAGAL PATHWAY OF REGULATION OF ENDOCRINE PANCREAS AND RELATED METABOLISM. I.G.Akmayev, O.V. Fidelina, O.S.Gorbatyuk, A.G.Reznikov*, V.G.Sergeyev, L.V.Tarasenko*. Institute of Experimental Endocrinology, Moscow, Russia and *Institute of Endocrinology and Metabolism, Kiev, Ukraine.

Long years of research have enabled us to prove the possibility of hypothalamic regulation of endocrine pancreas and related metabolism over the nerve pathway, originating in the neurons of the hypothalamic paraventricular nucleus (HPV) and synapsing on the neurons of the medullary dorsal vagal complex (DVC). It was also shown that neurons of this paraventriculo-vagal system were sex-dependent. The results of the present studies indicate that aromatase activity of the HPV and DVC neurons when determined in foetuses of diabetic rats increases, with its levels varying in males and females. The increase in aromatase activities of foetal HPV and DVC correlates with the gravity of maternal diabetes. Taking in consideration that gestational diabetes induce increase in foetal insulin levels it can be suggested that foetal insulin is capable of affecting the aromatase activity in the HPV and DVC neurons during the critical period of the brain sex differentiation.

P4.25

BOMBESIN-LIKE IMMUNOREACTIVITY AND BINDING SITES IN THE GOLDFISH HYPOTHALAMIC FEEDING AREA AND PITUITARY.

B.A. Himick[†*], S.R. Vigna[✠], R.E. Peter[†]. [†]Dept. Zoology, University of Alberta, Edmonton, Alberta, Canada, T6G 2E9 and [✠]Dept. Cell Biology, Duke University Medical Center, Durham, North Carolina, USA, 27710.

Recently we reported that bombesin (BBS) suppressed feeding in goldfish when administered into the third brain ventricle, and that associated with this decreased food intake were concomitant elevations in serum growth hormone (Physiol. Behav. 55: 65, 1994). To continue investigating the role(s) of BBS peptides in the fish CNS, we have examined the presence of BBS-like immunoreactivity (IR) and specific BBS binding sites in the goldfish hypothalamic feeding center and pituitary. Sparse, fine-beaded BBS/GRP-like IR fibres were detected in the ventro-posterior hypothalamus and hypothalamic inferior lobes, including the nucleus recessus posterioris, nucleus recessus lateralis, nucleus anterior tuberis, and the nucleus diffusus lobi inferioris. In the pituitary, IR fibres were localized in the neurointermediate lobe (NIL); occassionally cells and few fibres within the pars distalis contained BBS/GRP-like IR. Using ^{125}I-[Tyr^{4}] BBS-14, specific binding sites for BBS/GRP were localized by autoradiography in the forebrain and pituitary in areas which corresponded to the distribution of BBS/GRP-like IR. These data provide additional evidence that BBS-like peptides likely play a role in the central regulation of feeding behavior and pituitary hormone secretion in the goldfish.

P4.26

CCK IS DISTRIBUTED IN THE GOLDFISH CENTRAL NERVOUS SYSTEM AND ACTS TO REGULATE FOOD INTAKE AND ANTERIOR PITUITARY SECRETION.

R.E. Peter*, B.A. Himick. Dept. Zoology, University of Alberta, Edmonton, Alberta, Canada, T6G 2E9.

The presence of cholecystokinin (CCK) /gastrin-like immunoreactivity (IR) was investigated in the goldfish forebrain and pituitary. Intense CCK/gastrin-like IR was detected in fibres of the pituitary proximal pars distalis amongst the somatotrophes and gonadotrophes. In the forebrain, IR fibres and perikarya were localized to predominantly nuclei of the ventral telencephalon and diencephalon. The greatest concentration of CCK/gastrin-like IR material in the forebrain was consistently observed in nuclei of the ventro-posterior and inferior lobes of the hypothalamus, the previously established brain feeding center of fish. Exposure of goldfish pituitary fragments to three 5-minute pulses of 1.0 or 10 nM sulfated CCK8 (CCK8-s), at 55-minute interpulse intervals, resulted in an increase in both gonadotropin and growth hormone release. When injected either intraperitoneally (ip) or into the third brain ventricle of goldfish, CCK8-s acutely suppressed food intake. The nonsulfated form of CCK8 was not as effective as CCK8-s in suppressing feeding following ip injection. These studies are the first to document that CCK is capable of regulating anterior pituitary secretion, and acting both centrally and peripherally to suppress feeding behavior, in any lower vertebrate.

P4.27

RELATIONSHIPS BETWEEN THE HYPOTHALAMIC 3H-CLONIDINE BINDING SITES AND PLASMA TESTOSTERONE IN MICE.

G.T. Shishkina. Institute of Cytology and Genetics, Siberian Branch of the RAS, Novosibirsk, Russia, 630090.

Correlations between the specific binding of radiolabelled adrenoligands in frontal cortex and hypothalamus and plasma testosterone levels were investigated in inbred mouse strains. The binding values were brain region and genotype dependent. There were the significant negative intrastrain and interstrain correlations between the specific binding of imidazoline with alpha2-adrenergic receptor agonist specificity, 3H-clonidine, in hypothalamus and resting testosterone levels. Neither the alpha1 adrenergic receptor antagonist 3H-prazosin nor beta-adrenergic receptor antagonist 3H-dihydroalprenolol binding correlated significantly with the hormone concentrations. These data suggest the possible involvement of the hypothalamic 3H-clonidine binding sites in the regulation of testosterone-dependent processes, for example, in the feedback actions of steroid on gonadotropin secretion.

P4.28

AMYGDALA AS THE NEUROENDOCRINE CENTER.

L.B.Kalimullina*, A.W.Achmadeev. Dept. of Morphology and Physiology of Man and Animals, The Bashkir State University, The Bashkir State Medical Institute, Ufa,Russia,450074.

A hypothisis on structural-functional organization of amygdala as the neuroendocrine center which takes part in organizm's reproductional processis is suggested. It is based on the vast data obtained by the study of cytoarchitectonics, neuronal organization, hystophysiology, morphometrics and biochemistry of amygdala. It is supposed that the main locuses from which the influence of amygdala on hypothalamic centers of gonadotropines' secretion regulation is realized is dorsomedial nucleus, which is localized in the posterior part of amygdala, and nucleus corticalis anterior, which is localized in its anterior part. Both nuclei which take part in proccessing of specific and non-specific olfactory information are zones of sex dimorphizm. Both nuclei have neurons which react on sex steroids by changing their functional activity. This was established by the experimental study in conditions of gonadectomy, estrus cycle, by the level measurements of the estrogene cytoreceptors, and also by the activity of aromataze and reductaze enzym systems in rostral and caudal parts of amygdala. The character of interaction of above-mentional nuclei (which is realized through the medial nucleus) depens on sex and peculiarities of hormone background and is predetermined during the period of brain's sex determination. The information from amygdala to the brain stem and its higher centers goes through central and basolateral nuclei.

P4.29

EFFECTS OF PROGESTERONE AND ESTRADIOL 17β-BENZOATE ON SUPEROXIDE DISMUTASE ACTIVITY IN THE BRAIN OF MALE RATS. S.Pajović, *Z.S.Saičić, *M.B.Spasić, J.V.Martinović. Laboratory for Molecular Biology and Endocrinology, Vinča Institute for Nuclear Sciences, and *Department of Physiology, Institute for Biological Research, Belgrade, Yugoslavia.

Antioxidant enzymes superoxide dismutases (SOD) play an important role in defending the cells against free radical-mediated oxidative damage. We previously demonstrated that, in the female rat brain, progesterone (P) and estradiol 17β-benzoate (EB) suppress mitochondrial, manganese containing SOD (MnSOD) and do not affect cytoplasmic, copper-zinc containing SOD (CuZnSOD). In this study, the analysis of the ovarian steroid effects on SOD activity in the brain was extended to male rats. MnSOD and CuZnSOD were measured in appropriate brain homogenate fractions from intact and testectomized (TX) rats, non-treated or treated sc with 2 mg P and/or 5 μg EB 2h or 24h before sacrifice. Removal of the ovaries 10 days prior to experiments did not affect the enzyme activities, indicating no involvement of testicular hormones in the control of the rat brain SOD. On the other hand, both P and EB, alone or in combination with each other, were found to suppress MnSOD 2h after injection to either intact or TX rats. Suppressive effects of P and EB on MnSOD were also seen in TX rats 24h following treatment. At the same time, P and EB appeared to have no influence on CuZnSOD. These results suggest involvement of ovarian hormones in the control of mitochondrial SOD activity in the brain of male rats.

P4.30

GLUTATHIONE DEPENDENT ANTIOXIDANT ENZYME ACTIVITIES AND GLUTATHIONE CONTENT IN RAT BRAIN DURING DIFFERENT STAGE OF THE ESTROUS CYCLE. Z.S.Saičić, *S.Pajović, B.Korać, M.B.Spasić and *J.V.Martinović. Dept. of Physiology, Institute for Biological Research and *Laboratory for Molecular Biology and Endocrinology, Vinča Institute for Nuclear Sciences, Belgrade, Yugoslavia.

Involvement of the ovary in the control of enzymatic activity of glutathione peroxidase (GSH-Px), glutathione-S-transferase (GST), glutathione reductase (GR) and catalase (CAT) as well as glutathione (GSH) content in the rat brain was studied in order to check whether well documented central effects of ovarian hormones to alter neuronal properties and functions include modulation of antioxidative defense. GSH-Px, GST, GR, CAT activities and total glutathione (GSH + GSSG) content were measured in brain homogenates prepared from cycling rats at estrus, diestrus and proestrus, as well as from long-term ovariectomized (OVX) animals. GST and GR appeared to be stable during the cycle, whereas GSH-Px, CAT and GSH were suppressed at proestrus. Bilateral ovariectomy resulted three weeks later in an increase of GSH-Px, GST and CAT activities and had no effects on GR. At the same time removal of the ovaries decreased significantly the amount of GSH in comparison to values at estrus, diestrus and proestrus. These results suggest that ovarian hormones are involved in the control H_2O_2 content in the brain tissue by suppressing GSH-Px, GST, CAT and GSH content.

P4.31

THE OXYTOXIN-INDUCED MODULATION OF OXYTOXINERGIC HYPOTHALAMIC MAGNOCELLULAR NEURONS MAY INVOLVE A CONTROL OF INTRACELLULAR FREE CALCIUM. G. Dayanithi, R. C. Lambert, M.G. Desarménien*, F. Moos and Ph. Richard. Laboratoire de Neurobiologique Endocrinologique. URA CNRS 1197. Université Montpellier II. Place E. Bataillon 34095 Montpellier France

During lactation and parturition, oxytoxin (OT) is released from the neurohypophysis and conveyed by the blood stream towards its peripheral targets: mammary glands and uterus. In addition to this well known endocrine function, OT exerts a facilitatory action on OT neurons within the supraoptic and paraventricular nuclei; this is a prerequisite to the periodic bursting activity inducing pulsatile OT release.

The present study was designed to help understanding the mechanisms involved in this OT-induced regulation of OT neurons. To this aim, we have measured intracellular free calcium concentration ($[Ca^{2+}]_i$) in single, freshly isolated, supraoptic cells. Immunocytochemical identification demonstrates that, in such a preparation, roughly 50% of the cell population is oxytoxinergic and 50% is vasopressinergic.

In half the cells tested, OT (100 nM) induced a rapid and reversible increase in $[Ca^{2+}]_i$. This effect was dose-dependent within the range 1-1000 nM and was inhibited by the specific antagonist dOVT (100 nM). The facts that the response persisted in the absence of extracellular calcium but was blocked by pre-incubation with thapsigargin indicate that OT induces a release of calcium from intracellular stores.

P4.32

TETRODOTOXIN (TTX) BLOCKS OSMOTIC STIMULATED CENTRAL AND PERIPHERAL VASOPRESSIN (VP) RELEASE. M. Ludwig*, M.F. Callahan, G. Tsai, M. Morris. Department of Physiology and Pharmacology, Bowman Gray School of Medicine of Wake Forest University, Winston-Salem, North Carolina 27157-1083, USA.

VP is released within the hypothalamic nuclear region of the supraoptic nucleus (SON) in response to either direct or systemic osmotic stimulation. Experiments were performed to determine whether intranuclear VP release is modified by local TTX blockade of synaptic transmission. A microdialysis technique was used to administer TTX (10^{-4}M) bilaterally in the SON with simultaneous monitoring of central and peripheral peptide release in urethane anaesthetized rats. The osmotic stimuli were injected intraperitoneally (3.5M NaCl; 600μl/100g b.w.) or given via the microdialysis probe (1M NaCl-aCSF). TTX abolished the effect of central and peripheral osmotic stimulation on VP release into the SON and plasma. TTX also significantly lowered basal plasma VP levels (84% decrease). These results indicate that central peptide release is a physiological response mediated by neural input. The ability of TTX to abolish the stimulated intranuclear VP release suggests that VP release is axonal in origin. In addition, the SON seems to be a key mediator in regulating plasma VP under basal and osmotic stimulated conditions. (Supported by NIH HL 43178, M.L. is NIH/Fogarty International Fellow)

P4.33

CHOLECYSTOKININ-B/GASTRIN RECEPTOR SIGNALING PATHWAY INVOLVES TYROSINE PHOSPHORYLATION OF $p125^{FAK}$ and $p42^{MAP}$.
T. Taniguchi, T. Matsui, M.Ito, T. Murayama, T. Tsukamoto, Y. Katakami and K.Chihara. Third Division, Department of Medicine, Kobe University School of Medicine, Chuo-ku, Kobe 650, Japan.

The brain-gut peptide hormones, cholecystokinin (CCK) and gastrin have been suggested to have a trophic effect on gastro-intestinal tract *in vivo* as well as *in vitro*. In the present study, the human CCK-B/gastrin receptor was expressed in mouse NIH3T3 fibroblasts to investigate the molecular basis of signal transduction pathway of the guanine nucleotide regulatory protein (G protein)-coupled receptor. Human CCK-B/gastrin receptor expressed in NIH3T3 cells coupled efficiently to phosphoinositide hydrolysis and mobilization of intracellular Ca^{2+}, and transduced mitogenic signals assessed by $[^3H]$thymidine incorporation in a dose-dependent manner. Moreover, CCK-8 or gastrin I alone promoted the cell growth in serum-free medium. CCK-8 induced tyrosine phosphorylation of several protein species. Among them, mitogen-activated protein (MAP) kinase was tyrosine phosphorylated and activated in response to CCK-8, as was induced by platelet derived growth factor (PDGF). In contrast, tyrosine phosphorylation of $p125^{FAK}$ (focal adhesion kinase) was induced by CCK-8 but not by PDGF. CCK-8 as well as gastrin I induced the expression of early responsive genes such as c-*fos* and c-*myc*. These results suggest that CCK-B/gastrin receptors might transmit mitogenic signals by cross-talking with the tyrosine kinase cascades.

P4.34

POSSIBLE MECHANISM BY WHICH α-MELANOTROPIN ADVANCES THE TIME OF VAGINAL OPENING.
M. E. Celis*, P. E. Durando. Fisiología, Dept. of Farmacología, Fac. de Ciencias Químicas, Universidad Nacional de Córdoba, Córdoba, Argentina, 5016.

The aim of this work was to determine whether the acute administration of α-melanotropin (α-MSH) advances the time of vaginal opening (VO) by modifying the secretion of luteinizing hormone (LH), prolactin, growth hormone (GH), progesterone (P), oestradiol (E_2) and/or testosterone (T). Female rats received oestradiol benzoate (OB; 1 x 10^{-6} g/kg body weight, sc) on day 26 and 27 postnatal (PN). On day 28 PN, a third dose of OB was given together with either α-MSH (treated group) or 0.1 ml saline (control group)(ip). On day 32 PN, the animals were inspected for vaginal opening (VO) and were decapitated at hourly intervals between 12:00 and 18:00 h. Acute administration of α-MSH significantly advanced ($P < 0.001$) the day of VO compared to the control group. α-MSH treatment also increased serum LH levels ($P < 0.001$) in the period under study but had no significant effect on the other hormones analysed. LH profiles were determined between the day after α-MSH treatment (day 29 PN) and VO (day 33 PN). Blood samples were collected from the cannulated external jugular vein at 20 minutes intervals daily between 14 and 18 hours. α-MSH treatment did not significantly modify plasma LH levels on days 29 and 30 PN, although treated animals showed a sustained increase in LH on day 31 PN. On this day, mean LH levels of treated animals was significantly ($P < 0.05$) higher than the control group. On day 32 PN a transient surge-like rise ($P < 0.05$) in LH occurred in the treated animals which was not seen in the controls. Although a day latter (day 33 PN) this surge appeared in control group. These findings led us to propose that acute α-MSH administration advances the time of VO by accelerating the appearance of LH episodes of secretion.

P4.35

EFFECT OF SOMATOSTATIN-14 ON INOSITOL-1,4,5-TRISPHOSPHATE CONTENT AND PROTEIN KINASE C ACTIVITY IN THE VARIOUS AREAS OF THE BRAIN.
A. Lachowicz* and M. Pawlikowski. Institute of Endocrinology, Dep. of Experimental Endocrinology and Hormone Research, University of Medicine, Lódz, Poland.

The molecular mechanism of somatostatin action is connected with changes in cAMP and intracellular Ca^{2+} concentrations. The influence of this neuropeptide on phosphatidilinositol turnover has not been well documented. Inositol-1, 4, 5-triphosphate (IP_3), a product of phosphatidilinositol hydrolysis caused by phospholipase C, releases calcium from its intracellular stores. Protein kinase C, activated by second product of action of phospolipase C - DAG, phosphorylates may protein and thus can generate intra- or extracellular signals in cell. In this study we examined the effects of somatostatin-14 (SST) on IP_3 content and protein kinase C activity in rat anterior pituitary, hippocampus and cortex homogenates. The IP_3 concentration was determined using radioimmunoassay. The protein kinase C activity was determined using modified method by De Graan et al. It was found that somatostatin-14 increases IP_3 concentration in all these studied regions. The maximal increase of IP_3 content was found in pituitary homogenate, whereas in hippocampus and cortex IP_3 augmentation was lower. SST activated protein kinase C activity also in all these examinated regions. All these effects occurred only in short (1-3 min.) time of incubation and declined with the extended time of experiment. Our findings indicate that IP_3 and protein kinase C may play an important role in molecular action of somatostatin-14 in the brain.

P4.36

THE REGULATORY ROLE OF SUBSTANCE P ON THE CYCLOOXYGENASE AND LIPOXYGENASE PATHWAYS OF ARACHIDONATE CASCADE.
Zs. Mezei, B. Kis, Á. Gecse, G. Telegdy. Department of Pathophysiology Albert Szent-Györgyi Medical University of Szeged, Hungary, 6701, P.O.Box: 531.

The Substance P neuronal terminals are concentrated especially in the noradrenergic and dopaminergic neuron regions. Peptides with different structures might induce similar cellular reactions modifying same intracellular processes. One candidate of molecules for the intracellular messenger function might be the arachidonate cascade, which is present in all eukaryotic cells. It is well known, that the organelles and functions of platelets are very similar to the serotoninergic neurons, therefore the thrombocytes might be applied as modell cells of the central nervous system. The role of Substance P was investigated in vitro in rat platelets. The thrombocytes were incubated in Parker Medium 199 in the presence of 14C-arachidonic acid, then the Substance P was introduced into the Parker Medium in several concentrations (10-13 - 10-7 mol/L). The labelled cyclooxygenase and lipoxygenase arachidonate products were extracted with ethyl-acetate (three times), and the metabolites were separated either by overpressure layer chromatography and/or HPLC. The isolated and separated labelled arachidonate products were quantitatively determined by liquid scintillation in a Beckman LS 1800 scintillator. The cyclooxygenase pathway of platelets were significantly modified by Substance P in concentrations of 10-12 and 10-9 mol/L. The thromboxane B2 synthesis was inhibited by Substance P in a concentration of 10-12 mol/L, while the higher peptide concentration (10-9 mol/L) induced an increased formation of the vasoconstrictor metabolites of cyclooxygenase pathway.These concentrations of Substance P might be detected in the circulation both in physiologic and pathologic circumstances. The lipoxygenase pathway was stimulated by Substance P.
This work was supported by the grant (No 2683) of the National Scientific Research Foundation, Humgary.

P4.37

THE REGULATORY ROLE OF ENDOTHELIN 2 ON THE CYCLOOXYGENASE AND LIPOXYGENASE PATHWAYS OF ARACHIDONATE CASCADE OF RAT PLATELETS. **Á. Gecse, Zs. Mezei, B. Kis, *B. Penke and G. Telegdy. Dept. of Pathophysiology and *Dept. of Medical Chemistry Albert Szent-Györgyi Medical University of Szeged, Hungary, 6701, P.O.Box: 531.**

The organelles and functions of platelets are very similar to the serotoninergic neurones, therefore the thrombocytes might be applied as model cells of the central nervous system. Endothelins are a family of three peptides that act as local hormones released by the endothelium in each blood vessel type in all mammalian species. Endothelins bind to platelet membrane and interact with G proteins and stimulate protein kinase C. These may result in multiple activation of intracellular processes, governed by phospholipase C and/or phospholipase D. One other candidate of molecules for the intracellular messenger function is the arachidonate cascade, present in all eukaryotic cells. The role of endothelin 2 was investigated *in vitro* in rat platelets. The thrombocytes were incubated in Parker Medium 199 in the presence of ^{14}C-arachidonic acid, then the endothelin 2 was introduced into the Parker Medium in several concentrations (10^{-12} - 10^{-8} mol/L). The supernatants of control and endothelin 2 treated platelets were extracted with ethyl-acetate (three times), and the metabolites were separated either by overpressure layer chromatography and/or high-performance liquid chromatography. The isolated and separated labelled arachidonate products were quantitatively determined by liquid scintillation in a Beckman LS 1800 scintillator. The cyclooxygenase pathway of platelets were significantly modified by endothelin 2 in concentrations of 10^{-11} mol/L. The synthesis of thromboxane B_2 and PGD_2 were stimulated by endothelin 2 in a concentration of 10^{-11} mol/L. Endothelin (10^{-11} mol/L) induced an increased formation of the vasoconstrictor metabolites of cyclooxygenase pathway. These concentrations of endothelin 2 might be detected in the circulation both in physiologic and pathologic states.

This work was supported by the grant (No 2683) of the National Scientific Research Foundation, Hungary.

P4.38

INVOLVEMENT OF NEUROTRANSMITTERS IN THE "ANXIOLYTIC-LIKE" EFFECTS OF BRAIN NATRIURETIC PEPTIDE (BNP) IN RATS. É. Bíró *, G. Tóth#, G. Telegdy. Dept. of Pathophysiology and # Dept. of Medical Chemistry Albert Szent-Györgyi Medical University, szeged, Hungary, 6701.

In our department it has been shown that centrally administered $rANP_{1-28}$ is able to modulate learning and memory processes (Bidzseranova et al., 1991, Brain Res. Bul. 26, 1:177-180) and also the hypothalamo-pituitary-adrenal axis in rats (Bíró et al.,J of Psychpharm. A-273, 1992). Brain natriuretic peptide (BNP) is another member of natriuretic peptide family and in the present study an attempt was made to elicit the possible anxiolytic action of BNP in an elevated plus-maze test.

BNP given in the lateral brain ventricule was able to produce an "anxiolytic-like" action in dose dependent manner. The neurotransmitter systems involved in anxiolytic effect were investigated by using the pretreatment with specific receptor blockers, in doses which wouldn't influence the test per se. The β-adrenergic (propranolol) and cholinergic-muscarinergic (atropine) antagonists are able to inhibit the "anxiolytic-like" activity of BNP. The dopaminergic (haloperidol), α-adrenergic (phenoxybenzamine), serotoninergic (methysergide), and GABA-ergic (bicuculline) antagonists were ineffective.

These results indicate that a multiple neurotransmitters system activation might be responsible of BNP induced "anxiolytic-like" activity.

P4.39

THE EFFECT OF C-TYPE NATRIURETIC PEPTIDE (CNP) ON ANALGESIC ACTION OF MORPHINE IN MICE. E. Babarczy *, Z. Vízi, G. Telegdy. Dept. of Pathophysiology, Albert Szent-Györgyi Medical University, Szeged, Hungary, 6701.

Previously the effects of (atrial natriuretic peptide) ANP and (brain natriuretic peptide) BNP on the development of analgesic, tolerance and dependence action of morphine have been investigated. It was found that these peptides were able to diminish the development of acute and chronic morphine tolerance centrally administrated ANP and BNP. As a continuation of the former experiments we have studied the antinociceptive effect of CNP in mail CFLP mice. The different doses (0.2-200 ng) of CNP was administered into the lateral brain ventricule and morphine (5 mg/kg) was injected subcutaneously. The analgesic effect was measured by a tail-flick test. CNP administered centrally did not itself affect pain sensitivity, however, it depressed the acute nociceptive effect of a single subcutaneous dose of morphine (5 mg/kg) after 30 min icv (0.2 ng, 2 ng, 20 ng) CNP administration and 2 ng, 20 ng doses decreased this action after 60 min too. CNP in 0.2 ng, 200 ng doses blocked the development of acute tolerance to morphine 30 min and 200 ng 60 min after the administration of a test dose of morphine.

The data obtained indicate that CNP can modify the analgetic action of morphine in a dose-dependent manner. The action showes a similar profile as ANP and BNP.

P4.40

CEREBELLIN IN THE HUMAN BRAIN

F Satoh*, K Takahashi, K Totsune, M Ohneda, Y Mizuno#, O Murakami, M Sone, K Abe, H Sasano##, T Mouri##
The 2nd Dept of Int Med, #the Dept of Neurology and ##the 2nd Dept of Pathology, Tohoku Univ School of Medicine, Sendai, Japan

Cerebellin is a neuropeptide originally isolated from rat cerebellum. High concentrations of cerebellin are present in human cerebellum. But concentrations of immunoreactive(IR-) cerebellin in cerebellum obtained from patients with cerebellar diseases have not been studied.

In the present study, the distribution of IR-cerebellin was studied by RIA in brain tissues obtained at autopsy from patients without neurological diseases. IR-cerebellin concentrations were measured in the cerebellar hemisphere obtained from 4 patients with spino-cerebellar degeneration, and were compared with those from control subjects. The antiserum to cerebellin was raised in a rabbit by injecting cerebellin conjugated with bovine thyroglobulin by carbodiimide. The assay showed 100% crossreaction with des-Ser^1-cerebellin but less than 0.001% with other peptides such as NPY, VIP and CGRP. High concentrations of IR-cerebellin were found in cerebellar hemisphere (424 $\pm$ 13 pmol/g wet tissue, mean $\pm$ SEM, n=6) and cerebellar vermis (257 $\pm$ 31, n=6), followed by medulla oblongata (24.0 $\pm$ 8.4, n=4), thalamus (15.6 $\pm$ 5.6, n=5), hypothalamus (13.6 $\pm$ 5.6, n=6), pons (5.8 $\pm$ 1.2, n=6), and frontal cortex (3.8 $\pm$ 0.37). A significant decrease of IR-cerebellin concentrations was found in cerebellar hemisphere from patients with spino-cerebellar degeneration (178$\pm$47 pmol/g wet weight, n=4) compared with those from control subjects. Reverse phase HPLC showed that most of the IR-cerebellin (>95%) in the cerebellum was eluted in the position of synthetic cerebellin. These findings indicate that high concentrations of cerebellin are present thoughout in human brain, with the highest concentrations found in the cerebellum. Decreased concentrations of IR-cerebellin in cerebellar hemisphere from patients with spino-cerebellar degeneration suggest possible involvement of this peptide in the pathogenesis of this disorder.

P4.41

NEUROTHYRONINES: EVIDENCE FOR TRIIODOTHYRONINE AS A NORADRENERGIC NEUROMODULATOR IN ADULT BRAIN.
C.B.Rozanov and M.B.Dratman*. Department of Medicine, Medical College of Pennsylvania; Department of Psychiatry, University of Pennsylvania School of Medicine, and VA Medical Center, Philadelphia PA 19104

An association between thyroid hormones and adrenergic neurotransmitters has been established on the basis of clinical, physiologic, functional, and molecular evidence. The possibility that this association may be mediated through synaptic actions of iodothyronines within noradrenergic systems in the adult brain has been strengthened by recent evidence demonstrating both concentration and actions of T3 in nerve terminals. While many of these observations await confirmation, they conform with a growing trend in the neuroendocrine field which emphasizes the non-genomic as well as the genomic actions of the hormones related through the c-*erb*-A-based family of nuclear receptors. We now report several findings derived from T3 immunohistochemistry which greatly strengthen the case for association between T3 and norepinephrine in rat brain: (a) high concentrations of endogenous T3 in discrete neural systems strongly innervated by noradrenergic projections; (b) greatest accumulation of T3 reaction product over the nucleoplasm of those labeled neurons, together with strong labeling of their nerve cell processes and surrounding neuropil; (c) exceptionally high concentration and unique distribution of reaction product in locus coeruleus and all other noradrenergic brainstem nuclei with little or no labeling of the cell nuclei but with clumping in perikarya and beading in nerve cell processes (especially dendrites) indicating potential morphologic sites of non-genomic T3 and norepinephrine co-modulation.

P4.42

THE EFFECTS OF INTERACTION OF ADH AND CATECHOLAMINES ON MYOCARDIAL FUNCTION, BLOOD SUPPLY AND METABOLISM.
A.Khomazjuk, A.Nescheret.Dept.of Neuroendocrine Control of Circulation,Institute of Endocrinology & Metabolism, Kiev,Ukraine, 254114.

Catheterization, programmed extracorporal autoperfusion of coronary artery (CA) and continuous drainage of coronary sinus (CS) were performed in 32 closed-chest dogs under chloralose anaesthesia. Injection of ADH (arginine-vasopressin, 0.01-1.0 IU) into CA blood stream caused significant rise of CA resistance (CAR;+4.1±0.78 kPa), left ventricular dP/dt (+135.0 ±10.5 kPa/s), arterial blood pressure (ABP; +1.1 ±0.39 kPa) and release of FFA and glycerol into CS (1.3±0.65; 0.2±0.15 mmol/l,resp) This first part of the reaction was followed by the attenuation of CAR elevation, decrease of ABP, myocardial contractility and heart rate (-2.1±0.33 kPa; -160±15,55 kPa/s;-22.3±4.78/min,resp).Only the CAR increase was due to direct action of ADH. The changes of heart function and metabolism were due to increased sensitivity of myoocardial adrenoreceptors, their activation by endogenous catecholamines and were blocked by propranolol. The second part of the reaction was counterregulatory cholinergic and was blocked by atropine.

P4.43

ENDOCRINE RESPONSE TO STRESS IN DIFFERENT INBRED STRAINS OF RATS.
A. Armario*, A. Gavaldà, J. Martí. Departament de Biologia Cel.lular i de Fisiologia, Universitat Autònoma de Barcelona,
Ø8193 Bellaterra, Barcelona, Spain.

In order to characterize the emotional reactivity of five inbred strains of rats, their response to acute stress was assessed by measuring several endocrine variables well-accepted as indeces of stress: Pituitary-adrenal hormones, prolactin and glucose. The inbred strains studied were: Brown-Norway, Lewis, Fischer 344, Spontaneously Hypertensive Rats and Wistar-Kyoto. Our results are in good agreement with previous results from other laboratories. However, on the basis of the present data is not possible to rank the various inbred strains in terms of emotional reactivity because their position was different, depending on the endocrine variable taken as reference.

P4.44

ANXIOLYTIC EFFECTS OF INTERLEUKIN-1β IN THE RAT.
A. Montkowski *, B. Schöbitz, J.M.H.M. Reul, R. Landgraf. Max Planck Institute of Psychiatry, Clinical Institute, Munich, Germany, 80804

Interleukin-1β (IL-1β) is a key regulator of immune responses during infection and injury. Additionally, the cytokine exhibits prominent effects in the brain including behavioral alterations. There is increasing evidence that cytokines can also affect emotional reactions. We have analyzed the effects of various doses of IL-1β on anxious behavior, body temperature and behavioral responses which are typical for sick animals. Twenty minutes after intracerebroventricular (icv) injection of IL-1β or IL-6, adult male Wistar rats were tested in the elevated plus maze. The ratio of entries into the open arms to the total number of open-arm entries (RE) and the ratio of time spent in open arms to the total time spent in both types of arms (RT) were used as markers for the natural aversion of rodents to open space. IL-1ß significantly increased RT in a dose-dependent manner (dose range: 0, 0.001, 0.01, 0.1ng) with a maximum effect at 0.1ng ($p<0.01$) indicating an anxiolytic effect of IL-1β. Higher doses (1 and 10ng) were less effective than 0.1ng IL-1β. We additionally determined the effect of 0.1 ng on body temperature, locomotor activity, food and fluid intake. We found no effect on body temperature and locomotor activity 20 min after icv infusion. However, the low dose of 0.1 ng IL-1β evoked a fever response of more than 1°C between 3 and 5h after application and reduced locomotor activity between 9 and 21h. The same dose of IL-1β decreased food intake 12h after injection for about 24h, but did not influence fluid intake. In the plus maze test, 100ng IL-1ß markedly reduced RT and total number of entries into the closed arms reflecting depressed locomotor activity at this high dose. In contrast, 100ng IL-6 failed to alter overall activity and caused no anxiolytic effect suggesting effects specific for IL-1β. These data suggest, that IL-1β has anxiolytic properties at remarkably low doses, and that this effect is independent of fever and sickness behavior.
Supported by VW.

P4.45

CHANGES IN HYPOTHALAMIC-GROWTH HORMONE-SOMATOMEDIN (H-G-S) AXIS IN A STRESS-INDUCED DEPRESSION-MODEL IN RAT. K. Hamanaka*, H. Soya†, H. Yoshizato†, R. Okuyama, Y. Ishikawa, I. Kitayama and J. Nomura. Dept. of Psychiatry, Mie University School of Medicine, †Dept. of Health & Physical Education, Faculty of Education, Mie University, Tsu, Mie 514, JAPAN.

The aim of this study was to clarify pathophysiological changes in depression using a stress-induced depression-model animal which we have produced by exposing rats to a long-term intermittent walking stress. Many reports suggested abnormalities of the H-G-S axis in depressive patients, and we decided to study changes in the axis in our depression-model rats. We exposed rats to intermittent walking stress for 2 weeks, and gave them a rest and measured their spontaneous running activities (SRA) for another 2 weeks. Then we divided the rats into stress-induced depression-model group and recovery group by their SRA after the stress. Results were as follows;

1)Both somatostatin (SRIF) contents in the stalk-median eminences (SME) and growth hormone (GH) contents in the anterior pituitaries were decreased, but GH concentration in plasma was increased in depression-model group.

2)*In vivo* GH responses to GH-releasing factor (GRF) were enhanced in depression-model group.

3)*In vitro* GH responses to GRF in depression-model group were unchanged in comparison with both control group and recovery group.

Recovery group showed no significant changes in these three experiments.

These findings indicate that GH is hypersecreted at least in part in the depression-model group and that changes in GRF-GH responses may be due to some changes at extrapituitary level. Reduced SRIF contents in SME and enhanced GRF-GH responses *in vivo* may suggest that suppressive effects of SRIF on GH secretion are decreased in our depression-model animals.

P4.46

CENTRAL AMYGDALOID INVOLVEMENT IN NEUROENDOCRINE RESPONSES TO EMOTIONAL CONDITIONING. B. Roozendaal[1,2], J.L. McGaugh[2], B. Bohus*[1]. 1.) Dept. Animal Physiology, University of Groningen, P.O. Box 14, 9750 AA Haren, The Netherlands. 2.) Center for the Neurobiology of Learning and Memory, University of California, Irvine, CA 92717, U.S.A.

The purpose of this study was to examine the effects of bilateral electrolytic lesions in the central nucleus of the amygdala (CEA) on neuroendocrine responses during acute and conditioned emotional stress situations in the rat. Blood samples were repeatedly withdrawn via permanent heart catheters. Lesions in the CEA attenuated the magnitude of all hormonal responses (epinephrine, norepinephrine, corticosterone and prolactin) to the acute stress of a single inescapable footshock. In contrast to this general, nonselective role in acute neuroendocrine responses, there is a remarkable differential involvement of the CEA in the various hormonal correlates of conditioned stress, i.e., exposing the rats to the footshock environment a day after the stress of footshock. CEA lesions made before the footshock, but not posttraining intervention, abolished the conditioned elevations of circulating corticosterone and prolactin. However, CEA lesions, made either before or after the learning trial, failed to affect the conditioned sympathetic response of plasma epinephrine. Plasma levels of norepinephrine neither showed a conditioned stress effect, nor were influenced by lesioning. Altogether, these results indicate that the CEA is involved in the conditioning rather than the retention of neuroendocrine stress responses. The effects of pretraining lesioning of the CEA on conditioned responses can possibly be explained by a reduced feedback of all these neuroendocrine factors on the brain during or shortly after acquisition. Data will be presented showing that the amygdaloid complex is an important target area for these hormones on memory storage processes.

P4.47

INDEPENDENT SEGREGATION OF A HYPERACTIVE HYPOTHALAMIC-HYPOPHYSO-ADRENAL AXIS AND A REDUCED BEHAVIOURAL REACTIVITY IN PIGS. P. Mormède*, S. García-Belenguer, J. Dulluc, C. Oliver. INRA-INSERM U259, Université de Bordeaux II, 33077 Bordeaux, France.

When compared to European Large White, Chinese Meishan pigs have high levels of circulating ACTH and cortisol, and a reduced behavioural reactivity in various challenging situations such as exposure to a novel environment, two characteristic features of depression. We investigated whether this association is genetically built in or whether these psychobiological characteristics are fortuitously associated. Six-week old piglets from the segregating F2 crosses between the Meishan and Large White breeds were studied in a standardised protocol of novel environment exposure. As expected from the genetic diversity, a wide range of variation was recorded for behavioural reactivity (locomotion, vocalisations). ACTH, cortisol and glucose were measured in blood samples taken immediately before the test and at the end of the session. Again these measures varied considerably between animals, and the continuous distribution of the scores suggested that they are under control of numerous genes. Furthermore, no correlation could be found between neuroendocrine and behavioural measures. This result demonstrates that the association between high ACTH/corticosteroid levels and a low behavioural reactivity is not genetically controlled.

P4.48

SOCIAL STATE DEPENDENT REGULATORY CHANGES IN SQUIRREL MONKEY PITUITARY-ADRENAL ACTIVITY. D. Lyons, S. Levine*. Dept. of Psychiatry & Behavioral Sciences, Stanford University School of Medicine, Stanford, CA, USA 94305-5095.

Squirrel monkeys show unusually prolonged elevations in plasma cortisol when separated from social companions. Although this hypersecretion of cortisol is initially driven by acute elevations in plasma ACTH, monkeys that respond with greater elevations in cortisol 1-hr after separation subsequently show striking reductions in ACTH 1-day after separation. Moreover, while cortisol remains elevated in monkeys housed for 3-wk without companions, simultaneous ACTH measures remain significantly and consistently reduced. When challenged with a bolus infusion of exogenous ACTH, monkeys housed without companions also respond with significantly higher, more prolonged elevations in cortisol relative to monkeys housed in groups. These findings together suggest that sustained hypersecretion of cortisol in monkeys housed without companions is at least partly a consequence of enhanced adrenal responsiveness to low circulating levels of ACTH, and that low levels of ACTH in turn are maintained by robust glucocorticoid feedback effects. Similar peculiarities in pituitary-adrenal activity are evident during major depressive episodes in human beings.

P4.49

THE INFLUENCE OF PREGNENOLONE AND PENTOBARBITALUM ON THE PHOSPHORYLATION OF SYNAPTOSOMAL MEMBRANES PROTEINS FROM THE BRAIN CORTEX OF RAT BY PROTEIN KINASE A. **E. Rebas, T. Podkul, L. Lachowicz. Dept. of Biochemistry, Medical University of Lodz, Poland.**

Membrane proteins are good substrates for many protein kinases. A well known protein kinase is protein kinase A, the activity of which is regulated by cAMP. The degree of phosphorylation of these proteins may be modulated by compounds used in anesthesia, i.e. pentobarbitalum and pregnenolone, a neurosteroid intensifying the anesthetic effect. The mechanism of anesthetic effect of these compounds occurs by means of GABA-A receptors. The compounds may modulate various neuronal functions, including neurotransmission, which is connected among others, with phosphorylation of synapsins-proteins of synaptic vesicles. The aim of our study was the investigation of influence of pregnenolone and pentobarbitalum on the activity of protein kinase A "in vitro" and "in vivo". The phosphorylation of proteins was carried out in the presence of γ-p32 ATP, and the phosphorylated proteins were separated electrophoretically, simultaneously with the pattern proteins of molecular weights between 24 and 100 kDA. The analysis of the results was obtained by the densitometric assessment of the autoradiograms. The obtained results indicate that the studied compounds inhibit the phosphorylation of synapsins Ia and Ib of the rat brain cortex by protein kinase A, which justifies the hypothesis that the anesthetic effect of the studied compounds may occur this way.

P4.50

EFFECT OF ACUTE HALOPERIDOL ADMINISTRATION ON ALDOSTERONE SECRETION IN PSYCHIATRIC PATIENTS. P. Liberini, C. Turrina*, R. Caruso*, A. Ermentini*, C. Missale, P.F. Spano. Div. of Pharmacology, Dept. of Biomedical Sciences and Biotechnology, and *Institute of Psychiatry, University of Brescia, Brescia, Italy

Aldosterone secretion is under inhibitory control by dopamine. This effect is mediated by D-2 receptors located in the adrenal cortex and coupled to inhibition of adenyl cyclase.
This study was designed to investigate the effect of the D-2 antagonist haloperidol on plasma corticosteroid levels in previously unmedicated psychiatric patients. Seven young male normotensive subjects in metabolic balance received a single dose of haloperidol (2 mg i.m.). Blood samples were collected for the determination of plasma renin activity, cortisol and aldosterone concentration at baseline, 2h, 6h, 24h and 48h after injection. In five out of seven patients a significant, transient elevation of plasma aldosterone levels was observed within 24 hours from administration. In contrast, plasma renin activity and cortisol concentration were unchanged. The present investigation complements and extends previous research indicating that the aldosterone response to metoclopramide is mediated by a direct antagonist activity at adrenal dopamine D-2 receptors. The possibility that some early cognitive side effects associated to neuroleptic therapy might be mediated by aldosterone elevation (Mondadori et al., Psychopharmacology 1993, 108:11-15) should be considered in future neuropsychological studies.

P4.51

GROWTH HORMONE RESPONSE TO TRH STIMULATION IN DEPRESSIVES WITH DIFFUSE NONTOXIC GOITER. R.Bunevicius, Institute of Endocrinology, Eiveniu 2, 3007 Kaunas, Lithuania.

A most controversial finding among variety of neuroendocrin disturbances in depression is a paradoxical Growth hormone (GH) response to Thyrotropin - releasing hormone (TRH) stimulation. It is known that hypersecretion of GH may influence thyroid goiterogenesis. Relationship between the presence of diffuse nontoxic goiter (DNG) and GH response to TRH was the point of main interest in this study. In an endocrine clinic 22 women who have been found to have major depression were selected for TRH testing. Eleven had concomitant DNG and other 11 - autoimmune thyroiditis (AT). There were no differences between the two groups in basal GH level. Significant enhancement in GH release after TRH stimulation was observed in DNG group only 20 min. ($p<.05$) and 60 min. ($p<.05$) after I.V. 0.2 mg TRH injection. GH response was higher in depressives with DNG an hour after TRH administration (peak level) when compared to depressed patients with AT ($p<.05$). These results suggest that the presence of DNG may be related to the paradoxical GH response to TRH stimulation in depressives.

P4.52

NEUROENDOCRINE FUNCTION OF BRAIN MINERALOCORTICOID RECEPTORS. E.R. De Kloet, A. Cools*, A.D. Van Haarst, N.Y. Rots, D.T.W.M. van den Berg, E. Schönbaum and M.S. Oitzl, Division of Medical Pharmacology, Leiden/Amsterdam Center for Drug Research, University of Leiden, 2300 RA Leiden, The Netherlands. * University of Nijmegen.

Aldosterone (ALDO) -selective mineralocorticoid receptors (MR) occur in epithelial cells of the periventricular brain. Non-selective MR retain with high affinity ALDO as well as corticosterone (CORT) and prevail in limbic extra-hypothalamic circuits, particularly the hippocampus. The MR operates in coordination with co-localized GR sites that have lower affinity for CORT in control of cellular metabolism and excitability. These processes are stabilized via MR, while recovery of disturbed homeostasis requires simultaneous MR+GR activation.

Here we show that the "non-selective" brain MR despite its overwhelming occupancy by endogenous ligands (B, ALDO, DOC and PROG) operates as a dynamic regulatory component of the stress response system. These experiments include: (i) pulsatile and chronic exposure to exogenous MR-blocking agents, (ii) conditioning to hyperthermia and stress in order to attain variable endogenous MR occupancy, and (iii) the correlate of individual variations in MR properties with neuroendocrine reactivity determined in genetically selected rats. The data demonstrate that the brain MR system, including its ALDO-selective and non-selective components, tunes neural mechanisms aimed to control perception of stress and its sensitivity to autonomic and neuroendocrine responses. Supported by the Netherlands Organization for Scientific Research (NWO) 546-092/564-025.

P4.53

THE ACTION OF αCGRP-(8-37) AS ANTAGONIST OF ENDOGENOUS CALCITONIN GENE-RELATED PEPTIDE IN THE LEARNING AND MEMORY PROCESSES IN RATS.

A. Kovács, G. Telegdy. Department of Pathophysiology, A. Szent-Györgyi Medical University, Semmelweis u. 1. P.O.Box 531, H-6701 Szeged, Hungary

In previous studies we have shown that exogenously administered CGRP improved the learning and memory processes. The extinction of active avoidance response is delayed, the passive avoidance response is lengthened by the peptide in a dose dependent manner. I.c.v. injection of specific antiserum against CGRP showed an opposit effect to exogenously administered CGRP both in passive and active avoidance behaviour.

In the present work the action of αCGRP-(8-37) an antagonist of CGRP was tested in passive and active avoidance behaviour of rats.

Four doses (100 ng, 250 ng, 500 ng and 1 μg) of αCGRP-(8-37) was given i.c.v. immediatelly after the last learning trial in passive avoidance experiments. The peptide decreased the avoidance latency in a dose dependent manner, but only the 1 μg dose caused significant results.

250 ng, 500 ng and 1 μg of peptide were used in active avoidance tests. αCGRP-(8-37) facilitated the extinction of active avoidance learning in a dose of 500 ng and 1 μg.

The present data completed our previous experiments and confirmed that the endogenous CGRP plays some role in the organization of memory processes.

P4.54

BEHAVIORAL DEPRESSION AND ALTERED BRAIN CORTICOSTERONE RECEPTOR SITES FOLLOWING NEONATAL DEXAMETHASONE TREATMENT.

K. Felszeghy, E. Gáspár, C. Nyakas. Centr. Res. Lab., Haynal University of Health Sciences, Budapest, Hungary, H-1389 POB 112.

Depression, also in humans, is closely related to the abnormal hormonal state of pituitary-adrenocortical axis. Brain corticosteroid receptors are known regulatory factors of pituitary-adrenal function and their cellular expression can be influenced by hormonal treatments. Since neonatal hormonal manipulations exert long-term modulation on adaptive behavior on rats we studied the effect of neonatal dexamethasone (DEX) treatment on adult behavior related to the corticosteroid receptor biochemistry in different regions of the brain. Newborn rats were treated s.c. with 1 μg/g DEX on postnatal day 1, 3 and 5. The psychomotor activity was tested in adult age in different situations: water immersion test (Porsolt), open- and closed-field tests. Cytosolic [3H]corticosterone (CORT) binding was assayed in hippocampus, corpus striatum, hypothalamus and pituitary gland in 3 weeks old and adult animals. Corticosteroid receptor types (I and II) were quantified using a selective glucocorticoid ligand RU 28362. The behavioral results showed that DEX treatment resulted in behavioral depression in the Porsolt's as well as other activity tests. [3H]CORT binding capacity significantly decreased in all brain areas, which was due to a selective reduction in type II receptors. In summary, neonatal DEX treatment-induced behavioral depression and the long-term selective reduction of type II corticosteroid receptors are suggested to be functionally interrelated.

P4.55

SUBDIAPHRAGMATIC VAGOTOMY BLOCKS EFFECTS OF LIPOPOLYSACCHARIDE ON SOCIAL BEHAVIOUR IN RATS

R.-M. Bluthé*, V. Walter, P. Parnet, J. Lestage, D. Verrier, S. Poole, B.E. Stenning, K.W. Kelley, R. Dantzer. INRA-INSERM U 394, Domaine de Carreire, Rue Camille Saint-Saëns, 33077 Bordeaux Cedex, FRANCE.

Intraperitoneal (IP) injection of lipopolysaccharide (LPS), the active component of endotoxin induces changes in behaviour which are similar to those occurring during infection and inflammation. These effects are mediated by proinflammatory cytokines such as interleukin-1 (IL-1), IL-6 and tumor necrosis factor α released from activated macrophages and monocytes. To test the possibility that peripheral immune stimuli act on the brain via activation of primary sensory afferents (Kent *et al*, Trends Pharmacol Sci, 1992, **13**, 24-28), we compared the effects of LPS injected IP in vagotomized and sham operated rats. After a 3-week recovery period, male Wistar rats were injected IP with 1.25 mg/kg LPS (phenol extract from E. coli 0127:B8, Sigma) or saline immediately after a baseline session of social exploration consisting of a 4-min exposure to a social juvenile conspecific. LPS depressed exploration measured 2, 4 and 6 hr later in sham-operated but not in vagotomized rats. Since vagotomy could have impaired recruitment and activation of macrophages in the abdominal cavity, we measured macrophage content of IL-1β and plasma levels of IL-1β in vagotomized and sham-operated rats killed 2 h after IP injection of LPS or saline, using an ELISA assay. Vagotomy had no effect on the LPS-induced increases in IL-1β. These results suggest that peripheral immune stimuli alter brain functions indirectly via activation of primary afferent nerves.

P4.56

COMPRESSION OF THE PITUITARY STALK ELICITS LONG TERM INCREASE IN AGGRESSION.

G.B. Makara[1], J. Haller[1], M. Vecsernyés[2], I. Barna[1], K. Kovács[1]. [1]Institute of Experimental Medicine, Hungarian Academy of Sciences, Budapest, PO Box 67, H-1450. [2]Szent-Györgyi Albert University, Dept. of Endocrinology, Szeged, P.O. Box 744, H-6720.

Vasopressin has long been implicated in the regulation of aggressive behavior. The recently developed stereotaxic method for the pituitary stalk compression (Makara, 1993) diverts vasopressin secretion site from the posterior pituitary to the pituitary stalk and the median eminence and may chronically increase cerebrospinal fluid (CSF) vasopressin levels. Three month old Wistar rats were subjected to sham operation or pituitary stalk compression one week and one month before behavioral testing and CSF sampling from the cistaerna magna. Stalk compression caused lasting diabetes insipidus and a several fold increase in the CSF vasopressin contents. When operated rats were tested against an intruder, the stalk compression increased the number of biting attacks 4-5 folds over that observed in the sham operated rats one and four weeks after surgery, respectively. The latency to the first attack was reduced with 50%. Only minor effects were noticed in other behaviors. The increase in attack frequency and the decrease in the latency to the first attack showed a strong correlation both with the vasopressin content of the CSF and the water consumption of the animals. The CSF vasopressin and water consumption also showed strong positive correlation. We suggest that a chronic increase in brain exposure to vasopressin via CSF elicits a chronic increase in the aggression of rats.

P4.57

THE INVOLVEMENT OF STRESS HORMONES IN THE CONTROL OF AGGRESSION. J. Haller. Institute of Experimental Medicine, Hungarian Academy of Sciences, Budapest, PO Box 67, H-1450

The effects of adrenergic activation by means of alpha-2 adrenoceptor blockers on aggressiveness and the aggression induced endocrine changes were tested in rats. In the resident-intruder paradigm intraperitoneal injections of yohimbine, idazoxan and CH-38083 (α_2 adrenoceptor antagonist) produced a several fold increase in clinch fighting and mutual upright scores. The effect was dose-dependent: all the substances increased aggression at 0.5 and 1 mg/kg; at 2 mg/kg the effect of idazoxan and yohimbine disappeared, while with CH-38083 an additional increase was obtained. Experiments which were conducted in order to check the validity of the results revealed that the effects of the α_2 adrenoceptor blockers were also dependent upon the behavior of the opponent. Aggressive opponents triggered the full manifestation of CH-38083 effects, while the treated animals were passive against passive intruders. CH-38083 also enhanced ACTH and corticosterone responses to aggression. Indomethacin, a potent inhibitor of the catecholamine-induced ACTH release completely abolished the effects of the α_2 adrenoceptor antagonist CH-38083. Both the aggression-enhancing and ACTH-stimulating effects of the α_2 adrenoceptor blocker disappeared. It is concluded that a catecholaminergic activation may affect the animals' responsiveness to the actions of the opponent, possibly indirectly via ACTH and corticosterone.

P4.58

TIME COURSE OF HYPOTHALAMO-PITUITARY-ADRENAL (H-P-A) ADAPTATION TO RUNNING EXERCISE TRAINING IN RAT. H. YOSHIZATO*, H. SOYA, †K. HAMANAKA, H. HANAI, Y. KITAZAWA, N. YONEKAWA. Dept. of Health & Physical Education, Faculty of Education, Mie University, †Dept. of Psychiatry, Mie University School of Medicine, Tsu, Mie 514, JAPAN.

The aim of the present study was to clarify adaptive changes in the H-P-A axis due to exercise training at 0m/min (C, control), 10m/min (10T, below the lactate threshold; LT) or 30m/min (30T, above the LT), 5days/weeks (W) for 4W or for 10W. We examined *in vivo* ACTH responses to CRH and AVP (CRH, AVP- ACTH responses) and also *in vitro* CRH and AVP-ACTH responses. Rats were forced to run on a treadmill for 4W or 10W. At least two days after training, the right jugular vein of rats were cannulated under anesthesia for successive blood sampling during running or resting state. Significant muscle hypertrophy and decrease in blood lactate and glucose concentrations during a graded running test(every 10min speed is increased 10m/min to a maximum of 30m/min) that demonstrate training effects were observed only in 30T. It showed that in the 4w-training group, CRH and AVP-ACTH responses were significantly attenuated in 30T *in vivo* but unchanged in vitro by training. The plasma corticosterone (Cor) concentration significantly increased at rest in 30T of this period. On the other hand, in the 10w-training group, the *in vivo* CRH-ACTH response was unchanged but the AVP-ACTH response was decreased in 30T. *In vitro* CRH and AVP-ACTH responses were unchanged by 10w-training. The Plasma Cor concentration returned to the normal level. These results indicated that CRH and AVP-ACTH responses are attenuated by a negative feed-back system in 4w-training when the Cor level increased in peripheral blood. These endocrinological changes might disappear if training is continued for 10W when the Cor concentration returns to the normal level. The results *in vitro* suggested that the sensitivity of corticotophs in pituitaries to CRH or AVP is not influenced by this running training.

P4.59

ADAPTIVE CHANGES DUE TO EXERCISE TRAINING IN HYPOTHALAMO-GROWTH HORMONE-IGF-I (H-G-I) AXIS IN GROWING MALE RATS.
H. Soya, K. Nakao, †K. Hamanaka, H. Yoshizato. Dept. of Health & Physical Sci., Fac. of Education, †Dept. of Psychiatry, School of Med., Mie University, Tsu, Mie 514, Japan

The aim of the present study was to delineate adaptive changes in the H-G-I axis due to prolonged endurance running training in growing male rats. Rats were forced to run on a treadmill at 0 m/min (C, control), 10m/min (10T, beneath the lactate threshold; LT) or 30m/min (30T, above the LT), 5days/wk for 8wks. At least two days after the training, the right jugular veins of the rats were cannulated under anesthesia for successive blood samplings during the running test or in the resting state. Significant muscle hypertrophies and decreases in blood glucose or lactate concentrations during a graded running test (every 10min speed is increased 10m/min to a maximum of 30m/min) that demonstrate training effects were observed only in 30T. Significant increases in GH amplitude, the peak area and integrated concentration of GH in endogenous pulsatile GH secretions (3h every) were observed only in 30T. But no differences in GH responsiveness to GHRH or KCl in vitro perifusion were observed within groups. It was noted that in vivo GH responsiveness to GHRH (i.v.) in 30T decreased greatly in comparison with other groups. There were no changes in the IGF-I concentration in the groups. These results suggest that suprathreshold intensity (above the LT) of endurance training that is beneficial to physical and physiological adaptations amplifies the pulsatile release of GH. Reduced GH responsiveness in vivo, no changes in vitro GH responsiveness and the plasma IGF-I concentration in 30T suggest that the site of adaptation to exercise training with suprathreshold is on the suprapituitary level (cf. hypothalamic somatostatin neurons).

P4.60

DIAMETRICALLY OPPOSITE EFFECTS OF ESTROGEN ON SUBSETS OF FEMALE RAT PREOPTIC NEURONS WITH AXONS TO THE MIDBRAIN LOCOMOTOR REGION. Y. Sakuma[*1], S. Tashiro[1], T. Takeo[2]. [1]Dept. Physiol. I, Nippon Medical School, Bunkyo, Tokyo 113, and [2]Dept. Physiol. I, Hirosaki Univ. School of Medicine, Hirosaki 036, Japan.

Antidromic action potentials (n=252) were recorded from the preoptic region following electrical stimulation of the midbrain locomotor region (MLR) in 76 urethane-anesthetized ovariectomized female rats, which received either estrogen (n=33) or no treatment (n=43) prior to recordings. Histological distribution of the antidromically activated neurons centered in the medial preoptic area (MPO) and scattered dorsally toward the anterior commissure and laterally into the medial part of the lateral preoptic area (mLPO). The potentials had stable latencies in a range 1.8-33.5 ms. All-or-none thresholds were 60-1550 μA and relative refractory periods were 1.3-5.0 ms. Their wave form was positive-negative biphasic, with peak-to-peak amplitudes at 0.4-12.0 mV. The overall duration of each potential was 0.7-4.4 ms. Except for the threshold and refractory period, estrogen had no effects on these parameters. Across cells, the amplitude and the duration distributed unimodally, whereas the probability distribution for the antidromic activation latency was bimodal with a dividing value at 12.0 ms. In 121 neurons with latencies below or at 12.0 ms, estrogen decreased antidromic activation threshold ($P<0.02$). On the other hand, in 131 neurons with latencies exceeding 12.0 ms, estrogen increased the threshold ($P<0.005$) and prolonged relative refractory period ($P<0.02$). The two groups of neurons localized differently albeit with certain overlapping, with many shorter-latency neurons localized in the mLPO, lateral to the longer-latency neurons in the dorsal part of the MPO. MPO stimulation has been shown to interrupt locomotion, while that of the mLPO initiates it. The differential effects of estrogen on the excitability of the MPO and mLPO efferents to the MLR may provide neurophysiological basis for the increased locomotor activity in the female rats in estrus, that has been associated with enhanced sexual motivation.

P4.61

EFFECTS OF DORSAL RAPHE NUCLEUS LESION ON SUPPRESSION OF LORDOSIS BY BACLOFEN IN FEMALE AND MALE RATS.

M. Kakeyama and K. Yamanouchi. Neuroendocrinology, Department of Basic Human Sciences, School of Human Sciences, Waseda University, Tokorozawa, Saitama 359, Japan.

The GABAergic neural system and the dorsal raphe nucleus have been reported to play an inhibitory role in regulating lordosis in rats. In this experiment, to clarify the functional relationships between GABA neurons and the dorsal raphe nucleus, the effect of lesion of the dorsal raphe nucleus (DRL) on lordosis behavior suppressed by the $GABA_B$ receptor agonist, baclofen (BAC) was examined in female and male rats. BAC (10 mg/kg b.w.) was injected into estrogen-treated ovariectomized or orchidectomized rats with DRL and lordosis behavior was observed. In female control rats without brain surgery, vehicle treated animals showed a high score of lordosis quotient (LQ), while BAC-treated rats did not display lordosis. In contrast, even when treated with BAC, all DRL rats showed lordosis, and the LQs were similar to those of both female and male vehicle treated rats. Thus, the suppressive effect of BAC on lordosis was not shown in DRL rats. These results suggest that GABA neurons work, depending on the dorsal raphe nucleus in regulating lordosis in rats.

P4.62

SOCIAL RECOGNITION IS REGULATED BY NEUROHYPOPHYSEAL HORMONES PRESENT IN VARIOUS BRAIN AREAS.

Tj.B. van Wimersma Greidanus* and C. Maigret. Rudolf Magnus Institute, Utrecht University, 3584 CG Utrecht, The Netherlands.

Endogenous vasopressin and oxytocin affect various behaviors in which learning and memory functions are involved. It appeared that hippocampal vasopressin plays a physiological role in social recognition/memory. The present study was designed to further explore the role of endogenous vasopressin and oxytocin in social recognition/memory. Young male rats were exposed two times for 5 min, to older male rats with an interval of 30 min in the anti-vasopressin serum experiments and with an interval of 120 min in the anti-oxytocin serum experiments. The time spent by the older rats with social investigation of the younger animal was scored during the two encounters. In placebo-treated animals the time spent on social investigation of the younger animal during the second encounter at 30 min is significantly shorter than during the first one (social recognition). However, local application of anti-vasopressin serum in the dorsal septal area, results in similar periods of time spent for social investigation during the two encounters. Thus, endogenous vasopressin in the dorsal septal region plays a physiological role in social recognition/memory. In placebo-treated rats the time spent on social investigation of the younger animal during the second encounter at 120 min is similar to that during the first encounter. However, local administration of anti-oxytocin serum in the ventral hippocampus (but not in the dorsal hippocampus or dorsal septal area) results in shorter investigation times during the second encounter. Thus, taken together the presence/local release of vasopressin and oxytocin in the ventral hippocampus and that of vasopressin (but not oxytocin) in the dorsal hippocampus and dorsal septal area are of physiological importance for social recognition/memory.

P4.63

NEUROENDOCRINE REGULATION OF SEXUAL BEHAVIOR OF MALE RATS WITH STREPTOZOTOCIN-INDUCED DIABETES. **V.N. Babichev, T.V. Yelseva, Ye. I. Adamskaya, T.A. Peryshkova. Lab. of Physiology, National Research Endocrinology Center, Moscow, Russia, 117036**

The characteristics of the sexual behavior and the associated changes of LH-RH and of sex hormone receptor concentrations were studied in hypothalamic regions involved in the regulation of sexual behavior activity and hypophyseal gonadotropic function of rats with streptozotocin-induced diabetes. The activities of both motivational and copulative components of such rats were found reduced. These changes were parallelled by LH-RH reduction in the median eminence and in the synaptosomal fraction of the anterior preoptic and mediobasal regions. An increased concentration of estradiol nuclear receptors was found in the anterior preoptic region, that may be responsible for the male feminization in diabetes and for weaker male sexual activity parameters. Blood levels of LH and FSH in experimental rats were virtually the same as in the reference animals, whereas prolactin and testosterone levels were reduced in the presence of elevated estradiol content. The majority of the hormonal shifts and sexual characteristics normalized after compensatory insulin therapy.

P4.64

MORPHOMETRICAL ANALYSIS OF TESTOSTERONE-INDUCED ULTRASTRUCTURAL CHANGES IN NEURONS OF MALE QUAIL MEDIAL PREOPTIC NUCLEUS. G.C.Panzica, C.Castagna, N.Aste, J.Balthazart°, C.Viglietti-Panzica. Dept. Hum. Anat. & Physiol., Torino (Italy), °Lab. Biochem., Liège (Belgium).

The dorsolateral neurons of the medial preoptic nucleus (POM) of male Japanese quail are sensitive to the plasma levels of testosterone (T): their volume and optical density in Nissl-stained sections increase in castrated (CX) birds treated with T. We applied here a morphometrical approach to describe the ultrastructural variations induced by T in these neurons. The study was performed on 10 castrated male quail treated with Silastic implants filled with T (CX+T, n=5), or left empty (CX, n=5). Five additional gonadally intact male birds were included as controls (I, n=5). Frontal 200 µm-thick Vibratome sections were stained with toluidine blue to identify the POM region. They were flat embedded and ultrathin sections were taken from the dorsolateral portion of the POM (identified on semithin sections) in a region immediately anterior to the commissura anterioris. Printed pictures of randomly photographed neurons (15-30 per each bird) were analyzed at a final enlargement of 21,300x with the aid of a multipurpose grid. The ultrastructure of neurons was very different in CX birds and in the other two groups. Quantitative evaluations demonstrated a statistically significant decrease in CX of the rough endoplasmic reticulum (RER), of free polysomes, of Golgi complexes, and of dense bodies. These changes in the ultrastructure paralleled the decrease in the cell size. Treatment of CX birds with T restored the cell size and the percentage of volume occupied by the previously listed organelles to the values observed in I. These ultrastructural changes of dorsolateral neurons in the male quail POM are similar to those observed in neuronal targets for other gonadal hormones (estradiol, progesterone). The presence of high plasma levels of T stimulates the development of cytoplasmatic structures involved in protein synthesis and secretion. *This work was supported by MURST, FNRS, ESF.*

P4.65

UNCONTROLLED HYPERSEXUALITY AFTER "SUCCESSFUL" TREATMENT OF A PROLACTINOMA IN A MALE PATIENT.O. Jürgensen, B. Bardé, E. Jungmann. Dept. Endocrinology.University 60596 Frankfurt. FRG.

The case of a 51 years old teacher is presented who was referred to the dept. of endocrinology because of matrimonial impotence of 25 years' duration and a B4 gynecomastia. Diagnostic follow-up revealed a o,4cm prolactinoma. Within a few weeks bromocriptine- treatment lead to a spectacular normalization of body-shape, libido and potency. But the patient was overwhelmed by uncontrollable destructive sexual drives which broke up his marriage, drove his wife into attempted suicide and made him spend a fortune with expensive prostitutes. He also jeopardized his professional career by seducing young female pupils. Psychotherapy revealed that the prolactinoma was the equivalent of an organic fixation of longstanding infantile and adolescent psychosexual pathology. At the age of 51 he could not cope with his awakening late puberty. The consequences of unreflected medical therapy are discussed.

P4.66

BALANCING ROLE OF OUABAIN IN THE REGULATION OF ALDOSTERONE PRODUCTION OF ISOLATED RAT ZONA GLOMERULOSA CELLS. K.Sz. Szalay, E. Stark, D. Szabó. Institute of Experimental Medicine, Hungarian Academy of Sciences, H-1450 Budapest, P.O.Box 67. Hungary.

The fact that the endogenous Na-K-ATPase inhibitor is ouabain itself and is produced by the adrenal cortex raised the question: what is its role in aldosterone regulation and how does it interact with the other regulators of aldosterone synthesis. 10^{-4} M ouabain increased aldosterone production of collagenase dispersed rat adrenocortical zona glomerulosa cells at 3.6 and 5.4 mM K^+ concentrations, whereas at high K^+ concentration (7 mM) even lower concentration of ouabain (10^{-8} M) decreased it. There was a strong interaction between the effects of ouabain and potasssium. Corticosterone production of zona fasciculata cells was not affected by ouabain.

10^{-11}-10^{-7} M ANP decreased dose-dependently the stimulating effect of 10^{-4} M ouabain. 10^{-9} M ANP decreased (60±5.1, 54±6.2 and 26±3.2%), 10^{-8} M A-II increased (476±23, 168±12 and 86±7.2%) aldosterone production at 3.6, 5.4 and 8.3 mmol K^+ concentration. 10^{-4} M ouabain inhibited the stimulatory effect of A-II at all K^+ concentrations (23±2.2, 68±4.5 and 85±7.6%) and further decreased the aldosterone production if added together with ANP (59±5.6, 63±7.8 and 78±6.5%). A strong interaction was shown between the effect of ouabain, K^+, ANP and A-II. In the multifactorial regulation of aldosterone production A-II is always stimulatory, ANP is always inhibitory and ouabain plays a balancing role depending on the K^+ concentration.

P4.67

INSULIN RECEPTORS IN ADRENAL GLAND - CHARACTERIZATION AND EFFECT OF STARVATION AND IMMOBILIZATION STRESS. S. Zorad*, M. Rusnak, M. Fickova, R. Kvetnansky and L. Macho. Institute of Experimental Endocrinology, Slovak Academy of Science, Bratislava, Slovakia, 833 06.

Insulin receptors (IR) in rat adrenal gland (A) are not well studied. Using membrane binding technique and ^{125}I-(Tyr-A14)insulin we revealed insulin (I) specific binding in plasma membranes from both adrenal medulla (AM) and cortex. I binding reached equilibrium after 5 hr at 10 °C. The binding was displaced by unlabeled I similarly as in liver membranes (Kd in nM range). The specific I binding was two times higher in AM than in cortex. The possible function of adrenal IR was assessed by their response to 16 hr starvation and immobilization (IMO) stress. Starvation upregulated the adrenal IR consistently with decreased plasma I levels. A single IMO for 2 hr also upregulated the adrenal IR despite of increased I levels. IMO also increased plasma glucose and corticosterone. Under the same conditions, IR in adipocytes were downregulated. Our results demonstrate the presence of IR in rat A, especially in the AM. The atypical changes of adrenal IR evoked by IMO imply their possible direct involvement in response of A to this stressor.

P4.68

HETEROLOGUE REGULATION OF PLACENTAL β-ADRENERGIC RECEPTORS BY STEROID HORMONES. I.Földesi, G.Falkay Dept. of Obstetrics and Gynaecology, A. Szent-Györgyi Med. Univ., Szeged, Hungary

Human placenta is a rich source of β-adrenergic receptors. They may play an important role in the regulation of placental vascular tone. These receptors are regulated by steroid hormones especially progesterone corticosteroids and estrogens. We have investigated the effect of cortisol, estradiol and the antiprogestogen RU 486 on the affinity and density β-adrenoceptors in human placental explant experiments for studying the hormonal regulation of placental adrenergic receptors. After the incubation the crude membrane fractions were prepared from tissue samples and the β-adrenergic receptors were measured by in vitro radioligand binding techniques using [^{3}H]-dihydroalprenolol as radioactive compound. From our study it could be concluded that RU 486 treatment decreases the β-adrenoceptor binding sites in a dose-dependent fashion. This effect may be resulted from the antiglucocorticoid property of RU 486.

P4.69

ONTOGENY OF ADRENERGIC RECEPTORS IN HUMAN PLACENTA K. Melis, G. Falkay Dept. of Obstetrics and Gynaecology, A. Szent-Györgyi Med. Univ., Szeged, Hungary

α_2- and β-adrenergic receptors have been investigated in human placental membranes in early stage of pregnancy (7-12 weeks of gestation) and at term by saturation analysis, using radioligands [^{3}H]-RX 821002 and [^{3}H]-dihydroalprenolol respectively. The major finding presented here is that the β-adrenoceptor density in term placentas is about 2-fold higher than those of early placentas. The α_2-adrenoceptor density only slightly increases during pregnancy. We found a correlation between the α_2- and β-adrenergic receptor concentrations in the placenta at term (r=0.76) and in early stage of pregnancy (r=0.62). It suggests that the α_2/β-adrenoceptor balance may play an important role in regulation of the placental vascular bed. Determination of the α_2/β ratio may help towards an understanding of the contractility of the placental vascular muscles.

P4.70

EVIDENCE FOR THE PRESENCE OF A NOVEL GnRH PEPTIDE OR COMPOUNDS WITH GnRH-LIKE ACTIVITY IN THE OVARY OF GOLDFISH. D. Pati*, H.R. Habibi. Department of Biological Sciences, University of Calgary, Calgary, Alberta, Canada, T2N 1N4

In addition to the primary regulation of the pituitary gonadotropin (GTH) release, gonadotropin-releasing hormone (GnRH) or compounds with GnRH-like activity are produced in the vertebrate ovary and may directly influence ovarian function. In goldfish, the physiological significance of GnRH or compounds with GnRH-like activity as a modulator of ovarian function has been reinforced by our recent demonstration of 1) GnRH receptors in the ovary and 2) direct GnRH actions on oocyte meiosis and steroidogenesis. In this study we investigated the presence of ovarian compounds with GnRH-like activity in the goldfish ovary. Extracts were prepared using an acetone/HCl/ether extraction mixture, and was purified further using Waters C18 Sep-Pak columns. The ovarian extract stimulated GTH release from the goldfish pituitary in vitro, which was inhibited in the presence of a GnRH antagonist. In addition, the goldfish ovarian extract stimulated germinal vesicle breakdown (GVBD) in prophase-I arrested follicle enclosed goldfish oocytes and influenced GTH-induced production of testosterone, in vitro. Furthermore, serially diluted ovarian extracts displaced ^{125}I-sGnRH-A from both high and low affinity GnRH binding sites in the goldfish pituitary and ovary. HPLC analysis of the goldfish ovarian extract revealed the presence of two fractions that bind specifically to goldfish ovary, release GtH from cultured goldfish pituitary and cross react with various GnRH antibodies. These fractions include an early eluting peak that does not correspond with the retention time of known GnRH forms in addition to a fraction that co-elutes with the lamprey GnRH. These findings suggest the presence of a novel form of GnRH peptide or compound with GnRH-like activity in the goldfish ovary.

Supported by Natural Sciences and Engineering Research Council grant to H.R.H. and an Alberta Minister of Advanced Education International Education studentship to D.P.)

P4.71

THE ACTIVITY OF THYMIDINE KINASE IN THE TISSUE OF RAT THYROID LOBES, FOLLOWING THE EXPOSURE TO CERTAIN NEUROPEPTIDES (VIP, SP, NPY, ANP). A. Lewiński*, M. Karbownik, E. Skowrońska-Jóźwiak, P. Biliński, M. Klencki, D. Słowińska-Klencka, J. Kunert-Radek[1], H. Modrzejewska[2], J. Greger[2]. Dept. of Thyroidology, [1]Clinic of Endocrinology and [2]1st Dept. of Biochemistry, The University School of Medicine, 91-425 Łódź, Poland.

We have measured the activity of thymidine kinase (TK - EC 2.7.1.21), the enzyme responsible for catalyzing the phosphorylation of thymidine and functioning as a part of the pyrimidine salvage pathway involved in DNA synthesis; the activity of that enzyme increases in proliferating tissues. Male Wistar rats were donors of thyroid lobes. The thyroid tissue was incubated for 4 hours in RPMI 1640 medium (Gibco), containing Hepes buffer, 15% FCS and the examined neuropeptides - vasoactive intestinal polypeptide (VIP), substance P (SP), neuropeptide Y (NPY) and atrial natriuretic peptide (ANP); the presence of those neuropeptides was previously demonstrated by other authors in the thyroid gland. The TK activity was measured by means of Cheng and Prusoff's method [Biochemistry 13, 1179, 1974] in modification by Greger and Dramiński [Z. Naturforsch. 44c, 985, 1989]. The reaction products were separated by ascending chromatography. It was shown that the effect of VIP on TK activity was dose-dependent; the peptide used in high concentrations (10^{-7}M and 10^{-5}M) suppressed, whereas when studied in the lower concentrations (10^{-15}M, 10^{-13}M, 10^{-11}M, 10^{-9}M) - enhanced TK activity. Substance P exerted a reverse effect - the lowest concentration of SP (10^{-12}M) decreased and the highest one (10^{-6}M) - slightly increased TK activity. In case of NPY, the lowest (10^{-14}M) and the highest (10^{-6}M) examined concentrations decreased the activity of the enzyme in question. In turn, ANP increased TK activity in the concentration of 10^{-5}M, while in lower concentrations (10^{-13}-10^{-7}M) no significant effects of ANP were recorded. Our results suggest the possibility of involvement of the examined neuropeptides in the control of DNA synthesis in the rat thyroid tissue.

Author Index

Numbers refer to Abstracts No.